VITAMINS AND HORMONES

VOLUME 34

VITAMINS AND HORMONES

ADVANCES IN RESEARCH AND APPLICATIONS

Edited by

PAUL L. MUNSON
University of North Carolina
Chapel Hill, North Carolina

EGON DICZFALUSY
Karolinska Sjukhuset
Stockholm, Sweden

JOHN GLOVER
University of Liverpool
Liverpool, England

ROBERT E. OLSON
St. Louis University
St. Louis, Missouri

Consulting Editors

ROBERT S. HARRIS
32 Dwhinda Road
Newton, Massachusetts

KENNETH V. THIMANN
University of California, Santa Cruz
Santa Cruz, California

JOHN A. LORAINE
University of Edinburgh
Edinburgh, Scotland

IRA G. WOOL
University of Chicago
Chicago, Illinois

Volume 34
1976

ACADEMIC PRESS   New York   San Francisco   London
A Subsidiary of Harcourt Brace Jovanovich, Publishers

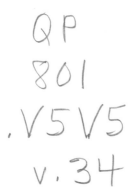

ACADEMIC PRESS, INC.
111 Fifth Avenue, New York, New York 10003

United Kingdom Edition published by
ACADEMIC PRESS, INC. (LONDON) LTD.
24/28 Oval Road, London NW1

LIBRARY OF CONGRESS CATALOG CARD NUMBER: 43–10535

ISBN 0–12–709834–8

PRINTED IN THE UNITED STATES OF AMERICA

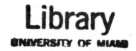

Contents

The Role of Vitamin B$_{12}$ and Folic Acid in Hemato- and Other Cell-Poiesis

VICTOR HERBERT AND KSHITISH C. DAS

Vitamin E

JOHN G. BIERI AND PHILIP M. FARRELL

The Biochemistry of Vitamin E in Plants

W. JANISZOWSKA AND J. F. PENNOCK

The Role of Prolactin in Carcinogenesis

UNTAE KIM AND JACOB FURTH

Evidence for Chemical Communication in Primates

RICHARD P. MICHAEL, ROBERT W. BONSALL, AND DORIS ZUMPE

Hormonal Regulation of Spermatogenesis

VIDAR HANSSON, RICARDO CALANDRA, KENNETH PURVIS, MARTIN RITZEN, AND FRANK S. FRENCH

A New Concept: Control of Early Pregnancy by Steroid Hormones Originating in the Preimplantation Embryo

ZEEV DICKMANN, SUDHANSU K. DEY, AND JAYASREE SEN GUPTA

Contributors to Volume 34

Numbers in parentheses indicate the pages on which the authors' contributions begin.

JOHN G. BIERI, *National Institute of Arthritis, Metabolism and Digestive Diseases, Bethesda, Maryland* (31)

ROBERT W. BONSALL, *Department of Psychiatry, Emory University School of Medicine, and Georgia Mental Health Institute, Atlanta, Georgia* (137)

RICARDO CALANDRA, *Institute of Pathology, Rikshospitalet, Oslo, Norway* (187)

KSHITISH C. DAS, *Hematology and Nutrition Laboratory, Bronx Veterans Administration Hospital, and Departments of Pathology and Medicine, Columbia University College of Physicians and Surgeons, New York, New York* (1)

SUDHANSU K. DEY, *Department of Gynecology and Obstetrics, and Ralph L. Smith Human Development Research Center, University of Kansas Medical Center, Kansas City, Kansas* (215)

ZEEV DICKMANN, *Department of Gynecology and Obstetrics, and Ralph L. Smith Human Development Research Center, University of Kansas Medical Center, Kansas City, Kansas* (215)

PHILIP M. FARRELL, *Neonatal and Pediatric Medicine Branch, National Institute of Child Health and Human Development, Bethesda, Maryland* (31)

FRANK S. FRENCH, *Department of Pediatrics, Laboratory of Reproductive Biology, University of North Carolina, Chapel Hill, North Carolina* (187)

JACOB FURTH, *Institute of Cancer Research, and Department of Pathology, Columbia University College of Physicians and Surgeons, New York, New York* (107)

VIDAR HANSSON, *Institute of Pathology, Rikshospitalet, Oslo, Norway* (187)

VICTOR HERBERT, *Hematology and Nutrition Laboratory, Bronx Veterans Administration Hospital, Departments of Pathology and Medicine, Columbia University College of Physicians and Surgeons, New York, New York, Department of Medicine, Brooklyn Veterans Administration Hospital, and Department of Medicine, State University of New York Downstate Medical Center, Brooklyn, New York* (1)

W. JANISZOWSKA,* *Department of Biochemistry, University of Liverpool, Liverpool, England* (77)

UNTAE KIM, *Department of Pathology, Roswell Park Memorial Institute, New York State Department of Health, Buffalo, New York* (107)

RICHARD P. MICHAEL, *Department of Psychiatry, Emory University School of Medicine, Atlanta, Georgia* (137)

J. F. PENNOCK, *Department of Biochemistry, University of Liverpool, Liverpool, England* (77)

KENNETH PURVIS, *Institute of Pathology, Rikshospitalet, Olso, Norway* (187)

MARTIN RITZEN, *Pediatric Endocrinology Unit, Karolinska Sjukhuset, Stockholm, Sweden* (187)

JAYASREE SEN GUPTA, *Department of Gynecology and Obstetrics, and Ralph L. Smith Human Development Research Center, University of Kansas Medical Center, Kansas City, Kansas* (215)

DORIS ZUMPE, *Georgia Mental Health Institute, Atlanta, Georgia* (137)

---

* Present address: Department of Biochemistry, University of Warsaw, Warsaw, Poland.

Preface

The Editors of *Vitamins and Hormones* take pleasure in presenting this volume, the thirty-fourth in an annual series of reviews of timely topics in vitamin and hormone research.

The present volume contains three reviews on vitamins and four on hormones. The role of vitamin B_{12} and folic acid in hemato- and other cell-poiesis is reviewed by Herbert and Das. There are two separate chapters on vitamin E, one focused on its importance for humankind (Bieri and Farrell), the other on the biochemistry of vitamin E in plants (Janiszowska and Pennock). The next four chapters cover diverse subjects all related to endocrinology: prolactin in carcinogenesis (Kim and Furth), chemical communication in primates (Michael, Bonsall, and Zumpe), hormonal regulation of spermatogenesis (Hansson, Calandra, Purvis, Ritzen, and French), and a new, still controversial, concept that the pre-implantation embryo synthesizes steroid hormones important for the maintenance of early pregnancy (Dickmann, Dey, and Sen Gupta).

Thus we are indebted to nineteen authors for the time and scholarship they devoted to the preparation of this volume. These authors are located in fourteen universities and institutes in five countries (England, Norway, Poland, Sweden, and the United States). If the countries of origin of the authors are added an even wider geographic distribution would be indicated.

PAUL L. MUNSON
EGON DICZFALUSY
JOHN GLOVER
ROBERT E. OLSON

The Role of Vitamin B_{12} and Folic Acid in Hemato- and Other Cell-Poiesis*

VICTOR HERBERT† AND KSHITISH C. DAS‡

* The work of the authors' laboratory is supported in part by United States Public Health Service grant AM15163.

† Hematology and Nutrition Laboratory, Bronx Veterans Administration Hospital, Departments of Pathology and Medicine, Columbia University College of Physicians and Surgeons, New York, New York, and Department of Medicine, Brooklyn Veterans Administration Hospital, and Department of Medicine, State University of New York Downstate Medical Center, Brooklyn, New York

‡ Hematology and Nutrition Laboratory, Bronx Veterans Administration Hospital, and Departments of Pathology and Medicine, Columbia University College of Physicians and Surgeons, New York, New York.

1

I. Introduction

Vitamin B_{12} and folic acid are essential for normal growth and proliferation of all human cells (Blakley, 1969; Pratt, 1972; Herbert, 1975b; Babior, 1975). In addition, vitamin B_{12} functions through currently unknown biochemical mechanisms to maintain myelin throughout the nervous system.

Deficiency of either vitamin B_{12} or folic acid produces a clinical disorder in man known as megaloblastic (large germ cell) anemia, characterized by increased size and slowed DNA synthesis in all proliferating cells in the body. Although this same clinical picture of megaloblastosis may result from any of a staggering variety of drugs and agents that may damage DNA synthesis (Herbert, 1975a), in the vast majority of cases it results from a vitamin deficiency of B_{12} or folic acid, brought about through decreased ingestion, absorption, or utilization, or due to increased requirement, or excretion, or destruction of the vitamin (Herbert, 1973, 1975a).

Clinical investigation by hematologists has demonstrated an apparent reciprocity in therapeutic responses to either of these vitamins in patients suffering from deficiency of either or even both vitamins. Large pharmacological doses of folic acid almost invariably cause at least temporary or partial hematological remission in vitamin B_{12}-deficient patients (Marshall and Jandl, 1960); and, conversely, large doses of vitamin B_{12} may elicit partial hematological response (reticulocytosis) in patients with folate-deficiency megaloblastic anemia (Zalusky et al., 1962). The urinary excretion of formiminoglutamic acid (FIGLU) and aminoimidazole carboxamide (AIC), both intermediary metabolites of folate-dependent reactions, are increased not only in patients with folate deficiency, but also in many patients with vitamin B_{12} deficiency (Herbert, 1959; Herbert and Zalusky, 1962; Herbert et al., 1964a,b; Chanarin, 1964). Essentially similar cytokinetic and cytogenetic aberrations, found in the bone marrow and lymphocytes of patients with megaloblastic anemia due to deficiency of either vitamin (Heath, 1966; Menzies et al., 1966; Das and Aikat, 1967; Das, 1971, 1974; Yoshida et al., 1968), are consistent with the fact that a final common defect (inadequate conversion of deoxyuridylate to thymidylate) leads to slowing of DNA synthesis per unit time in the affected cells (Herbert, 1959; Metz et al., 1968; Das and Hoffbrand, 1970b; Beck, 1975).

The clinical and therapeutic overlap, as well as the morphological and biochemical similarities at the cellular level, suggest closely interrelated metabolic roles of these two vitamins in the pathogenesis of megaloblastic anemia. The metabolic interactions of vitamin B_{12} and folic acid have been the subject of many extensive recent reviews (Stokstad and Koch, 1967; Sullivan, 1967; Chanarin, 1969, 1974; Herbert, 1971, 1973, 1975b; Hoffbrand, 1971, 1972; Babior, 1975). The present review outlines and updates this information on the metabolic roles and interrelations of vitamin B_{12} and folate.

II. Metabolism of Vitamin B_{12} and Folate

Neither vitamin B_{12} (cyanocobalamin) nor folic acid (pteroylglutamic acid) occurs as such in significant quantity in the human body, microorganisms, or the various food materials from which these vitamins are isolated. They are present in living organisms and foods as metabolically active reduced coenzyme forms, usually conjugated in peptide linkage either to specific protein binders (vitamin B_{12}) or to glutamates (folic acid). These naturally occurring labile active forms are oxidized to the stable forms, cyanocobalamin and folic acid, during the extraction procedure and are liable (particularly folates) to oxidative degradation in this process.

A. Vitamin B_{12}

The structural formula of vitamin B_{12} (cyanocobalamin) is shown in Fig. 1. The two major portions of the molecule are the corrin nucleus (a planar structure), and a "nucleotide" lying at right angles to the corrin nucleus and linked to it by D-1-amino-2-propanol. The "nucleotide" consists of a base, 5,6-dimethylbenzimidazole, attached to ribose 3-phosphate by an α-glycoside linkage. The corrin ring contains a cobalt atom in the center, which is linked to the four reduced pyrrole rings and to an anionic ligand (-R group). A second bond between the two major parts of the molecule is the coordinate linkage of the cobalt atom to one of the nitrogen atoms of the nucleotide. The permissive term "cobalamin" (or B_{12}) is used to describe the vitamin B_{12} molecule without the anionic ligand. Commercially available stable forms of vitamin B_{12} for therapy are cyanocobalamin and hydroxycobalamin. The two forms of vitamin B_{12} coenzymes (5-deoxyadenosylcobalamin and methylcobalamin) are unstable in light and undergo photolysis with formation of aquocobalamin, and in the presence of cyanides they are converted to cyanocobalamin. In cyano- and hydroxycobalamin, the cobalt is trivalent. In the biosynthesis of the coenzyme forms of vitamin B_{12}, the cobalt atom is reduced in two steps from a trivalent to a monovalent state before the organic

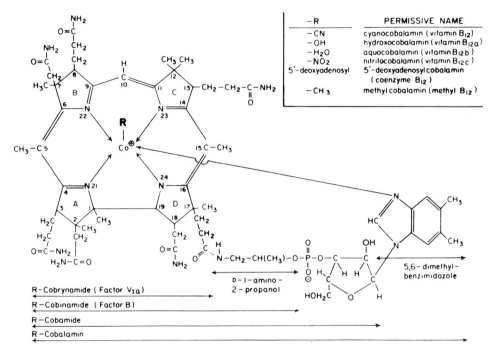

FIG. 1. Structural formula of vitamin B_{12} (cyanocobalamin). The numbering system for the corrin nucleus is made to correspond to that of the porphin nucleus by omitting the number 20. The corrin nucleus is in the plane of the page. The R anionic ligand is above it; the rest of the molecule is below it. MDR, adult minimum daily requirement from exogenous sources to sustain normality. From Herbert (1975b).

anionic ligands are attached to the molecule enzymically (Mahoney and Rosenberg, 1970) (Fig. 2). Methylcobalamin is the major form of B_{12} in the plasma and 5-deoxyadenosylcobalamin in the liver, and probably also in other tissues (Stahlberg, 1967; Linnell et al., 1969, 1971).

B. ENZYMIC FUNCTIONS OF VITAMIN B_{12}

Vitamin B_{12} is the generic descriptor for all forms of the vitamin, including the two classes of cobamides that serve as coenzymes: the adenosylcobamides and the methylcobamides. The enzymic reactions in which they function in bacteria are summarized in Table I. Only two of these reactions have so far been demonstrated unequivocally in man and other mammals: (1) methylmalonate–succinate isomerization; (2) methylation of homocysteine to methionine.

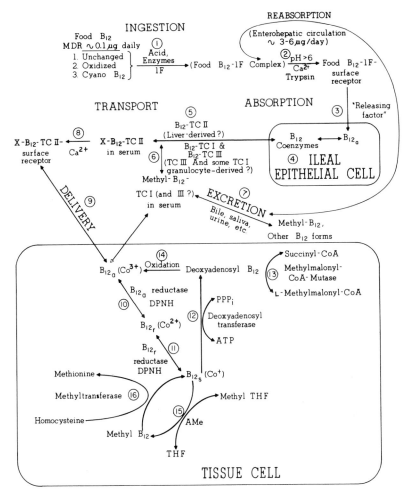

FIG. 2. Flow chart of vitamin B$_{12}$ metabolism TC, transcobalamin. From Herbert (1975a).

1. *Methylmalonate–Succinate Isomerization*

In man and most other animals, the major pathway of propionyl-CoA metabolism is via methylmalonyl-CoA to succinyl-CoA. Methylmalonyl-CoA may be formed from propionate, isoleucine, or valine. Propionyl-CoA undergoes carboxylation to the D-isomer of methylmalonyl-CoA, which is then racemized to its L-isomer. L-Methylmalonyl-CoA is metabolized to succinyl-CoA by an intramolecular change, catalyzed by the enzyme methylmalonyl-CoA mutase, which requires 5'-deoxyadenosyl-B$_{12}$ (co-

TABLE I

REACTIONS REQUIRING A COBALAMIN[a]

Order of discovery	Reaction	Pathway	Organism
Requiring 5'-deoxyadenosylcobalamin (coenzyme B_{12})			
1	Glutamate mutase	Glutamic acid fermentation	*Clostridium tetanomorphum*
2	Methylmalonyl-CoA mutase	Propionate oxidation	*Propionibacterium shermanii*, animals, man
3	Dioldehydrase	Glycol metabolism	*Aerobacter aerogenes*
		Glycerol metabolism	*Lactobacillus* (unidentified)
4	Ribonucleotide reductase	Deoxyribonucleotide formation	*Lactobacillus leichmannii*
5	Ethanolamine deaminase	Ethanolamine fermentation	Choline-fermenting *Clostridium*
6	β-Lysine isomerase	Lysine fermentation	*Clostridium sticklandii*
Requiring methylcobalamin (methyl B_{12})			
1	N^5-Methyltetrahydrofolate:homocysteine methyltransferase	Methionine synthesis	*Escherichia coli*, pig, man
2	Methane synthesis	Methanol fermentation	*Methanosarcina barkeri*
3	Acetate synthesis	Carbon dioxide metabolism	*Clostridium thermoaceticum*

[a] From Herbert (1971).

enzyme B_{12}) as an essential cofactor (Fig. 2) (Huennekens, 1968; Weissbach and Taylor, 1968, 1970). Succinyl-CoA enters the citric acid cycle, and is either completely metabolized to CO_2 or provides a pathway for gluconeogenesis via oxaloacetate to phosphoenol pyruvate. This B_{12}-dependent pathway forms a link between lipid and carbohydrate metabolism, and has allowed considerable speculation regarding its possible role in the biosynthesis of myelin, whose synthesis is deranged in B_{12} deficiency. In vitamin B_{12} deficiency, urinary excretion of methylmalonic acid increases. This may be of great importance in ruminants, such as sheep, because these animals get much of their energy requirements from the metabolism of short-chain fatty acids, such as propionic acid. Vitamin B_{12} deficiency is known to occur in sheep grazing on cobalt-deficient pastures (Dawbarn *et al.*, 1958). As vitamin B_{12}-deficient subjects are unable to metabolize propionate in the absence of vitamin B_{12}, methylmalonic acid is excreted in urine in excess. Such excretion is an ancillary diagnostic test for the existence of vitamin B_{12} deficiency, particularly after a loading dose of valine (Cox and White, 1962; Gompertz *et al.*, 1967; Gompertz, 1968; Herbert, 1971, 1975a).

2. *Methylation of Homocysteine to Methionine*

The methylation of homocysteine to methionine is catalyzed by the enzyme 5-methyltetrahydrofolate–homocysteine transmethylase, which requires methyl B_{12} as a cofactor (Fig. 2). Other cofactors involved in this reaction are 5-adenosylmethionine and reduced flavin adenine dinucleotide ($FADH_2$). The methyl group probably passes from 5-methyltetrahydrofolate to vitamin B_{12} and then to homocysteine (Weissbach and Taylor, 1970). Since methionine is available also from dietary sources, the main importance of this reaction is probably not as a source of methionine, but as a means of regeneration of tetrahydrofolate from 5-methyltetrahydrofolate (Buchanan, 1964).

In *Escherichia coli*, there is an additional B_{12}-independent pathway for the conversion of homocysteine to methionine, in which 5-methyltetrahydrofolate diglutamate is the methyl donor (Hatch *et al.*, 1961; Foster *et al.*, 1964). The preliminary reports of Foster (1966) and Wang *et al.* (1967), suggesting that a similar B_{12}-independent pathway exists in the liver of man and rats, which utilizes 5-methyltetrahydrofolate triglutamate as a methyl donor, remain unconfirmed. As of the present time, therefore, the only proven homocysteine methyltransferase enzyme pathway in man is B_{12} dependent.

C. Ribonucleotide Reductase

This enzyme catalyzes the reduction of uridine (uridine monophosphate) to deoxyuridine (deoxyuridine monophosphate) in bacteria and mammals. This reaction is B_{12} dependent in *L. leichmannii*, but not in *E. coli* or most other species (Babior, 1975). It is not yet certain that ribonucleotide reductase in man and mammals does not require vitamin B_{12}, but the best available evidence is against such a requirement (Fujioka and Silber, 1969; Hopper, 1972). *In vitro* DNA synthetic studies in human bone marrow cells suggest that this enzyme does not require vitamin B_{12} in man (Metz *et al.*, 1968; Silber and Moldow, 1970).

D. The Metabolism of Folate

The Commission on Biochemical Nomenclature (IUPAC–IUB Commission, 1966) designated both folic acid and "folate" as generic terms for any member of the family. However, in much of the literature, the term folic acid has been also used as a synonym for pteroylglutamic acid. In this review, we shall follow this usage to avoid confusion in terminology. Because all folate metabolism may be generally deranged in severe B_{12} deficiency, it is necessary to here discuss folate metabolism at some length.

The structural formula of the parent compound pteroylglutamic acid and the major coenzymically active forms are illustrated in Fig. 3. The major portions of the molecule are the pteridine moiety linked by a methylene bridge to *p*-aminobenzoic acid, which itself is joined in amide linkage to glutamic acid. Folate in circulating blood and tissue fluids is a monoglutamate (usually 5-methyltetrahydrofolate); but intracellular folate occurs as conjugates of 2–7 glutamic acid residues (pteroylpolyglutamate) (Lavoie *et al.*, 1975; Hoffbrand, 1975). The α-amino group of the second glutamic acid molecule is linked with the γ-carboxyl group of the proximal molecule. This γ-glutamyl chain structurally resembles that of a cation-exchange resin, and cations probably bind to it (Cooper, 1973). The polyglutamate forms of folate are resistant to the action of trypsin, but are hydrolyzed to mono- or diglutamate by conjugases found in plasma and in other tissues.

Pteroylglutamic acid, the parent compound, is not normally found in foods or in the human body in significant concentration. It is not biochemically active, but becomes so after reduction (in positions 5, 6, 7, and 8), and substitution of one-carbon adducts on the N^5 and/or N^{10} positions (Fig. 3). The enzymic reduction of pteroylglutamic acid is catalyzed by dihydrofolate reductase, which is inhibited by various folate

	R	OXIDATION STATE
N 5-formyl-THFA	-CHO	formate
N 10-formyl-THFA	-CHO	formate
N 5-formimino-THFA	-CH=NH	formate
N 5,10-methenyl-THFA	>CH	formate
N 5,10-methylene-THFA	>CH$_2$	formaldehyde
N 5-methyl-THFA	-CH$_3$	methanol

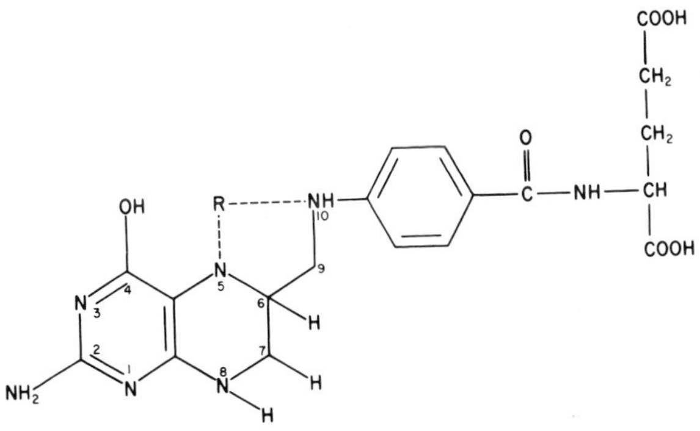

5,6,7,8-Tetrahydrofolic Acid (THFA)(FH$_4$)(R=—H)

FIG. 3. Structures and nomenclature of folate derivatives. The table above the formula lists some of the possible one-carbon adducts with THFA. Dashed lines indicate the N^5 or N^{10} site of attachment of various one-carbon units for which THFA acts as a carrier. From Herbert (1975b).

antagonists which bind to it, such as methotrexate, aminopterin, pyrimethamine, and triamterene. Tetrahydropteroylglumatic acid is the basic reduced folate compound ("one-carbon acceptor") concerned in the transfer of single carbon units in different states of reduction required for a variety of biosynthetic reactions. These include formyl (CHO-), methenyl (=CH-), methylene (-CH$_2$), formimino (-CHNH), and methyl (-CH$_3$), the most reduced form (Fig. 3). The series of interrelated enzymic reactions that lead to the formation of the various folate coenzymes

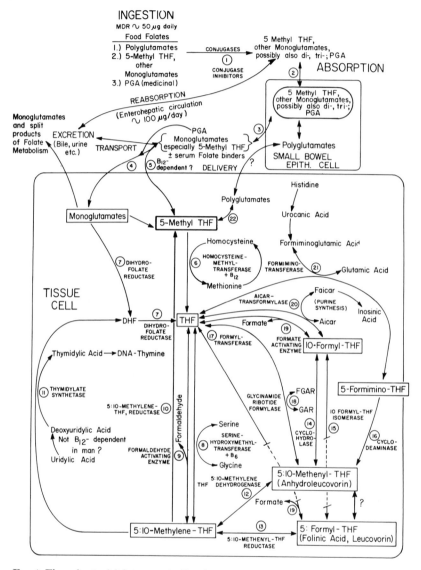

FIG. 4. Flow chart of folate metabolism in man. Circled numbers identify individual steps in folate metabolism. THF, tetrahydrofolate; DHF, dihydrofolate; PGA, pteroylglutamic acid; AICAR, aminoimidazole carboxamide ribotide; MRD, adult minimum daily requirement from exogenous sources to sustain normality. From Herbert (1975a).

is illustrated in Fig. 4. These folate coenzymes may be identified spec-
trophotometrically, fluorometrically, or by their affinity for anion-ex-
change column or absorption on Sephadex or cellulose (Chanarin, 1969;
Blakley, 1969). They may also be identified by microbiological assay
(Table II).

E. Role of Folate Coenzymes in One-Carbon-Unit Transfers

The one-carbon-unit transfer reactions in which various folate coenzymes participate include the following (Fig. 4): (1) *de novo* purine synthesis; (2) pyrimidine nucleotide biosynthesis; (3) amino acid interconversions; (4) utilization and generation of formate.

1. *Purine Biosynthesis*

The introduction of carbon-2 and -8 in the purine ring involves two
folate-dependent reactions (Hartman and Buchanan, 1959). In the first
reaction, formylation of glycinamide ribonucleotide by 5,10-methenyl-
tetrahydrofolate provides carbon-8. The second reaction involves the
formylation of aminoimidazolecarboxamide ribotide by 10-formyltetra-
hydrofolate to add carbon-2, which closes the purine ring to form inosinic
acid. There is increased excretion of aminoimidazole carboxamide (AIC)
in deficiencies of either folate or vitamin B$_{12}$ in rats and man (Herbert
et al., 1964b; Middleton *et al.*, 1964; McGeer *et al.*, 1965). The effect of

TABLE II
Folic Acid Activity for Microorganisms of Various Folic Acid Analogs[a]

Analog	*P. cerevisiae* (*Leuconostoc citrovorum*)	*Streptococcus faecalis*	*Lactobacillus casei*
Reduced pteroylmonoglutamates (except N^5-methyl)	+	+	+
Pteroylmonoglutamic acid	−	+	+
Pteroyldiglutamates[b]	−	+	+
N^5-Methylfolate-H$_2$	−	−	+
N^5-Methylfolate-H$_4$	−	−	+
Pteroyltriglutamates[b]	−	−	+
Pteroic acid	−	+	−

[a] From Herbert and Bertino (1967).
[b] *S. faecalis* does not grow well on some diglutamates; *L. citrovorum* may grow well
on some reduced di- and triglutamates.

vitamin B_{12} deficiency is probably indirect, via B_{12}-dependent pathways of folate metabolism, i.e., the homocysteine methyltransferase reaction.

2. *Pyrimidine Synthesis*

The methylation of uridylate to thymidylate is a rate-limiting step in cellular DNA synthesis (Fig. 5). The enzyme thymidylate synthetase transfers a methylene group from 5,10-methylenetetrahydrofolate to uridylate, and the methylene group is simultaneously reduced to methyl group, forming thymidylate. In the process, 5,10-methylenetetrahydrofolate is not only demethylated, but also reduced to dihydrofolate, which requires dihydrofolate reductase for reconversion to tetrahydrofolate for further participation in one-carbon-transfer reactions (Friedkin, 1957). Folate antagonists block this latter reductive process, thus interfering with thymidylate synthesis.

3. *Amino Acid Conversions*

a. Interconversion of Glycine and Serine. Serine may serve as a source of one-carbon units. The conversion of serine to glycine is catalyzed by serine transhydroxymethylase, which requires tetrahydrofolate and pyridoxal 5-phosphate (vitamin B_6) as cofactors, tetrahydrofolate acting as

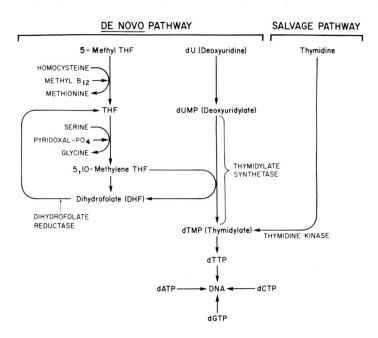

FIG. 5. DNA synthetic pathways in man.

one-carbon acceptor. This reaction is reversible and may account for the reported toxicity of glycine in rats and chickens, which is corrected by folic acid (Dinning et al., 1949; Machlin et al., 1951), and for the fact that glycine may make human megaloblastosis worse (Waxman et al., 1970).

b. *Catabolism of Histidine.* Formiminoglutamic acid (FIGLU) is an intermediate enzymic degradation product of histidine. Formiminotransferase catalyzes the further breakdown of this product to glutamic acid, which is then excreted in urine. Tetrahydrofolate acts as cofactor and accepts the formimino group, forming formiminotetrahydrofolate. Deficiency or metabolic abnormality of folate interferes with the removal of the formimino unit of formiminoglutamic acid, which consequently is excreted unchanged in large amount in the urine. Elevated urinary FIGLU levels are considered a sign of folic acid deficiency.

c. *Conversion of Homocysteine to Methionine.* This reaction in the mammalian system involves a B$_{12}$-dependent enzyme, homocysteine-5-methyltetrahydrofolate transmethylase, and is thus of particular interest in the metabolic interrelationship of vitamin B$_{12}$ and folate. This has been discussed above.

4. *Utilization and Generation of Formate*

Formate is activated enzymically in the presence of ATP and tetrahydrofolate, generating 10-formyltetrahydrofolate, which is then converted to 5,10-methenyltetrahydrofolate by acidification. The reverse reaction producing formate from 10-formyltetrahydrofolate is also known to occur in mammals (Osborne et al., 1957).

III. EVIDENCE FOR THE "METHYLTETRAHYDROFOLATE (METHYL-THF) TRAP" HYPOTHESIS

The conversion of methylene-THF to 5-methyl-THF by methylene-THF reductase is essentially an irreversible reaction (Katzen and Buchanan, 1965), leaving only one pathway for the transfer of the methyl group from 5-methyl-THF to regenerate THF for one-carbon-unit transfer reactions. This occurs by the B$_{12}$-dependent homocysteine-5-methyl-THF transferase reaction.

Herbert and Zalusky (1961, 1962) showed that *L. casei* active material, subsequently identified as 5-methyl-THF (Herbert et al., 1962) accumulated in the sera of patients with vitamin B$_{12}$ deficiency (Fig. 6). The "pile up" of this major form of circulating folate was suggested to reduce the available pool of folate coenzymes including THF and methylene-

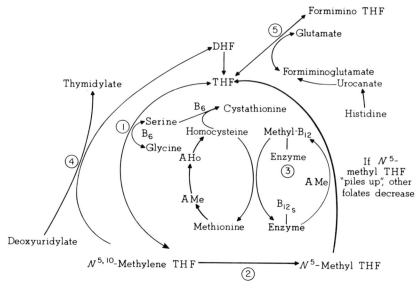

FIG. 6. Interrelationships of vitamin B_{12} and folate. DHF, dihydrofolate; THF, tetrahydrofolate. From Herbert (1971).

THF required for single-carbon transfer reactions, since 5-methyl-THF could not be converted either to THF by the homocysteine–methionine pathway, owing to vitamin B_{12} deficiency, or to methylene-THF, because the reverse reaction is not known to occur significantly in man (Herbert et al., 1964a). This metabolic trapping of folate as 5-methyl-THF leading secondarily to folate deprivation was put forth as a "methylfolate trap" hypothesis in the pathogenesis of megaloblastic erythropoiesis in vitamin B_{12} deficiency (Herbert and Zalusky, 1962; Noronha and Silverman, 1962). A large body of clinical and biochemical evidence provides substantial support to this hypothesis. Recently it has been shown that the uptake of 5-methylfolate by PHA-stimulated lymphocytes (Das and Hoffbrand, 1970a; Lavoie et al., 1974) and bone marrow cells (Tisman and Herbert, 1973) of vitamin B_{12}-deficient patients is impaired, and can be corrected by addition of vitamin B_{12}. These observations expand the concept of the "methylfolate trap" to include both folate trapped outside of cells due to the mechanism for cellular uptake of methylfolate being dependent on vitamin B_{12}, and also folate trapped inside cells due to inadequate conversion of methylfolate to THF by the B_{12}-dependent homocysteine–methionine reaction. However, these two processes may not be independent, since it is not yet ruled out that the failure of transport of methylfolate into cells or its retention in cells in vitamin B_{12} deficiency is secondary to the block in the further metabolism of methyl-THF. For example, it is possible that a cell membrane-bound transport protein for methylfolate constitutes a B_{12}-dependent mechanism for cellular transport of this form of folate (Tisman and Herbert, 1973) and that vitamin B_{12} removes the methyl group from methylfolate at the cell wall to promote its entry into cells (Herbert, 1971).

It is of interest that a unique megaloblastic anemia, resistant to vitamin B_{12} and folate therapy, has been described in a Japanese child who had a congenital defect in the homocysteine-transmethylase reaction probably due to deficiency of the pertinent apoenzyme (Arakawa, 1970). This patient also had mental retardation, marked dilatation of cerebral ventricles, and abnormally high serum and red cell level of 5-methyl-THF (*L. casei* active folate). This condition represents an example of congenital "methylfolate trap" syndrome resulting in megaloblastic erythropoiesis, virtually identical in effect to that due to vitamin B_{12} deficiency. The fact that the apoenzyme deficiency is associated with a high intracellular methylfolate, but the coenzyme (i.e., B_{12}) deficiency is not, tends to support the concept that the B_{12}-dependent transport of methylfolate across cell walls is unrelated to homocysteine transmethylase.

The clinical and biochemical events in vitamin B_{12}-deficient megaloblastic anemia will now be reviewed to assess how they fit into the above hypothesis in the interrelationship of vitamin B_{12} and folate metabolism.

A. SERUM FOLATE LEVEL IN VITAMIN B_{12} DEFICIENCY

As stated earlier, the initial clues to the "methylfolate trap" in vitamin B_{12} deficiency were the twin findings of accumulation of an *L. casei* active folate compound, 5-methylfolate, in the sera of vitamin B_{12}-deficient patients and its relatively slow or delayed clearance from the plasma of these patients (Herbert and Zalusky, 1961, 1962). Study of 100 consecutive patients with vitamin B_{12} deficiency revealed that 17 had initial serum folate levels for *L. casei* of 25 ng/ml or more, 9 had values of 16–24.9 ng/ml, 34 had 7–15.9 ng/ml, despite frequent or protracted anorexia, and the remaining patients with serum folate level of 6.9 ng/ml or less had debilitating complications, such as chronic urinary tract infection, alcoholism, or marked neurological disability, causing anorexia and inadequate folate ingestion (Herbert and Zalusky, 1962). Of 107 patients with pernicious anemia described by Waters and Mollin (1963), 24 had high serum *L. casei* activity, and the majority of these patients had minimal anemia, but often with neurological complications. Thus, it appears that high serum folate level, active for *L. casei* but not for *S. faecalis* (i.e., presumptively due mainly to 5-methyl-THF), occurs more often in the least anemic patients with B_{12} deficiency, who do not suffer from anorexia or other gastrointestinal dysfunction, and therefore, ingest adequate amounts of dietary folate. These observations also support the concept that anemia in vitamin B_{12} deficiency is precipitated by deficiency of metabolically available folate coenzyme. The high serum folate in patients with B_{12}-deficient megaloblastic anemia falls to normal following therapy with vitamin B_{12} (Herbert and Zalusky, 1962; Waters and Mollin, 1963). Although optimal hematological response is obtained in such patients with vitamin B_{12} therapy, the morphological correction of megaloblastic marrow to normoblastic may be more rapid when large doses of folic acid are added to the therapeutic regime (Gutstein et al., 1973; Dawson et al., 1975). 5-Methyl tetrahydrofolate alone is ineffective (Metz et al., 1968; Gutstein et al., 1973). These findings are consistent with the view that vitamin B_{12} deficiency produces functional folate deficiency, which can be attributed to metabolic blockade of the utilization of 5-methyl-THF.

B. Serum Folate Clearance in Vitamin B_{12} Deficiency

The "methylfolate trap" hypothesis would be supported by delayed clearance of circulating serum 5-methyl-THF and more rapid clearance of folate compounds other than methyl folates. There is general agreement that following intravenous injections of folic acid (PGA), folate activity measured by S. faecalis (serum folate other than 5-methyl-THF) in fact does disappear more rapidly from the circulation both in folate-deficient and vitamin B_{12}-deficient patients than in normal subjects (Chanarin et al., 1958; Herbert and Zalusky, 1961, 1962; Mollin et al., 1962; Chanarin and McLean, 1967; Herbert, 1971, 1973). It has been further observed that the greater the anemia, the more rapid is the clearance rate of S. faecalis activity from the serum after intravenous injection of folic acid in patients with pernicious anemia (Foster et al., 1964). These findings support the concept that in vitamin B_{12}-deficient patients, the anemia is dependent on deficiency of folate coenzymes other than 5-methyl-THF.

Herbert and Zalusky (1961, 1962) showed that after intravenous injection of folic acid (PGA), 5-methyl-THF (measured by the difference between L. casei and S. faecalis activity for as long as 24 hours after the injection) was cleared slowly from the sera of patients with vitamin B_{12} deficiency. Chanarin and Perry (1968), however, reported being unable to demonstrate delayed serum clearance of methylfolate measured only for 90 minutes, after intravenous administration of this folate compound to patients with pernicious anemia. In a study of 3 patients with pernicious anemia, Mollin et al., (1962) observed initial rapid disappearance of methylfolate, which became slower than normal after the first 30 minutes.

The most recent study demonstrating the accumulation of 5-methylfolate in the serum in vitamin B$_{12}$ deficiency is the report by Nixon and Bertino (1972), who observed that after intravenous administration, radioactive methyl-THF was cleared from the serum to tissues of B$_{12}$-deficient subjects half as fast as after the same subject had received vitamin B$_{12}$ therapy. They further showed that this blockade in utilization could not be demonstrated when too large a dose of methylfolate was injected. It is most likely that the use of larger doses of methylfolate prevented investigators such as Chanarin and Perry (1968) from confirming the phenomenon of delayed clearance. Thus, slow clearance of injected 5-methylfolate from serum, demonstrated under appropriate conditions of dose and time sequence, indicates that in fact there is abnormal accumulation in serum of this form of folate in vitamin B$_{12}$ deficiency, supporting the "methylfolate trap" hypothesis. The recent work of Chello and Bertino (1973) in cultures of L5178Y murine leukemic cell line provides further support. They showed that 5-methyl-THF failed to maintain cell growth in cultures in the absence of added vitamin B$_{12}$, with or without transcobalamin II, whereas folic acid (pteroylglutamic acid) in large quantity and folinic acid (N^5-formyl-THF) in relatively small doses were able to do so. This further indicates the dependence on vitamin B$_{12}$ of 5-methyl-THF for its metabolic participation in the promotion of cell growth *in vitro*.

C. EFFECT OF VITAMIN B$_{12}$ DEFICIENCY ON FORMIMINOGLUTAMIC ACID (FIGLU) AND OTHER METABOLITES

Urinary excretion of FIGLU after a histidine load is almost invariably increased in folate deficiency owing to lack of reduced folate (THF) coenzyme as acceptor of the formimino group (Luhby and Cooperman, 1964; Chanarin, 1964; Herbert, 1959, 1968, 1973). However, this may occur in other forms of metabolic blockade involving folate coenzyme or formiminotransferase, the enzyme that catalyzes the transfer of the formimino group to THF (H$_4$PteGlu). The majority of patients with untreated vitamin B$_{12}$-deficiency megaloblastic anemia also show increased urinary excretion of this intermediary metabolite of histidine catabolism (Herbert, 1959; Herbert and Sullivan, 1963; Chanarin, 1960, 1964; Chanarin and McLean, 1967). Some investigators observed the highest FIGLU excretion in the most anemic patients with vitamin B$_{12}$ deficiency (Knowles and Prankerd, 1962). Vitamin B$_{12}$ therapy results in a decline of FIGLU excretion in these patients; a similar decline also occurs in B$_{12}$-deficient patients after administration of folic acid in large doses (Chanarin, 1963), methionine, or glycine, but not serine (Herbert and Sullivan, 1963); the therapeutic effects of glycine and serine are not always consistent. However, the oxidation of the β-carbon of serine into respiratory CO_2 and the incorporation of [^{14}C]formate into serine by lymphocytes are clearly decreased in B_{12}-deficient as well as folate-deficient patients (DeGrazia et al., 1969; Ellsgaard and Esmann, 1973a,b). It is probable that vitamin B_{12} acts by relieving the metabolic blockade of methylfolate to make THF available for transfer of the formimino group from FIGLU. The response to folic acid is explained by its conversion to THF.

The greater part of the formimino group of FIGLU enters the single-carbon-unit pool as active formate, and a small, but significant amount appears in the expired air as CO_2 (Borsook et al., 1950). The administration of [2-^{14}C]histidine is followed by rapid appearance of $^{14}CO_2$ in the expired air. Thenen, Gawthorne, and Stokstad (1971) observed that $^{14}CO_2$ expired by rats on a basal diet containing 5 mg of folate per kilogram, in 1 hour after injection of [2-^{14}C]histidine, was 3-fold that after [5-^{14}C]H-THF injection. Such rats, when deprived of dietary B_{12}, had no decrease in $^{14}CO_2$ production from [5-^{14}C]H$_3$-THF, although $^{14}CO_2$ production from histidine was reduced. The rate of transfer of ^{14}C[2-^{14}C] from histidine into expired CO_2 was found to be markedly reduced in folate-deficient patients and mildly reduced in vitamin B_{12}-deficient patients as compared to normal subjects (Fish et al., 1963), indicating a block in folate metabolism brought about by deficiency of B_{12}.

Aminoimidazole carboxamide (AIC), an intermediary in purine synthesis, is formylated as the ribotide to inosinic acid, and this reaction is folate dependent. Folate deficiency or metabolic block-depleting reduced folate coenzymes interferes with the above reaction, and causes increased excretion of the intermediary product (AIC). Increased urinary excretion of AIC has been found in megaloblastic anemia owing to either vitamin B_{12} or folate deficiency (Herbert et al., 1964b), again indicating a metabolic interrelationship relevant to the methylfolate trap.

D. Cellular Folate Stores and Pteroylpolyglutamate Synthesis in Vitamin B_{12} Deficiency

Intracellular folate constitutes the major part of the total body pool of folate and occurs predominantly as reduced pteroylpolyglutamate. It is uncertain whether these are largely storage forms of the vitamin or participate as active coenzymes in biochemical reactions requiring folates. Although it has been suggested that pteroylpolyglutamates may be active intracellular coenzymes in some systems (Foster et al., 1964; Curthoys and Rabinowitz, 1972; Waxman et al., 1969; Weissbach and Taylor, 1970; Lavoie et al., 1975), no direct evidence to support this possibility exists in mammalian systems (Blakley, 1969; Herbert, 1974).

There are important changes in intracellular folate in vitamin B_{12} deficiency. Red cell folate content has been shown to be reduced in vitamin B_{12}-deficient patients (Niewig et al., 1954; Herbert and Zalusky, 1962; Hansen, 1964; Cooper and Lowenstein, 1964; Jeejeebhoy et al., 1965; Hoffbrand et al., 1966). This reduction is corrected after vitamin B_{12} therapy, the rise being coincidental with the reticulocyte response (Herbert and Zalusky, 1962; Hoffbrand et al., 1966; Butterworth et al., 1966). This is consistent with the fact that active transport of folate occurs in the reticulocytes and erythroid precursor cells of the bone marrow, but not in mature erythrocytes (Izak et al., 1968; Corcino et al., 1971). The polyglutamate forms of erythrocyte folate are decreased in quantity in patients with vitamin B_{12}-deficient anemia, whereas the quantity of monoglutamates (L. casei active) remains relatively normal (Chanarin et al., 1974) or mildly (Jeejeebhoy et al., 1965), and possibly only as a technical aberration (Scott et al., 1974), increased.

Similar to the situation in human blood cells, decreased pteroylpolyglutamates with an increase in the ratio of methylated to nonmethylated folates has been shown to occur in livers of vitamin B_{12}-deficient rats (Thenen and Stokstad, 1973; Vidal and Stokstad, 1974), with little or no decrease of the monoglutamate forms of folate. Administration of vitamin B_{12} or methionine restores the pteroylpolyglutamate level with corresponding increase of the nonmethylated form. There is a paucity of studies on liver folate in human subjects with vitamin B_{12}-deficient megaloblastic anemia, except that hepatic folate level was described as "normal" in pernicious anemia in a report by Waters and Mollin (1963). Lavoie et al., (1974) reported that the transfer of methyl group from 5-methyl-THF to nonfolate compounds including proteins is decreased in PHA-stimulated lymphocytes of patients with B_{12}-deficient megaloblastic anemia, and that the defect was corrected in vitro by added vitamin B_{12}. They further showed that the conversion of methyl-THF to THF was an important condition antecedent to intracellular pteroylpolyglutamate synthesis, because THF rather than methyl-THF appears to be the preferred substrate for the biosynthesis of folate polyglutamates in mammalian cells.

The evidence cited above in animals and man indicates that the methylated form of folate polyglutamate increases in vitamin B_{12}-deficient cells owing to failure of methyl transfer from 5-methyl-THF by the B_{12}-dependent homocysteine methyltransferase reaction. The resulting reduced availability of tetrahydrofolate, which is probably the preferred substrate for polyglutamate synthesis, results in decrease of total cellular pteroylpolyglutamates, and therefore reduced total intracellular folate.

Current evidence in PHA-stimulated lymphocytes (Lavoie et al., 1974) showing that PGA makes polyglutamate equally well in the normal and the B_{12}-deficient cell, tends to refute the speculation of Chanarin *et al.* (1974) that vitamin B_{12} is involved in the biosynthesis of pteroylpolyglutamate from monoglutamate by mammalian cells. The impaired cellular entry of 5-methyl-THF together with the failure of the transmethylase reaction offer adequate explanation for the reported diminution of tissue stores of pteroylpolyglutamate in vitamin B_{12}-deficient man and animals.

E. Molecular Basis of Megaloblastosis in Vitamin B_{12} and Folate Deficiency

A unified concept of megaloblastic anemias as the morphological expression of any biochemical defect leading to slowing of deoxyribonucleic acid (DNA) synthesis per unit time has been presented (Herbert, 1959, 1965; Stebbins *et al.*, 1973).

Cellular DNA synthesis depends on the availability of the four nucleotide triphosphate building blocks (triphosphates of deoxyadenosine, deoxyguanosine, deoxycytosine, and deoxythymidine) (Fig. 5) (Werner, 1971; Fridland, 1973). The synthesis of thymidine triphosphate is of particular interest, since it plays a key role in DNA synthesis owing to the specificity of the thymine base for DNA. This is achieved in most cell systems by the conversion of uridylate to deoxyuridylate (dUMP) by the iron-dependent enzyme ribonucleotide reductase, and the subsequent methylation of deoxyuridylate to thymidylate (dTMP) by the enzyme thymidylate synthetase. This is a rate-limiting step in mammalian DNA synthesis, and requires the folate coenzyme, 5,10-methylene-THF as an essential cofactor (Friedkin, 1963). Deoxyuridine can be taken up by proliferating cells and then phosphorylated to deoxyuridylate (dUMP) to act as a substrate for *de novo* synthesis of thymidylate and thymidine triphosphate. This constitutes the major pathway of thymine-DNA synthesis in most mammalian cells. However, almost all cells also contain the enzyme thymidine kinase for cellular uptake of preformed thymidine, which provides a "salvage pathway" of thymine-DNA synthesis. This alternative pathway may be of particular significance in the bone marrow for the possible reutilization of thymidine available from the breakdown products of cells (Rabinowitz and Wilhite, 1969). Cellular DNA synthesis appears to be regulated by feedback mechanisms involving these pathways. For example, the incorporation of [³H]thymidine into DNA by the "salvage pathway" is inhibited by the *de novo* synthesis of thymidylate (dTMP and dTTP) from deoxyuridine added to cultures of normal proliferating cells (Ives *et al.*, 1963; Bresnik and Karjala, 1964). dGTP allosterically inhibited thymidine kinase, thereby blocking uptake and phosphorylation of TdR.

Studies on bone marrow from patients with both folate-deficient and vitamin B$_{12}$-deficient megaloblastic anemia have shown a defect in the folate-dependent *de novo* pathway of thymine-DNA synthesis. Killman (1964) reported that excess of deoxyuridine added to cultures of normal bone marrow suppressed the incorporation of [^{3}H]thymidine into DNA, but failed to do so in bone marrows of patients with vitamin B$_{12}$-deficient megaloblastic anemia, thus suggesting that thymine-DNA synthesis might require vitamin B$_{12}$ in mammalian systems. Metz *et al.* (1968) extended these studies to show that vitamin B$_{12}$ was not directly involved in *de novo* thymidylate synthesis in human bone marrows and the impaired thymine-DNA synthesis in vitamin B$_{12}$-deficient marrows was mediated by a blockade in folate metabolism. These investigators demonstrated that the defective *de novo* synthesis of thymidylate (impaired "dU suppression" of [^{3}H]thymidine incorporation into DNA) was partially corrected by added vitamin B$_{12}$ in the bone marrow cultures of B$_{12}$-deficient, but not of folate-deficient subjects, although in both types of deficiencies, this defect was completely corrected by large doses of folic acid (pteroylmonoglutamic acid), and smaller doses of folinic acid (5-formyltetrahydrofolic acid). Further, the corrective effects of vitamin B$_{12}$ and folate in B$_{12}$-deficient marrows and of folate in folate-deficient marrows was blocked by the folate antagonist methotrexate. A crucial piece of evidence, supporting the "5-methyl-THF trap" hypothesis in vitamin B$_{12}$ deficiency, is provided by the differential behavior of 5-methyltetrahydrofolate when used to try to correct *de novo* thymine DNA synthesis in folate- and vitamin B$_{12}$-deficient bone marrows, 5-Methyltetrahydrofolate, the main folate coenzyme in plasma, which has been shown to "pile up" in the plasma of patients with vitamin B$_{12}$ deficiency, corrects the abnormal "dU suppression" in folate-deficient marrows, but fails to do so in B$_{12}$-deficient marrows unless vitamin B$_{12}$ too is added to the *in vitro* culture system (Metz *et al.*, 1968; Herbert *et al.*, 1974). Essentially similar abnormalities in DNA synthesis have been shown to occur in "megaloblastic lymphocytes," created by PHA-stimulation, of patients with vitamin B$_{12}$ and folate deficiencies (Das and Hoffbrand, 1970b). Thus, in deficiency of vitamin B$_{12}$ or folate, the defective cellular synthesis of thymine-DNA is due to reduced availability of the folate coenzyme 5,10-methylene-THF, and the reported increased activity of thymidylate synthetase is consistent with these observations (Sakamoto *et al.*, 1975). In vitamin B$_{12}$ deficiency, the reduced activity of the pertinent folate coenzyme results from a block in the utilization of 5-methyl-THF due to failure of the B$_{12}$-dependent homocysteine–methyl-THF transmethylase reaction.

Beck (1975) reported that nonradioactive thymidine fails to decrease the incorporation of [^{3}H]UdR (radioactive deoxyuridine) into DNA by normal bone marrow cells, and that these findings cast doubt on the validity of "dU suppression test" as a biochemical index of megaloblastosis.

This reported failure may be a reflection of the minor role of the "salvage pathway" in providing thymidine for DNA synthesis in normal cells, the major pathway being the *de novo* synthesis of thymidylate (dTMP) from deoxyuridine. However, in our own laboratory, nonradioactive TdR decreased the incorporation of [^{3}H]UdR into DNA of phytohemagglutinin-stimulated human lymphocytes by more than 98% (K. C. Das and V. Herbert, unpublished). Several experiments have shown that radioactive deoxyuridine is actively incorporated into DNA by normal marrow and neoplastic cells (Metz *et al.*, 1968; Tisman *et al.*, 1973) and this process is inhibited in megaloblastic marrow cells (Metz *et al.*, 1968), and by methotrexate in PHA-stimulated normal lymphocytes, leukemic cells (Hoffbrand *et al.*, 1973), and tumor cells (Tissman *et al.*, 1973).

It remains uncertain exactly how the morphological peculiarities of megaloblastic transformation relate to defective DNA synthesis. The modal DNA content of nuclei of interphase erythroblasts and lymphocytes of patients with vitamin B_{12} and folate-deficient megaloblastic anemia has been reported to be diploid (2C), although a significant proportion of cells appear to contain an intermediate amount of DNA between diploid (2C) and tetraploid (4C) quantities (Beck, 1964, 1972; Wickramasinghe *et al.*, 1968; Yoshida *et al.*, 1968; Das and Hoffbrand, 1970b) with possible arrest of cells at all phases of the cell cycle. Although disturbance in the balance of deoxyribonucleotide synthesis has been postulated, no qualitative or quantitative difference in the base composition of DNA in megaloblastic bone marrow has been detected (Hoffbrand and Pegg, 1972; Hoffbrand and Tripp, 1972). An explanation for the finely reticulated appearance of nuclear chromatin in interphase megaloblasts is lacking. It has been recently reported that the biosynthesis, acetylation, and methylation of arginine-rich histone is impaired in B_{12}-deficient megaloblastic bone marrows (Kass, 1973, 1974). However, it is possible that these abnormalities are secondary to defective DNA synthesis. Further, the relationship between vitamin B_{12} and folate in histone biosynthesis and metabolism cannot be determined from the available data, since the studies were limited to patients with pernicious anemia. The possible role of folate deficiency in the causation of such abnormalities cannot be ruled out in view of the biochemical evidences that folate coenzymes are required in methylation and acetylation reactions in mammalian and bacterial cells, as reviewed elsewhere in this chapter.

F. Effect of Methionine in Vitamin B_{12} Deficiency

The administration of methionine appears to markedly influence the metabolism of folate in animals and man. Silverman and Pitney (1958) first observed that methionine decreased the elevated urinary excretion of FIGLU in rats either deficient in vitamin B$_{12}$ or in folate. Subsequent studies confirmed these observations, and further showed that the depleted liver folates in vitamin B$_{12}$-deficient rats were increased by the administration of methionine or vitamin B$_{12}$ or both with reduction in the ratio of methylated to nonmethylated forms of reduced folate (Kutzbach et al., 1967; Gawthorne and Stokstad, 1971; Thenen and Stokstad, 1973; Vidal and Stokstad, 1974). Similar effect of methionine was also reported in vitamin B$_{12}$-deficient sheep (Dawbarn et al., 1958; Smith and Osborne-White, 1973; Gawthorne and Smith, 1974; Smith et al., 1974). The "profolate" influence of methionine in vitamin B$_{12}$-deficient animals was attributed to its effect on the metabolism of folate coenzymes. As described above, in vitamin B$_{12}$ deficiency, 5-methyl-THF, formed by the essentially irreversible methylene-THF reductase reaction (Kutzbach and Stokstad, 1971) is metabolically trapped due both to a block in the vitamin B$_{12}$-dependent 5-methyl-THF homocysteine–transmethylase reaction and to reduced cellular uptake. The administered methionine is metabolized to 5-adenosylmethionine, an inhibitor by negative feedback of 5,10-methylene-THF reductase in rat liver. That inhibition reduces methylfolate, thus increasing the levels of nonmethyl-reduced folate in rat liver (Kutzbach and Stokstad, 1971; Kutzbach et al., 1967).

In patients with vitamin B$_{12}$-deficient megaloblastic anemia, the administration of methionine reduces the elevated urinary excretion of FIGLU, but appears to have an "antifolate" effect, in that it aggravates megaloblastosis in the bone marrow. The studies of Waxman et al. (1969) show that methionine aggravates the defective synthesis of thymine-DNA from deoxyuridylate (dUMP) in bone marrow cultures of patients with vitamin B$_{12}$-deficient megaloblastic anemia, just as Rundles and Brewer (1958) had shown that methionine made bone marrow megaloblastosis worse. This could be explained by a dominant end-product inhibition effect of methionine on the homocysteine transmethylase reaction (Fig. 6) resulting in further accumulation of 5-methyl-THF, with minor or no negative feedback inhibition of bone marrow, 5,10-methylene-THF reductase. Alternatively, the apparent discrepancy in the effect of methionine on B$_{12}$-deficient animals as compared to man may be due to species difference, since vitamin B$_{12}$ deficiency does not seem to produce megaloblastic change in rats and sheep. The recent report of Cheng et al. (1975) appears to support the former possibility. They have shown that methionine exerts a "profolate" effect in the liver and an "antifolate" effect in the bone marrow of vitamin B$_{12}$-deficient rats. In bone marrow, methionine reduced the folate-dependent methylation of dUMP and increased the levels of 5-methyl-THF at the expense of THF and N^{10}-formyl-THF, but this did not happen in liver. It is possible that methionine plays a more important role in the feedback inhibition of the homocysteine–methyltransferase reaction than of the methylene-THF reductase reaction in bone marrow cells and the reverse (i.e., greater effect on the latter reaction) in the liver cells.

G. Neurological Lesions in Vitamin B_{12} Deficiency

The biochemical basis of the neurological lesions of vitamin B_{12} deficiency is one of the least understood aspects of B_{12} metabolism. Clinical observations, associating neurological symptoms with folate deficiency have been reported without any evidence of organic damage of the myelin sheath (Luhby and Cooperman, 1967; Reynolds et al., 1973). Patients with pernicious anemia who present with neurological lesions may often have minimal anemia and higher serum folate levels (L. casei active) than normal (Waters and Mollin, 1963). Damage to the myelin sheath is the most obvious organic lesion in B_{12}-deficient neuropathy. The biochemical basis for the myelin damage is obscure. It has been proposed that the neurological damage may be related to the deoxyadenosyl-B_{12} requirement for the propionate–methylmalonate–succinyl conversion, but this is unlikely because infants with congenital methylmalonic aciduria lacking the apoenzyme for the conversion do not have myelin damage (Dillon et al., 1974) and the abnormalities reported in the lipids of myelin in vitamin B_{12}-deficient subjects have not been shown to produce neurological damage (Frenkel, 1973; Frenkel et al., 1973; Burton and Frenkel, 1975; Kishimoto et al., 1973). This reaction links fat and carbohydrate metabolism via the Krebs tricarboxylic acid cycle, but there is as yet no clear evidence that it has a role in vitamin B_{12} deficiency nerve damage (Herbert and Tisman, 1973).

IV. Concluding Remarks

The "5-methyltetrahydrofolate trap hypothesis," which postulates that vitamin B_{12} deficiency is largely a conditioned folate deficiency, offers a satisfactory explanation for most of the clinical and biochemical similarities of vitamin B_{12} and folate deficiency in man. The trap has two facets: inadequate or impaired conversion of 5-methyl-THF to THF by the B_{12}-dependent homocysteine methyltransferase reaction, and defective cellular uptake of 5-methyl-THF in vitamin B_{12} deficiency. These two facets explain both the reduced folate stores and impaired synthesis of intracellular folate polyglutamates in vitamin B_{12}-deficient man and animals (Thenen and Stokstad, 1973; Vidal and Stokstad, 1974; Lovoie et al., 1974). The coenzyme forms involved in the conversion of homocysteine to methionine include 5-methyl-THF, methyl-B$_{12}$, S-adenosylmethionine, and reduced flavin adenine dinucleotide (FADH$_2$), as mentioned earlier in this chapter (Fig. 6). Several investigators have shown reduced homocysteine-methyltransferase activity in vitamin B$_{12}$-deficient chickens (Dickerman et al., 1964), rats (Kutzbach et al., 1967), and sheep (Gawthorne and Smith, 1974). Direct measurements of homocysteine methyltransferase in man are lacking, although indirect biochemical evidences of their reduced activity have been referred to above.

S-Adenosylmethionine has been suggested to inhibit, in vitamin B$_{12}$-deficient rats, the essentially irreversible methylene-THF reductase reaction, responsible for the synthesis of 5-methyl-THF from methylene-THF (Kutzbach and Stokstad, 1967, 1971), and thus to reduce the trapping of 5-methyl-THF. Methionine is available in the cells at least partly from the vitamin B$_{12}$-dependent homocysteine-methyltransferase reaction, and the "methylfolate trap" in B$_{12}$ deficiency would in turn limit the inhibitory effect of S-adenosylmethionine on the synthesis of 5-methyl-THF. However, the recent report of Cheng et al. (1975) appears to indicate that the regulation of folate coenzyme synthesis in bone marrow cells may be different than that in the liver cells. The feedback inhibition of the methylene-THF-reductase reaction due to S-adenosylmethionine may be overwhelmed by the end-product inhibition of homocysteine-transmethylase reaction by methionine in the bone marrow of B$_{12}$-deficient man (Waxman et al., 1969) and rats (Cheng et al., 1975). This is suggested by the fact that added methionine aggravates the defective in vitro synthesis of thymine-DNA by the bone marrow cells of B$_{12}$-deficient man and rats. Thus the importance of the homocysteine-methyltransferase reaction in the bone marrow cells is probably not as a source of methionine, but as a means of regeneration of THF from 5-methyl-THF to provide adquate supply of the main one-carbon acceptor to the tissues.

It is yet to be proved that there exist alternative pathways not requiring vitamin B$_{12}$ for the transfer of the methyl group from 5-methyl-THF in mammalian cells. Preliminary reports suggesting that methylation of homocysteine may occur at least to some extent by a B$_{12}$-independent mechanism in man (Foster, 1966) [i.e., a possible "escape hatch" from the folate trap (Waxman et al., 1969)] and rats (Wang et al., 1967) are yet to be confirmed. Two reports suggested a methyl transfer involving biogenic amines (Laduron et al., 1974; Leysen and Laduron, 1974). However, this proved to be transfer of one-carbon units other than the methyl group of 5-methyl-THF in livers of chick and rat (Mandel et al., 1974; Wyatt et al., 1975; Meller et al., 1975). Furthermore, the possibility of these being degradation products exists, and their relevance, if any, to the regulation of folate coenzymes in vitamin B_{12}-deficient mammalian bone marrows is uncertain. It is possible these reactions do generate THF (Boarder, 1975), and thus constitute part of an "escape hatch" from the folate trap. It should be noted that the possible existence of an "escape hatch" from the "folate trap" does not weaken the theoretical importance of the trap itself; it simply means that the trap is relative rather than absolute.

Evidence available at present supports the "methyl-THF trap" hypothesis as the most plausible mechanism for the pathogenesis of megaloblastic anemia in vitamin B_{12} deficiency. The neurological manifestations that occur in vitamin B_{12}-deficient patients appear to be mediated by as yet unknown, probably nonfolate-related, pathways, which may or may not relate to the fatty acid biochemical lesions noted by Frankel (1973; Burton and Frenkel, 1975) in human nerve tissue in B_{12} deficiency.

The most recent reported researches continue to present new evidence consistent with the "folate trap" hypothesis (Shin et al., 1975; Robertson et al., 1976).

REFERENCES

Arakawa, T. (1970). Am. J. Med. 48, 594.

Babior, B. M., ed. (1975). "Cobalamin: Biochemistry and Pathophysiology." Wiley, New York.

Beck, W. S. (1964). Medicine (Baltimore) 43. 715.

Beck, W. S. (1972). In "Hematology" (W. J. Williams et al., eds.), pp. 249–297. McGraw-Hill, New York.

Beck, W. S. (1975). In "Cobalamin: Biochemistry and Pathophysiology" (B. M. Babior, ed.), pp. 403–450. Wiley, New York.

Blakley, R. L. (1969). "The Biochemistry of Folic Acid and Related Pteridines." Wiley, New York.

Boarder, M. R. (1975). Lancet 2, 982.

Borsook, H., Seasy, C. L., Haagen-Smit, A. J., Keighley, G., and Lowy, P. H. (1950). J. Biol. Chem. 187, 839.

Bresnick, E., and Karjala, R. J. (1964). Cancer Res. 24, 841.

Buchanan, J. M. (1964). Medicine (Baltimore) 43, 697.

Burton, W. C., and Frenkel, E. P. (1975). Biochim. Biophys. Acta 398, 217.

Butterworth, C. E., Jr., Scott, C. W., Magnus, E., Santini, R., and Sempsey, H. (1966). Med. Clin. N. Am. 50, 1627.

Chanarin, I. (1960). Proc. Eur. Soc. Haematol., 7th, 1959 Vol. 2, p. 52.

Chanarin, I. (1963). Br. J. Haematol. 9, 141.

Chanarin, I. (1964). Proc. R. Soc. Med. 57, 384.

Chanarin, I. (1969). "The Megaloblastic Anaemias." Blackwell, Oxford.

Chanarin, I. (1974). In "Advanced Haematology" (R. G. Huntsman and G. C. Jenkins, eds.), pp. 87–107. Butterworth, London.

Chanarin, I., and McLean, A. (1967). Clin. Sci. 32, 57.

Chanarin, I., and Perry, J. (1968). *Br. J. Haematol.* **14**, 297.

Chanarin, I., Mollin, D. L., and Anderson, B. B. (1958). *Br. J. Haematol.* **4**, 435–446.

Chanarin, I., Perry, J., and Lumb, M. (1974). *Lancet* **1**, 1251.

Chello, P. L., and Bertino, J. R. (1973). *Cancer Res.* **33**, 1898.

Cheng, F. W., Shane, B., and Stokstad, E. L. R. (1975). *Br. J. Haematol.* **31**, 323.

Cooper, B. A. (1973). *Clin. Haematol.* **2**, 461.

Cooper, B. A., and Lowenstein, L. (1964). *Blood* **24**, 502.

Corcino, J., Waxman, S., and Herbert, V. (1971). *Br. J. Haematol.* **20**, 503.

Cox, E. V., and White, A. M. (1962). *Lancet* **2**, 853.

Curthoys, N. P., and Rabinowitz, J. C. (1972). *J. Biol. Chem.* **247**, 1965.

Das, K. C. (1971). *Proc. Cong. Asian-Pac. Div. Int. Soc. Haematol., 2nd, 1971,* pp. 11–13.

Das, K. C. (1974). *Proc. Symp. Nutr. Anaemias, Silver Jubilee Conf. Indian Assoc. Pathol. Microbiol., 1974,* pp. 22–23.

Das, K. C., and Aikat, B. K. (1967). *Proc. Cong. Asian Pac. Soc. Hematol., 4th, 196 ,* p. 14.

Das, K. C., and Hoffbrand, A. V. (1970a). *Br. J. Haematol.* **19**, 203.

Das, K. C., and Hoffbrand, A. V. (1970b). *Br. J. Haematol.* **19**, 459.

Dawbarn, M. C., Hine, D. C., and Smith, J. (1958). *Aust. J. Exp. Biol. Med. Sci.* **36**, 541.

Dawson, D. W., Lewis, M. J., and Wadsworth, L. D. (1975). *Br. J. Haematol.* **31**, 77.

DeGrazia, J. A., Fish, M. B., Pollycove, M., Wallerstein, R. O., and Hollander, L. (1969). *J. Nucl. Med.* **10**, 329.

Dickerman, H., Redfield, B. G., Bieri, J. G., and Weissbach, H. (1964). *J. Biol. Chem.* **239**, 2545.

Dillon, M. J., England, J. M., Gompertz, D., Goodey, P. A., Grant, D. B., Hussein, H. A.-A., Linnell, J. C., Matthews, D. M., Mudd, S. H., Newns, G. H., Seakins, J. W. T., Uhlendorf, B. W., and Wise, I. J. (1974). *Clin. Sci. Mol. Med.* **47**, 43.

Dinning, J. S., Keith, C. K., Day, P. L., and Totter, J. R. (1949). *Proc. Soc. Exp. Biol. Med.* **72**, 262.

Ellsgaard, J., and Esmann, V. (1973a). *Scand. J. Clin. Lab. Invest.* **31**, 9.

Ellsgaard, J., and Esmann, V. (1973b). *Br. J. Haematol.* **24**, 571.

Fish, M. B., Pollycove, M., and Feichtmeir, T. V. (1963). *Blood* **2**, 447.

Foster, M. A. (1966). *In* "Proceedings of a Symposium on Folic Acid" (V. Anderson, ed.), p. 79. Glaxo Laboratories Ltd., Greenford, Middlesex, England.

Foster, M. A., Tejerina, G., Guest, J. R., and Woods, D. D. (1964). *Biochem. J.* **92**, 476.

Frenkel, E. P. (1973). *J. Clin. Invest.* **52**, 1237.

Frenkel, E. P., Kitchens, R. L., and Johnston, J. M. (1973). *J. Biol. Chem.* **248**, 7540.

Fridland, A. (1973). *Nature (London), New Biol.* **243**, 105.

Friedkin, M. (1957). *Fed. Proc., Fed. Am. Soc. Exp. Biol.* **16**, 183.

Friedkin, M. (1963). *Annu. Rev. Biochem.* **32**, 185.

Fujioka, S., and Silber, R. (1969). *Biochem. Biophys. Res. Commun.* **35**, 759.

Gawthorne, J. M., and Smith, R. M. (1974). *Biochem. J.* **142**, 119.

Gawthorne, J. M., and Stokstad, E. L. R. (1971). *Proc. Soc. Exp. Biol. Med.* **136**, 42.

Gompertz, D. (1968). *Clin. Chim. Acta* **19**, 477.

Gompertz, D., Hywel-Jones, J., and Knowles, J. P. (1967). *Lancet* **1**, 424.

Gutstein, S., Bernstein, L. H., Levy, L., and Wagner, G. (1973). *Am. J. Dig. Dis.* **18**, 142.

Hansen, H. A. (1964). "On the Diagnosis of Folic Acid Deficiency," p. 49. Almqvist & Wiksell, Stockholm.

Hartman, S. C., and Buchanan, J. M. (1959). *J. Biol. Chem.* **234**, 1812.

Hatch, F. T., Larrabee, A. R., Cathou, R. E., and Buchanan, J. M. (1961). *J. Biol. Chem.* **236**, 1095.

Heath, C. W. (1966). *Blood* **27**, 800.

Herbert, V. (1959). "The Megaloblastic Anemias." Grune & Stratton, New York.

Herbert, V. (1965). *Dis.-Mon.*, August.

Herbert, V. (1968). *Vitam. Horm. (N.Y.)* **26**, 525.

Herbert, V. (1971). *In* "The Cobalamins" (H. R. V. Arnstein and R. J. Wrighton, eds.), pp. 1–16. Churchill, London.

Herbert, V. (1973). *In* "Modern Nutrition in Health and Disease: Dietotherapy" (R. S. Goodhart and M. E. Shils, eds.), 5th ed., pp. 221–243. Lea & Febiger, Philadelphia, Pennsylvania.

Herbert, V. (1974). *Lancet* **2**, 834.

Herbert, V. (1975a). *In* "Textbook of Medicine" (P. B. Beeson and W. McDermott, eds.), 14th ed., pp. 1404–1413. Saunders, Philadelphia, Pennsylvania.

Herbert, V. (1975b). *In* "The Pharmacological Basis of Therapeutics" (L. S. Goodman and A. Gilman, eds.), 5th ed., pp. 1324–1349. Macmillan, New York.

Herbert, V., and Bertino, J. R. (1967). *In* "The Vitamins (Chemistry, Physiology, Pathology, Methods)" (P. György and W. N. Pearson, eds.), Vol. 7, pp. 243–269. Academic Press, New York.

Herbert, V., and Sullivan, L. W. (1963). *Proc. Soc. Exp. Biol. Med.* **112**, 304.

Herbert, V., and Tisman, G. (1973). *In* "Biology of Brain Dysfunction" (G. Gaull, ed.), Vol. 1, pp. 373–392. Plenum, New York.

Herbert, V., and Zalusky, R. (1961). *Clin. Res.* **9**, 161.

Herbert, V., and Zalusky, R. (1962). *J. Clin. Invest.* **41**, 1263.

Herbert, V., Larrabee, A. B., and Buchanan, J. M. (1962). *J. Clin. Invest.* **41**, 1134.

Herbert, V., Sullivan, L. W., Streiff, R. R., and Friedkin, M. (1964a). *Nature (London)* **201**, 196.

Herbert, V., Streiff, R., Sullivan, L., and McGeer, P. (1964b). *Fed. Proc., Fed. Am. Soc. Exp. Biol.* **23**, 188.

Herbert, V., Tisman, G., Go, L.-T., and Brenner, L. (1974). *Br. J. Haematol.* **24**, 713.

Hoffbrand, A. V. (1971). *In* "Recent Advances in Haematology" (A. Goldberg and M. C. Brain, eds.), pp. 1–76. Churchill, London.

Hoffbrand, A. V. (1972) *Br. J. Haematol.* **23**, Suppl., 109.

Hoffbrand, A. V. (1975). *Prog. Hematol.* **9**, 85.

Hoffbrand, A. V., and Pegg, A. E. (1972). *Nature (London), New Biol.* **235**, 187.

Hoffbrand, A. V., and Tripp, E. (1972). *Br. Med. J.* **1**, 140.

Hoffbrand, A. V., Newcombe, B. F. A., and Mollin, D. L. (1966). *J. Clin. Pathol.* **19**, 17.

Hoffbrand, A. V., Tripp, E., Catovsky, D., and Das, K. C. (1973). *Br. J. Haematol.* **25**, 497.

Hopper, S. (1972). *J. Biol. Chem.* **247**, 3336.

Huennekens, F. M. (1968). *In* "Biological Oxidations" (T. P. Singer, ed.), p. 439. Wiley (Interscience), New York.

IUPAC-IUB Commission. (1966). *J. Biol. Chem.* **241**, 2991.

Ives, D. H., Morse, P. A., Jr., and van Potter, R. (1963). *J. Biol. Chem.* **238**, 1467.

Izak, G., Rachmilewitz, M., Grossowicz, N., Galewski, K., and Kraus, S. H. (1968). *Br. J. Haematol.* **14**, 447.

Jeejeebhoy, K. N., Pathare, S. M., and Noronha, J. M. (1965). *Blood* **26**, 354.

Kass, L. (1973). *Blood* **41**, 549.

Kass, L. (1974). *Blood* **44**, 125.

Katzen, H. M., and Buchanan, J. M. (1965). *J. Biol. Chem.* **240**, 825.

Killman, S. A. (1964). *Acta Med. Scand.* **175**, 485.

Kishimoto, Y., Williams, M., Moser, H. W., Hignite, C., and Biemann, K. (1973). *J. Lipid Res.* **14,** 69.

Knowles, J. P., and Prankerd, T. A. J. (1962). *Clin. Sci.* **22,** 233.

Kutzbach, C., and Stokstad, E. L. R. (1967). *Biochim. Biophys. Acta* **139,** 217.

Kutzbach, C., and Stokstad, E. L. R. (1971). *Biochim. Biophys. Acta* **250,** 459.

Kutzbach, C., Galloway, E., and Stokstad, E. L. R. (1967). *Proc. Soc. Exp. Biol. Med.* **124,** 801.

Laduron, P. M., Gommeren, W. R., and Leysen, J. E. (1974). *Biochem. Pharmacol.* **23,** 1599.

Lavoie, A., Tripp, E., and Hoffbrand, A. V. (1974). *Clin. Sci. Mol. Med.* **47,** 617.

Lavoie, A., Tripp, E., Parsa, K., and Hoffbrand, A. V. (1975). *Clin. Sci. Mol. Med.* **48,** 67.

Leysen, J. E., and Laduron, P. M. (1974). *Adv. Biochem. Psychopharmacol.* **11,** 65.

Linnell, J. C., Mackenzie, H. M., Wilson, J., and Matthews, D. M. (1969). *J. Clin. Pathol.* **22,** 545.

Linnell, J. C., Hoffbrand, A. V., Peters, T. J., and Matthews, D. M. (1971). *Clin. Sci.* **40,** 1.

Luhby, A. L., and Cooperman, J. M. (1964). *Adv. Metab. Disord.* **1,** 263.

Luhby, A. L., and Cooperman, J. M. (1967). *Abstr., Am. Pediatr. Soc., 77th Meet.* p. 387.

McGeer, P. L., Seu, N. P., and Grant, D. A. (1965). *Can. J. Biochem.* **43,** 1307.

Machlin, L. J., Denton, C. A., and Bird, H. R. (1951). *Fed. Proc., Fed. Am. Soc. Exp. Biol.* **10,** 388.

Mahoney, M. J., and Rosenberg, L. E. (1970). *Am. J. Med.* **48,** 584.

Mandel, I. R., Rosegay, A., Walker, R. W., VandenHeuvel, W. J. A., and Rokach, J. (1974). *Science* **186,** 741.

Marshall, R. A., and Jandl, J. H. (1960). *Arch. Intern. Med.* **105,** 352.

Meller, E., Rosengarten, H., Friedhoff, A. J., Stebbins, R. D., and Silber, R. (1975). *Science* **187,** 171.

Menzies, R. C., Crossen, P. E., Fitzgerald, P. H., and Gunz, F. W. (1966). *Blood* **28,** 581.

Metz, J., Kelly, A., Swett, V. C., Waxman, S., and Herbert, V. (1968). *Br. J. Haematol.* **14,** 575.

Middleton, J. R., Coward, R. F., and Smith, P. (1964). *Lancet* **2,** 253.

Mollin, D. L., Waters, A. H., and Harris, E. (1962). *In* "Vitamin B$_{12}$ and Intrinsic Factor" (H. C. Heinrich, ed.), p. 737. Enke, Stuttgart.

Niewig, H. O., Faber, J. G., DeVries, J. A., and Kroese, W. F. S. (1954). *J. Lab. Clin. Med.* **44,** 118.

Nixon, P. F., and Bertino, J. R. (1972). *J. Clin. Invest.* **51,** 1431.

Noronha, J. M., and Silverman, M. (1962). *In* "Vitamin B$_{12}$ and Intrinsic Factor" (H. C. Heinrich, ed.), p. 728. Enke, Stuttgart.

Osborne, M. J., Hatefi, Y., Kay, L. D., and Huennekens, F. M. (1957). *Biochim. Biophys. Acta* **26,** 208.

Pratt, J. M. (1972). "Inorganic Chemistry of Vitamin B$_{12}$." Academic Press, New York.

Rabinowitz, Y., and Wilhite, B. A. (1969). *Blood* **33,** 759.

Reynolds, E. H., Rothfeld, P., and Pincus, J. H. (1973). *Br. Med. J.* **1,** 398.

Robertson, J. S., Hsia, Y. E., and Scully, K. J. (1976). *J. Lab. Clin. Med.* **87,** 89.

Rundles, W. R., and Brewer, S. S. (1958). *Blood* **13,** 99.

Sakamoto, S., Niina, M., and Takaku, F. (1975). *Blood* **46,** 699.

Scott, J. M., O'Broin, J. D., and Weir, D. G. (1974). *Lancet* **2,** 906.

Shin, Y. L., Buehring, K. U., and Stokstad, E. L. R. (1975). *Mol. Cell. Biochem.* **9,** 97.

Silber, R., and Moldow, C. F. (1970). *Am. J. Med.* **48**, 549.

Silverman, M., and Pitney, A. L. (1958). *J. Biol. Chem.* **233**, 1179.

Smith, R. M., and Osborne-White, W. S. (1973). *Biochem. J.* **136**, 279.

Smith, R. M., Osborne-White, W. S., and Gawthorne, J. M. (1974). *Biochem. J.* **142**, 105.

Stahlberg, K. G. (1967). *Scand. J. Haematol., Suppl.* **1**.

Stebbins, R., Scott, J., and Herbert, V. (1973). *Semin. Hematol.* **10**, 235.

Stokstad, E. L. R., and Koch, J. (1967). *Physiol. Rev.* **47**, 85.

Sullivan, L. (1967). *Newer Methods Nutr. Biochem.* **3**, 365.

Thenen, S. W., and Stokstad, E. L. R. (1973). *J. Nutr.* **103**, 363.

Thenen, S. W., Gawthorne, J. M., and Stokstad, E. L. R. (1971). *Proc. Soc. Exp. Biol. Med.* **134**, 199.

Tisman, G., and Herbert, V. (1973). *Blood* **41**, 465.

Tisman, G., Herbert, V., and Edlis, H. (1973). *Cancer Chemother. Rep., Part 1* **57**, 11.

Vidal, A. J., and Stokstad, E. L. R. (1974). *Biochim. Biophys. Acta* **362**, 245.

Wang, F. K., Koch, J., and Stokstad, E. L. R. (1967). *Biochem. Z.* **346**, 458.

Waters, A. H., and Mollin, D. L. (1963). *Br. J. Haematol.* **9**, 319.

Waxman, S., Metz, J., and Herbert, V. (1969). *J. Clin. Invest.* **48**, 284.

Waxman, S., Corcino, J. J., and Herbert, V. (1970). *Am. J. Med.* **48**, 599.

Weissbach, H., and Taylor, R. T. (1968). *Vitam. Horm. (N.Y.)* **26**, 395.

Weissbach, H., and Taylor, R. T. (1970). *Vitam. Horm. (N.Y.)* **28**, 415.

Werner, R. (1971). *Nature (London), New Biol.* **233**, 99.

Wickramasinghe, S. N., Cooper, E. H., and Chalmers, D. G. (1968). *Blood* **31**, 304.

Wyatt, R. J., Erdelyi, E. D., Amaral, J. R., Elliott, G. R., Renson, J., and Barchas, J. D. (1975). *Science* **187**, 853.

Yoshida, Y., Todo, A., Shirakawa, S., Wakisaka, G., and Uchino, H. (1968). *Blood* **31**, 292.

Zalusky, R., Herbert, V., and Castle, W. B. (1962). *Arch. Intern. Med.* **109**, 545.

Vitamin E

JOHN G. BIERI AND PHILIP M. FARRELL

*National Institute of Arthritis, Metabolism and Digestive Diseases, and
Neonatal and Pediatric Medicine Branch, National Institute of Child Health
and Human Development, Bethesda, Maryland*

I. INTRODUCTION

In the past several years in the United States, a preoccupation with vitamin E by the public has forced many nutritional scientists to become involved in areas of nutrition and health that they usually avoid. This increased interest in vitamin E has led to a reexamination of many of the "basic tenets," so to speak, concerning this vitamin as the debate on its role in human health has surged and waned. Although the importance of vitamin E to many species of animals has been accepted for twenty or more years, it was only in 1968 that the Food and Nutrition Board of the U.S. National Research Council decided that vitamin E should be included as a quantified nutrient for man (Food and Nutrition Board, 1968). Prior to this, there were many individuals who questioned whether vitamin E was essential for man. No doubt, the paucity of *bona fide* demonstrations of either deficiency symptoms attributed to the vitamin or of medical benefits from therapeutic doses of vitamin E, contributed to the skepticism surrounding this nutrient. Events in the past ten years have removed doubts about the essentiality of vitamin E for man, but controversy has continued on the amount that is desirable in the diet. Furthermore, there are still claims being made for the efficacy of vitamin E in a variety of clinical conditions, most of which have not been experimentally verified but add to the public's uncertainty and preoccupation with this vitamin. This review will attempt to deal largely with these more or less applied aspects of vitamin E in nutrition and medicine.

Although interest in the biochemical functions of vitamin E has continued unabated, advances on this front have been slow with no definitive evidence to explain many of the biochemical derangements evoked by a deficiency of the vitamin in animals. Several new postulates of the site of action of vitamin E have been proposed, but the supporting evidence has not been forthcoming. Although the primary role of α-tocopherol in preventing lipid peroxidation in tissues is accepted by practically all investigators in this field, this action does not adequately explain some biochemical abnormalities observed in vitamin E deficiency.

A role for vitamin E in medicine has only begun to emerge during this decade partly because tocopherol deficiency in man secondary to nutritional deprivation is a rare occurrence in developed countries. It is difficult, in fact, to produce vitamin E deficiency under experimental conditions in adult man because of the considerable tissue storage leading to an extended period of diminished intake before depletion occurs (Horwitt, 1960). On the other hand, deficiency does occur in association with intestinal malabsorption syndromes of various etiologies. In addition, prematurely delivered infants, who begin life with marginal stores at best and who also exhibit transient malabsorption, are commonly subject to vitamin E deficiency.

The elusive search for clinical correlates of tocopherol deficiency in man has been aided by studies of the manifestations of vitamin E deficiency in lower animals. The most notable features of vitamin E deficiency in lower animals are the marked degree of species specificity and the great diversity of tissue and organ functions affected by diminished antioxidant levels (Mason and Horwitt, 1972). In many instances, particularly in rapidly growing animals, disorders such as muscular degeneration and encephalomalacia occur in an acute fashion over a matter of several days to a few weeks. In man, however, rapid development of tocopherol deficiency does not apparently occur owing to the resistance of tissue stores to depletion as well as the wide distribution of the vitamin in foodstuffs. Thus, it seems improbable that all of the animal deficiency syndromes will be found in man.

Because of the pronounced differences in nutritional status of animals under study and humans available for clinical investigations of vitamin E deficiency, it has become necessary to search for insidious pathological processes in man, leading to subclinical manifestations. Nonetheless, the ongoing efforts of investigators to uncover specific clinical signs of human tocopherol deficiency have met with frustration in many instances. In view of this unsettled picture, it is not at all surprising that a diversity of opinion exists with respect to efficacy of treatment with vitamin E.

In order to discuss the role of vitamin E in medicine, it becomes necessary to divide nutritional observations into two broad categories: (1) findings in patients with chemically proven vitamin E deficiency and (2) those on subjects who possess normal circulating tocopherol levels but have been placed on therapeutic trials ("megavitamin E" supplementation) because of diseases perceived by some physicians to be associated with antioxidant deficiency. Especially emphasized in previous reviews (Horwitt, 1960, 1962, 1974; Mason and Horwitt, 1972; Gordon and Nitowsky, 1968) is the so-called "Elgin Project," in which a limited number of adult male volunteers nutritionally depleted for three years were found to show low plasma tocopherol levels but little in the way of symptoms. In addition, many reviews tend to stress data obtained from the study of small populations of human subjects with secondary vitamin E deficiency.

In this review, we make a deliberate attempt to put all the information on vitamin E requirement, absorption, metabolism, and function in both animals and man in better perspective. The large clinical trials in which vitamin E was given at pharmacological levels for presumed medical indications, as well as trials of vitamin E for *bona fide* deficiency disease in man, will be extensively reviewed.

II. Nutritional Aspects

A. Dietary Intake

Improved analytical techniques in the past ten years not only have resulted in more accurate determinations of the α-tocopherol content of foods but have also permitted a more complete description of the content of other tocopherols and tocotrienols. Reports from several developed countries (Table I) indicate a range of about 4–9 mg of α-tocopherol (6–13.5 IU) in diets considered to be representative. If the activity of the other tocopherols, primarily γ-tocopherol in the United States and probably also in Japan, is added to these values by assuming that their combined activity is 20% of the activity of α-tocopherol (Food and Nutrition Board, 1974), then the total α-tocopherol equivalent for the United States and Japan diets calculated from the highest values in Table I would be about 11 and 7 mg (16 and 11 IU), respectively.

It can be calculated that in United States diets containing more than 10 mg of α-tocopherol equivalent, over one-half of the vitamin E activity

TABLE I

AVERAGE PER CAPITA DAILY INTAKES OF VITAMIN E AND POLYUNSATURATED
FATTY ACIDS (PUFA) IN VARIOUS COUNTRIES[a]

Country	α-Tocopherol (mg)	Other tocopherols (mg)	PUFA (gm)	Reference
Canada	6.4	—	12.4	Thompson *et al.* (1973)
England	3.9[b]	—	—	Smith *et al.* (1971)
Japan	5.2	7.0	12.4	Ikehata *et al.* (1968)
	5.9	26.9	12.5	Fukuba (1975)
United States	7.4	—	—	Bunnell *et al.* (1965)
	9.0	29.7[c]	21.2	Bieri and Evarts (1973)
	7.5	21.2[c]	19.5	Witting and Lee (1975)

[a] Dashes indicate that no analyses were made.
[b] Calculated from plotted data of 10 normal subjects.
[c] Predominantly γ-tocopherol.

is derived from vegetable oil, shortening, and margarine. Thus, relatively high intakes of vitamin E are possible only when dietary fat derived from vegetable oils is abundant. The tocopherol content of most bean and seed oils (soybean, corn, cottonseed, peanut, safflower, rapeseed) is much higher than that of animal fats (butter and lard). Olive oil and coconut oil, the predominant dietary fats in some countries, are relatively low in tocopherols. This means that vitamin E intake will be determined primarily by geographical considerations but also by economic factors, since vegetable oils are usually an expensive dietary component for low-income individuals, especially in many underdeveloped countries.

Very probably many diets throughout the world which are very low in vegetable fats and oils contain less than 5 mg of α-tocopherol equivalent (7.5 IU). For example, our calculation (unpublished) of the vitamin E content of typical rural diets in Bangladesh (Nutrition Survey of East Pakistan, 1966) where 400–500 gm of polished rice daily is the staple food, indicates at most 3.5–4 mg of α-tocopherol equivalent. In many of these low-income populations fat intake is very low, 10–15% of calories, so that most of the vitamin E in the diet comes from the staple grains. In other developing areas of the world, where tubers are the primary source of calories, similarly low intakes may exist.

In contrast to these largely vegetarian diets, Alaskan Eskimos who subsist largely on caribou meat and sea mammals have vitamin E intakes similar to those in the general United States diet (Wo and Draper, 1975). This is due to the high vitamin E content of seal meat and oil, items constituting a prominent portion of average native diets not yet modified by the use of processed foods.

Davis (1972) calculated the approximate vitamin E intake of infants up to one year of age, using published values for milk and formulas (Herting and Drury, 1969) and for infant formulas and cereals (Dicks-Bushnell and Davis, 1967). She concluded that, in order to obtain the recommended intake of 5 IU of vitamin E, the bulk would have to come from infant formulas. Formulas on the market at that time varied widely in their vitamin E content, but currently all formulas are fortified because of the infant's precarious position with respect to this vitamin (see Section IV, A).

Calculation of dietary vitamin E content is at present still inadequate owing to the failure of analysts to either separate the various tocopherols or report other vitamers in addition to α-tocopherol. Food items should be analyzed as consumed, since storage and cooking have been shown to lead to significant losses of the vitamin (Harris, 1962). Calculations should include corrections for losses of the various tocopherols during analysis, since these can be substantial under certain conditions (Bieri and Evarts, 1973; Evarts and Bieri, 1974).

B. Biological Activity

The determination by Bieri and Evarts (1973) that current United States diets may contain two to three times as much γ-tocopherol as α-tocopherol raised the possibility that the γ-compound may make a substantial contribution to the total vitamin E intake. Calculations of dietary vitamin E usually consider only the α-tocopherol in foods. Since literature values for the activity of γ-tocopherol relative to α-tocopherol ranged from 1 to 25%, a reevaluation was made. Using several different bioassay systems in rats, chicks, and hamsters, a range of 6 to 16% was found, which agrees well with the generally accepted value in the literature of 13% (Brubacher and Weiser, 1967). When γ-tocopherol was administered together with α-tocopherol, a slightly greater activity was apparent than could be accounted for by the summation of the two compounds given separately, suggesting a synergistic effect. This was studied in an *in vitro* system in which the two tocopherols separately or combined were incorporated into red cell membranes which were then subjected to the dialuric acid hemolysis test (Bieri *et al.*, 1976). γ-Tocopherol in the red cell membrane was 38% as active as α-tocopherol in preventing oxidative hemolysis, a value close to that of 30% first determined by Rose and György (1952) but considerably less than the 67% reported by Bunyan *et al.* (1960). No evidence was found for an interaction between the two tocopherols when present together in the red cell membrane. This result suggests that the possible synergistic effect noted in the whole-animal bioassays may have occurred during digestion and absorption. In comparing the antioxidant activities of tocopherols added to milk fat, Kanno *et al.* (1970) did not observe synergism between α- and γ-tocopherols. The marked difference in activity of γ-tocopherol versus α-tocopherol in nutrition assays, (10%), compared to the activity *in situ*, (38%), is probably due to the more rapid turnover of γ-tocopherol than α-tocopherol in tissues (Gloor *et al.*, 1966; Peake *et al.*, 1972).

C. Evaluation of Nutritional Status

The classic *in vitro* hemolysis of vitamin E-deficient red cells by hydrogen peroxide (Rose and György, 1952) has been criticized by various investigators as being influenced by factors other than the blood tocopherol content (Horwitt *et al.*, 1968). Poor correlation between the plasma α-tocopherol concentration and the degree of red cell hemolysis *in vitro* was found in both normal subjects and patients with malabsorption (Leonard and Losowsky, 1976), in patients with iron-deficiency anemia (Melhorn and Gross, 1969; Macdougall, 1972) as well as in anemias of other origin (Melhorn *et al.*, 1971). Patients with paroxysmal nocturnal hemoglobinemia had high peroxide hemolysis values despite normal plasma tocopherol levels (Mengel *et al.*, 1967). A partial answer to the poor correlation between the degree of hemolysis and the plasma α-tocopherol level may lie in the observation by Bieri and Evarts (1975a) that the distribution of α-tocopherol between red cells and plasma is influenced by the plasma lipid concentration. α-Tocopherol exchanges rapidly between the red cells and plasma (Silber *et al.*, 1969; Poukka and Bieri, 1970), and apparently the distribution is shifted in favor of plasma with increased lipid content of this compartment (Table II). The implications of this relationship on the usefulness of evaluating nutritional status of vitamin E from the blood tocopherol content are discussed below.

The reports above indicate that caution must be used in interpreting *in vitro* hemolysis tests. More reliable than the hemolysis test for routine screening is the plasma total tocopherol concentration using a value of 0.5 mg/dl as the lower limit of acceptability. For more accurate evaluations in experimental research, separation of the α-tocopherol from other tocopherols and carotenoids may be necessary (Bieri and Prival, 1965).

Interpretations of blood tocopherol concentration as it relates to body status of vitamin E has become complicated by observations that several factors besides the dietary intake can affect tissue tocopherol content. It is well documented that with normal intakes the plasma concentration

TABLE II
EFFECT OF PLASMA LIPID CONTENT ON DISTRIBUTION OF α-TOCOPHEROL BETWEEN
RED CELLS AND PLASMA[a]

Plasma total lipid (mg/dl)	Red cell:plasma ratio of α-tocopherol
474	0.221
975	0.132
1459	0.065
2200	0.059

[a] J. G. Bieri, unpublished data. Plasma from normal rats and from rats made hyperlipemic by injecting Triton WR-1339 were mixed to give the four lipid concentrations shown. [14C]α-Tocopherol was mixed with the plasmas, which were incubated with an equal volume of normal red cells for 5 hours. Average of two experiments.

of α-tocopherol correlates highly with the plasma concentration of total lipids (Rubinstein et al., 1968), cholesterol (Darby et al., 1949; Davies et al., 1969) and also β-lipoproteins (Kater et al., 1970). Weiss and Bianchine (1969) showed that patients with either hypertriglyceridemia or hypercholesterolemia had elevated serum tocopherol levels, which subsequently declined 20–68% when their hyperlipemia was lowered by drug therapy.

These observations have focused attention on the limited usefulness of the plasma tocopherol concentration in estimating the body's vitamin E status. Horwitt et al. (1972) have proposed that blood tocopherol determinations should always be accompanied by blood lipid values, either total lipids or cholesterol, in order to provide a more accurate interpretation of the blood tocopherol value. From a survey of bloods from infants and hospitalized adults, Horwitt et al. (1972) proposed that a ratio of 0.8 mg of total tocopherols per gram of total lipids be considered indicative of adequate nutritional status. Burk and Seely (1973) found in 14 normal adult men an average of 1.74 mg of α-tocopherol per gram of total lipids. Additional data relating these two blood components, together with information on the dietary vitamin E intake, would be desirable.

A further complicating factor in evaluating body status of vitamin E was introduced by the report of Bieri and Evarts (1975b) that the degree of adiposity affects the amount of the vitamin in organ tissues. When normal and genetically obese rats were fed the same amounts of α-tocopherol, the obese rats had lower concentrations of the vitamin in heart and lung than did normal rats. This difference occurred even though the obese rats, owing to hyperlipemia, had three times the plasma α-tocopherol of the normal animals. On the other hand, owing to their large adipose stores, the obese rats had about six times more total tocopherol in their bodies. This study indicates that organ stores of vitamin E are affected by body adiposity as well as by the plasma concentration of tocopherol.

In a related study, these investigators (Bieri and Evarts, 1975b) showed that in nonobese rats with depressed plasma lipids from feeding orotic acid, tissue stores of α-tocopherol were proportionately lower than in normal animals fed the same amount of the vitamin. These studies indicate that in animals with similar body composition, the tissue and total body storage are related to the plasma concentration of vitamin E, but that this relationship can be changed when adiposity is excessive. For practical purposes in human nutrition, at the present we may assume that vitamin E adequacy exists when plasma tocopherols exceed 0.5 mg/dl in individuals with normal body weight, but this may not be true for obese individuals.

D. RELATIONSHIP TO DIETARY POLYUNSATURATED FATTY ACIDS

Although the effect of dietary polyunsaturated fatty acids in increasing the vitamin E requirement is well documented for animals (Dam, 1962), this relationship is less clearly defined in human nutrition (Horwitt, 1962; Witting, 1972). Present evidence indicates that in diets with mixed types of fats from a variety of foodstuffs, such as occur in human diets, a single fixed ratio of milligrams of vitamin E to grams of polyunsaturated fatty acids (E:PUFA ratio) cannot be used to characterize vitamin E adequacy. Vogtmann and Prabucki (1971), using chickens, found no consistent relationship between dietary linoleic acid and liver storage of α-tocopherol when the linoleic acid was 0.3–1.1% of the diet, but at 6.5% level there was a depression in vitamin E storage. Similarly, Jager (1972) found that increased unsaturation in the diet affected the vitamin E requirement only at relatively high intakes of oils. In our studies with corn, soybean, and safflower oils (E:PUFA=0.49, 0.60, and 0.35, respectively) (Bieri and Evarts, 1975c), it was found, by all criteria of vitamin E sufficiency, that these oils produced satisfactory vitamin E status when fed at a level of 20% of the diet. Typical human diets in this country, presumably adequate in all nutrients, recently have been reported to have E:PUFA ratios averaging 0.43 (Bieri and Evarts, 1973) and 0.40 (Witting and Lee, 1975). In Japan a ratio of 0.53 was reported by Fukuba (1975). These data indicate that adequate vitamin E status in man can be achieved with diets providing an E:PUFA ratio of 0.4–0.5.

Probably of more importance than the E:PUFA ratio is the absolute dietary content of both components. This factor has been generally ignored in discussions of vitamin E and polyunsaturated acids, and few studies have been specifically designed to evaluate these relationships. Fukuba (1972) fed three different dietary fat intakes with three E:PUFA ratios and measured red cell hemolysis. He found that, for each E:PUFA ratio, the degree of hemolysis decreased with increasing dietary fat content (Table III), Similarly, we found that vegetable oils that gave significant hemolysis when fed at 5% of the diet gave insignificant hemolysis at a dietary level of 20% (Table III). These studies show that dietary oils with a relatively low E:PUFA ratio apparently become adequate when a sufficient amount is fed. This has particular relevance to human nutrition, where increased PUFA intakes must necessarily be accompanied by increased amounts of tocopherols. Horwitt (1974) has suggested a formula for calculating human dietary vitamin E requirements that considers both the percentage of PUFA in the dietary fat and the amount of PUFA consumed. This formula, α-tocopherol equivalents $= 0.25$ (% PUFA in dietary fat + grams of PUFA consumed) + 4 mg, gives values similar to the empirical values found from analyzing presumably adequate United

TABLE III

In Vitro RED CELL HEMOLYSIS IN RATS FED VARYING AMOUNTS OF FATS WITH FIXED E:PUFA RATIOS

Dietary fat (%)	E:PUFA[a]	Dietary α-tocopherol (mg/100 gm)	Hemolysis (%)
Fukuba (1972)			
Linoleic acid, 7	0.4	2	82
Linoleic acid, 16	0.4	4.6	52
Linoleic acid, 26	0.4	7.5	40
Linoleic acid, 7	0.6	3	22
Linoleic acid, 16	0.6	6.9	37[b]
Linoleic acid, 26	0.6	11.2	10
Linoleic acid, 7	0.8	4	9
Linoleic acid, 16	0.8	9.2	6
Linoleic acid, 26	0.8	15.0	7
Bieri and Evarts[c]			
Soybean oil, 5	0.38	0.8	76
Soybean oil, 20	0.38	3.2	2
Safflower oil, 5	0.34	1.3	12
Safflower oil, 10	0.34	2.6	8
Safflower oil, 20	0.34	5.2	2

[a] Milligrams of α-tocopherol per gram of PUFA.
[b] Anomalous result.
[c] Unpublished data.

States diets (Bieri and Evarts, 1973). Additional experimental testing of this formula is desirable.

This mechanism whereby PUFA increases the vitamin E requirement has been postulated to involve both absorption and storage. Increased deposition of PUFA in tissues of the rat leads to increased oxidation of α-tocopherol via accelerated fatty acid peroxidation (Witting and Horwitt, 1964). Much more tocopheryl quinone was found in depot fat of rats fed a diet high in linoleic acid than in the fat from rats fed a saturated fat (Weber and Wiss, 1966). These latter investigators also found a higher fecal excretion of labeled α-tocopherol in rats fed corn oil compared to cocoa fat (Weber et al., 1964), and tissue α-tocopherol was higher in animals ingesting the saturated fat. When the labeled α-tocopherol was given intraperitoneally to rats fed the two fats, no difference was found in tissue uptake after 2 days. These investigators concluded that PUFA interfered with the absorption of α-tocopherol and possibly also caused destruction of the vitamin. In contrast, Peake et al. (1972) found similar absorption of labeled α-tocopherol, based on lymph collection, when the compound was given in an emulsion made with lard or with corn oil. Other experiments in the author's laboratory indicate that PUFA at moderate dietary levels did not interfere with tocopherol utilization (Bieri and Poukka, 1970a). Thus, in diets containing 5 or 10% of fat and with increasing linoleic acid contents (0, 0.23, 1.1, 2.75% of the diet), plasma α-tocopherol levels generally *increased* with increasing dietary PUFA. When linoleic acid was raised to 5.5% of the diet, a decrease in plasma α-tocopherol was noted. In other experiments in which a low dietary level of α-tocopherol was fed in order to possibly maximize differences, increased dietary PUFA slightly depressed plasma levels of α-tocopherol only at the highest intake (Table IV). Concentrations in lung, heart, and liver showed slight, nonsignificant decreases with increased PUFA. Thus, a 4-fold change in E:PUFA ratio had only a minor effect on tissue tocopherol levels. Although additional studies of these relationships are needed, the authors concluded that dietary PUFA at usual intakes do not interfere significantly with α-tocopherol utilization. The data described above provide additional evidence that the relationship between dietary PUFA and α-tocopherol does not vary in a simple, linear manner.

III. METABOLISM

A. ABSORPTION

As with other fat-soluble vitamins, the absorption of tocopherols is dependent on an animal's ability to digest and absorb fat. Recent studies

TABLE IV

Effect of Increased Linoleic Acid Intake on Plasma and Tissue Concentrations of α-Tocopherol[a]

Dietary fat (%)	Dietary linoleic acid (%)	E:PUFA[b]	α-Tocopherol[c]			
			Plasma (μg/dl)	Lung (μg/gm)	Heart (μg/gm)[c]	Liver (μg/gm)
Stripped lard, 16	1.6	1.25	283 ± 17	9.9 ± 1.2	11.4 ± 2.4	6.3 ± 0.2
Stripped lard, 11 + stripped corn oil, 5	3.85	0.52	260 ± 18	9.4 ± 0.7	10.5 ± 1.2	5.9 ± 0.6
Stripped lard, 5 + stripped corn oil, 11	6.55	0.31	236 ± 12[d]	8.3 ± 1.5	9.2 ± 1.1	5.5 ± 0.6

[a] J. G. Bieri, unpublished data.
[b] Calculated using the d-α-tocopherol equivalent (20 mg/kg).
[c] Mean ± standard error of six rats fed the diets, all containing 30 mg of dl-α-tocopheryl acetate per kilogram for 8–10 weeks.
[d] Significantly different from group 1 ($p < 0.05$). Differences between groups for lung, liver, and heart were not significant.

have centered on the physical form in which it reaches the intestine, its location within the mucosal cells, the efficiency of absorption, and the effect of dietary fat unsaturation on absorption or intestinal destruction.

Tocopherol in the mucosa during absorption was found about equally in the particulate matter and in the cytosol fraction bound to lipoproteins (Rajaram et al., 1974). The essentiality of bile for tocopherol absorption has been shown both in rats (Gallo-Torres, 1970; MacMahon and Thompson, 1970) and in man (MacMahon and Neale, 1970). α-Tocopheryl acetate was found to be almost completely hydrolyzed prior to absorption in rats (Gallo-Torres, 1970) and in man (Blomstrand and Forsgren, 1968). Studies of the efficiency of absorption in rats and man, however, have not shown such agreement.

Experiments in which absorption was determined from the radioactivity collected in lymph after a dose of labeled α-tocopherol have given lower values for absorption by some investigators than by others. Thus, Johnson and Pover (1962) recovered only 10% of a dose in the lymph of rats, and Gallo-Torres (1970) found a similar low absorption efficiency. In man, Blomstrand and Forsgren (1968) found 21 and 29% of orally administered labeled α-tocopheryl acetate and α-tocopherol, respectively, in lymph.

In contrast, in studies with both rats and man in which absorption was estimated from fecal excretion, considerably higher efficiencies of absorption were noted. In rats, Losowsky et al. (1972) claimed 60–75% absorption when the labeled α-tocopherol was administered in either arachis oil, a Tween emulsion, or alcohol. Vitamin E-deficient rats gave slightly better apparent absorption than did normal rats. These investigators also showed decreasing efficiency of absorption as the dose increased. Also in rats, Cheeke and Oldfield (1969) reported 48–68% absorption of α-tocopherol. On the basis of fecal excretion in normal human subjects, MacMahon and Neale (1970) found 55–79% absorption of a radioactive dose of α-tocopherol, and Kelleher and Losowsky (1970) found 51–86% using a similar procedure.

In the only study involving recovery of labeled α-tocopherol in lymph, bile, and feces, MacMahon and Thompson (1970) showed that with mixed micelles, but not with emulsions, α-tocopherol was absorbed via the lymph to the extent of 43% while 33% of the radioactivity appeared in feces and 3% in urine, with a total recovery of 81%. When the bile duct was also cannulated, then lymphatic absorption from the mixed micelles was reduced to 20%, but 8% of the activity appeared in bile, 55% in feces, and 2% in urine.

A similarly high lymphatic absorption of α-tocopherol, 46%, was found by Peake et al. (1972) with an emulsion containing Tween, lard, and serum albumin. Thus, under optimum conditions the absorption of α-tocopherol is about 45%. The small amount of radioactivity found in bile (Mac-Mahon *et al.*, 1970), about 8% of the dose, was characterized as being predominantly (85%) water-soluble metabolites of α-tocopherol. The bile thus would appear to be a more important excretory route of metabolites than urine, where 2–4% of the dose usually appeared. MacMahon *et al.* (1970) also measured the radioactivity simultaneously in portal and arterial plasma, and found a slightly higher concentration in the portal plasma. A high proportion of the portal activity, 34–70%, was not α-tocopherol, indicating that breakdown products formed in the intestine are absorbed via this route, as well as a small amount of unchanged tocopherol. In summarizing these studies, the predominant route of absorption is the lymph, in which about 45% of a dose appears almost entirely as unchanged α-tocopherol, 10% is absorbed via the portal vein but much of the tocopherol has been degraded, and the remainder, comprising 45–55%, appears in feces, primarily as degraded products (MacMahon and Neale, 1970).

The question of the magnitude of enterohepatic circulation of α-tocopherol appears not to be clearly established. Klatskin and Molander (1952) reported the α-tocopherol concentration of bile from four human subjects to be of the "same order of magnitude" as the plasma concentration, but gave no values. The bile concentration did not increase following the oral administration of α-tocopherol. Schmandke and Proll (1964) found a concentration of 40–130 μg/dl in bile from rats on a very low dietary intake (8 mg/kg), values probably not much lower than the expected plasma concentrations at this intake. Mellors and Barnes (1966) found an insignificant amount of radioactivity in 1-hour bile collections from rats 12 or 24 hours after an oral dose of labeled α-tocopherol. Blomstrand and Forsgren (1968) in studies with human subjects found the bile to be a significant excretory pathway for tocopherol. These various studies indicate that bile has a constant α-tocopherol concentration related to the blood level and that marked changes in dietary intake of the vitamin are not immediately reflected in the bile concentration. Clarification of the role of biliary excretion of α-tocopherol and its metabolites is necessary.

B. TRANSPORT AND DEPOSITION

Most tocopherol enters the blood stream via lymph where it is associated with chylomicrons and very low-density lipoproteins. Upon entering the blood, the tocopherol in chylomicrons rapidly equilibrates with the other plasma lipiproteins (Peake *et al.*, 1972). In studies *in vitro* in which rat chylomicrons containing labeled α-tocopherol were incubated with fasted rat plasma, redistribution to all lipoprotein fractions was complete in 2 hours. A similar rapid equilibration occurred when labeled chylomicrons were injected intravenously. In each case, the α-tocopherol was found in lipoprotein fractions in proportion to the total lipid in each fraction. About 85% of the α-tocopherol was associated with two fractions with densities of 1.035–1.063 and 1.063–1.21. These fractions include the high-density lipoproteins and contain the bulk of the total lipids in rat blood. These results indicate that there is no specific lipoprotein carrier for α-tocopherol.

In human blood, where high-density lipoproteins are proportionately less plentiful, α-tocopherol is found predominantly in the low-density lipoproteins (McCormick et al., 1960). In fourteen normal subjects, Burk and Seely (1973) found 65% of the total plasma α-tocopherol in low-density lipoproteins, 24% in high-density lipoproteins, and 8% in the very low-density fraction.

Circulating tocopherols are rapidly taken up by most tissues, maximum concentrations being reached 4–8 hours after oral dosing (Pearson and Barnes, 1970). At any given plasma level of α-tocopherol, a tissue concentration is established that is proportional to the logarithm of the blood concentration (Bieri, 1972; Bieri and Evarts, 1975c). Adipose tissue differs, however, in that it continually accumulates α-tocopherol. As noted above (Section II, C), excessive adiposity can result in reduced concentrations of tocopherol in some tissues even though blood levels are high (Bieri and Evarts, 1975b).

C. CELLULAR FUNCTION

This general area was thoroughly reviewed in 1972 in this series (Molenaar et al., 1972) and therefore only recent work bearing directly on the function of α-tocopherol at the cellular level will be included here. Although many biochemical abnormalities have been found as sequelae of vitamin E deficiency, the exact mechanism whereby tocopherol prevents these metabolic lesions still remains uncertain. There is good evidence that tocopherols have antioxidant activitiy in vivo in adipose tissue (Weber and Wiss, 1966), but evidence for peroxidative loss of unsaturated fatty acids and accumulation of products of lipid peroxidation in other tissues is not as definitive. Most support for an antioxidant action of tocopherol comes from studies in vitro, where both enzymic and nonenzymic lipid peroxidation can be inhibited by the vitamin (Molenaar et al., 1972). As emphasized by these reviewers, the feeding of tocopherol to animals may produce results different from the in vitro addition of the compound because metabolic incorporation of tocopherol into some unique relationship with subcellular membrane lipids may be necessary. Relatively high dietary levels of the vitamin may be necessary to demonstrate in vitro inhibition of enzymic peroxidation because of possible disruption of cellular relationships and also because of the usually higher oxygen tension *in vitro* than *in vivo*.

Although α-tocopherol may have to be incorporated into membranes in order to function, this does not necessarily imply that the compound performs a requisite structural function in membranes as proposed by· Lucy (1972). This theory must explain how such spatially different chromanol structures as α-tocopherol and *N*-methyl-γ-tocopheramine can show the same biological activity (Bieri, 1969), and also how the different configuration of side chains in the tocopherols and tocotrienols can perform similar structural functions. The most recent theory of vitamin E action, that it acts as a redox controller of selenium in membrane proteins (Diplock, 1974), needs further clarification.

Not many years ago it was fashionable to credit vitamin E with being THE *in vivo* antioxidant. As such, it was postulated that the vitamin kept lipid peroxidation in the tissues to a minimum and suppressed formation of such products as ceroid and lipofuscin. It is now apparent that other systems also perform this function in controlling free-radical attacks on oxidizable substrates. Two enzymes, glutathione reductase (Hoekstra, 1975) and *p*-phenylenediamine peroxidase (Armstrong *et al.*, 1973) may be more important than is α-tocopherol as interrupters of radical chain reactions at given cellular sites.

The observed changes in activity in a number of enzyme systems in vitamin E-deficient animals led to the postulate that vitamin E had a regulatory role in protein synthesis (Olson, 1967). This hypothesis has recently been extensively reviewed by Catignani (1976), so will be dealt with here only briefly.

The increase in DNA content of vitamin E-deficient rabbit muscle described by Dinning (1962), resulting from a marked acceleration of DNA synthesis, may have been the result of infiltration by leukocytes and macrophages. A 4-fold increase in ribosomal RNA content of deficient muscle in vitamin E-deficient rabbits (Olson, 1974) remains unexplained at the molecular level. The increased rate of muscle protein synthesis in vitamin E deficiency has generated conflicting evidence for the rates of amino acid incorporation and the changes in polysome profiles (De Villers *et al.*, 1973; Olson, 1974).

Among the large number of enzymes that undergo changes in activity during vitamin E deficiency, those receiving the most attention have been muscle creatine kinase and liver xanthine oxidase. Deficiency leads to a doubling of the turnover rate of creatine kinase (Olson, 1974), although the primary event may be increased destruction due to the absence of α-tocopherol. Extensive studies by Catignani *et al.* (1974) have demonstrated that the increase in liver xanthine oxidase activity in the vitamin E-deficient animals is due to an increased rate of synthesis *de novo*. These various studies on rates of enzyme synthesis suggest a role for α-tocopherol in the regulation of protein synthesis. Just how the vitamin may participate in this sequence of events is not known.

Relevant studies have described the binding of α-tocopherol to a nucleoprotein of rat liver (Patnaik and Nair, 1975), but evidence for specificity was lacking. Similar *in vivo* studies have shown the association of tocopherol with a supernatant lipoprotein from intestinal mucosa and liver (Rajaram *et al.*, 1974), but it is questionable if this represents specific binding. A low-molecular-weight protein that appears to have high specificity for α-tocopherol was reported by Catignani (1975) in rat liver supernatant. Perhaps these clues to the specific localization of α-tocopherol within the cell will clarify the functional role of the vitamin.

IV. CLINICAL ASPECTS

A. DEFICIENCY STATES

Prior to considering specific human deficiency states, it is worthwhile to review briefly the expected normal levels and the distribution of plasma vitamin E levels in the United States population. This will permit a definition, albeit an arbitrary one, of what constitutes "biochemical deficiency."

Unfortunately, data available from population surveys deal almost exclusively with plasma total tocopherol values without information on plasma lipids. The results of two such surveys in adults by Harris *et al.* (1961) and Bieri *et al.* (1964) are shown in Fig. 1. From these results, it may be concluded that the normal level of total tocopherols in plasma averages 1.05 mg/dl, but that the range is wide. The values essentially follow a normal distribution, the two standard-deviation range being 0.5–1.6 mg/dl serum. On the other hand, limited surveys on normal infants and children have disclosed relatively lower plasma tocopherol levels. In subjects of 4 months to 6 years of age, for instance, McWhirter (1975) found a mean total tocopherol of 0.64 mg and a range of 0.2–1.3 mg per deciliter of plasma.

Although the ratio between plasma tocopherols and lipids is clearly a better expression of vitamin E status than plasma tocopherols alone, most of the studies with deficient human subjects, even those published recently, have been based on the latter. Thus, in this review it is necessary to approach recorded observations in humans on the basis of blood tocopherol concentrations. For practical purposes, the authors will consider a level of

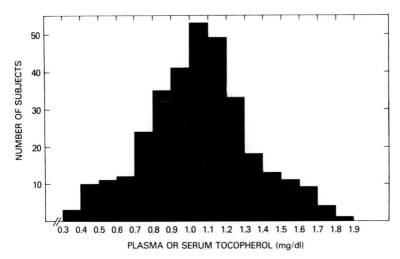

FIG. 1. The distribution of plasma or serum total tocopherol values in 327 normal adults as reported by Harris *et al.* (1961) and Bieri *et al.* (1964).

total tocopherols in serum or plasma less than 0.5 mg/dl as indicative of vitamin E inadequacy in adults with normolipemia whereas this level is only suggestive of chemical deficiency in infants and children. It must be kept in mind, however, that many of the studies of "vitamin E deficiency" states may contain subjects who, because of lower blood lipids, are in reality not deficient in vitamin E.

1. *Premature Infants*

Newborns delivered prematurely have been the subject of a number of human vitamin E-deficiency studies. These infants have been denied a full period of gestation and have not developed adequate tissue stores of various nutrients, nor have they attained maturity with respect to several important physiological functions relating to organ systems, such as the gastrointestinal tract. The crisis in care of the newborn associated with an alarming increase in retrolental fibroplasia (RLF) in the late 1940s provided the occasion for the first demonstration that neonates are biochemically deficient in vitamin E. Owens and Owens (1949) first called attention to this state of malnutrition when they reported that the serum total tocopherol concentration averaged 0.25 mg/dl in a group of 46 premature infants 2–8 weeks of age.

Subsequently, a number of investigators reported low blood tocopherol levels and abnormal erythrocyte hemolysis tests in prematures, as listed in Table V. The vitamin E deficiency state of premature infants over the

TABLE V
BLOOD TOCOPHEROL LEVELS REPORTED IN HUMAN VITAMIN E DEFICIENCY STATES

Condition	Mean plasma or serum tocopherol (mg/dl)	Range	Reference
A. Premature birth			
	0.25	—[a]	Owens and Owens (1949)
	0.22[b]	0.04–0.46	Moyer (1950)
	0.26[c]	0.02–0.56	Moyer (1950)
	0.28	—[c]	Wright et al. (1951)
	0.20	0.06–0.39	Mackenzie (1954)
	0.26[b]	—[a]	Nitowsky et al. (1956)
	0.20[c]	—[a]	Nitowsky et al. (1956)
	0.32	0.12–0.50	Hassan et al. (1966)
	0.25	0–0.41	Oski and Barness (1967)
	0.22	0.09–0.32	Oski and Barness (1968)
	0.25[d]	—[a]	Gross and Melhorn (1972)
	0.38[e]	—[a]	Gross and Melhorn (1972)
B. Cystic fibrosis			
	0.27	0.04–0.58	Filer et al. (1951)
	0.11	0.01–0.97	Goldbloom (1960)
	0.15	0–0.47	Nitowsky et al. (1962)
	0.44	0.05–0.90	Binder et al. (1965)
	0.22	—[a]	Harries and Muller (1971)
	0.24[f]	—[a]	Underwood and Denning (1972)
	0.30	0.1–0.6	Taylor et al. (1973)
	0.25	—[a]	Muller et al. (1974)
	0.13[f]	0.02–0.41	Farrell et al. (1975)
	0.24	0–0.74	McWhirter (1975)

[a] Data not reported.
[b] Blood samples obtained at birth.
[c] Blood samples obtained 2 days to 2 months postnatally.
[d] Blood obtained 3 weeks postnatally from premature infants of 28–32 weeks gestational age.
[e] Blood obtained 3 weeks postnatally from premature infants of 32–36 weeks gestational age.
[f] Plasma α-tocopherol levels determined after thin-layer chromatography.

first several weeks of life can be attributed to several factors including limited tissue storage at birth (Filer, 1968), relative dietary deficiency (Davis, 1972), intestinal malabsorption (Gordon and McNamara, 1940), and rapid growth. After development of mature digestive and absorptive capability, tocopherol absorption improves, as shown by Gross and Melhorn (1972), and blood vitamin E levels rise. It is noteworthy, however, that prematures of early gestational age weighing 1000–1250 gm at birth may show tocopherol malabsorption until 2–3 months of age. The severity of vitamin E loss by this group is such that even oral supplementation with large doses of water-miscible α-tocopherol fails to increase blood levels significantly (Barnes et al., 1968; Gross and Melhorn, 1972).

The discovery that prematures are chemically deficient in vitamin E rapidly led to a search for a corresponding vitamin E-deficiency syndrome that might bridge the gap between experimental studies in laboratory animals and practical application of vitamin E therapy in medicine. A number of clinical problems and pathological findings in newborns superficially resemble some of the manifestations of vitamin E deficiency as found in lower animals. Early attempts to uncover a counterpart in prematures of the animal syndromes focused on three disturbances: (1) encephalomalacia, (2) increased vascular fragility, and (3) retrolental fibroplasia. More recently, investigations have pursued hematological aspects of vitamin E deficiency. Studies addressing the first two possibilities have been unconvincing, and, to the authors' knowledge, neither of these possibilities is under active current study. On the other hand, a relationship between hypovitaminosis E and retrolental fibroplasia continues to be pursued to the present day.

Retrolental fibroplasia is a condition affecting the growth of immature retinal blood vessels and is characterized in severe stages by scar tissue formation and blindness. The presence of relatively large amounts of α-tocopherol in the retinal outer segment of vertebrate eyes has been documented by Dilley and McConnell (1970), and the possibility that vitamin E deficiency in prematures leads to or aggravates retrolental fibroplasia was explored shortly after the discovery of the deficiency state. Owens and Owens (1949) conducted the first such clinical trial using oral supplements of α-tocopheryl acetate. Their results, although promising at first, are difficult to interpret in retrospect because of inadequate controls, with particular regard to oxygen monitoring. Kinsey and Chisholm (1951) reevaluated the possible role of tocopherol therapy and after 3 years of investigation concluded that this treatment had little or no effect on the incidence of retrolental fibroplasia. In contrast to the disappointing results with tocopherol supplementation, reduced oxygen therapy caused a dramatic decrease in RLF incidence when it was realized that the disease was a manifestation of oxygen toxicity (Kinsey, 1956).

Interest in the possible relationship of vitamin E to retinal oxygen toxicity was rekindled in recent years by the advent of special-care nurseries which are largely designed to provide intensive respiratory care for prematures suffering from hyaline membrane disease. Such infants are commonly managed with assisted ventilation and receive high oxygen concentrations. Not surprisingly, the great need to provide adequate tissue oxygenation has led to excessive oxygen use in some instances, and thus an apparent resurgence in RLF occurred in the late 1960s (De Leon et al., 1970). Reawakening of interest in this disease and the possible role of vitamin E is evidenced by the recent planning of well-controlled clinical studies for the purpose of further characterizing RLF, determining the safe limits of oxygen, and evaluating potential therapeutic agents, such as tocopherol. Because the early vascular changes associated with hyperoxia are extremely subtle, more sophisticated instrumentation is being employed in present ophthalmoscopic examination, leading in turn to more frequent detection of early pathological changes.

The possible therapeutic use of vitamin E in preventing or ameliorating retrolental fibroplasia is currently under investigation by Johnson et al. (1974), who are utilizing a parenteral form of α-tocopheryl acetate in a water-miscible base. In their first report, the authors suggested that vitamin E reduces the incidence, severity, and duration of the early stages of RLF detected with the indirect ophthalmoscope. This conclusion, however, was entirely based on differences in 16 infants of less than 1.5 kg birth weight with the group of >1.5 kg showing no evidence of beneficial effects of tocopherol therapy. Because of the small number of patients and the unusually high RLF incidence (71%) in the control group, further information will be required to assess the significance of the findings initially reported by Johnson et al. (1974). Preliminary results from another study have recently been recorded by Curran et al. (1975), who concluded that no correlation could be established between vitamin E levels and retinal vascular changes.

Hemolytic anemia represents another reported manifestation of hypovitaminosis E in premature infants. Investigations dealing with this possibility must be viewed against the background of the rapidly changing hematological system of the newborn as reviewed by Oski and Naiman (1972). Profound alterations and hematological adjustments take place from birth until several months of age as the erythrocyte population undergoes a "switchover" from cells containing fetal hemoglobin to those predominantly composed of adult hemoglobin. As a result of these changes, prematures almost invariably develop anemia by 6–10 weeks of age, a state that is often referred to as "physiological anemia" (Stockman, 1975).

Although the possible relationship between vitamin E deficiency and hematological disturbances in prematures was first noted by Hassan et al. (1966), the studies of Oski and Barness (1967, 1968) have had the most significant impact on our assessment of the role vitamin E deficiency might play in prematures, if not generally in man. Oski and Barness (1967) initially recognized the association of anemia and vitamin E deficiency in 11 infants, all of whom were treated orally with tocopherol at 44–77 days of age. After treatment, serum tocopherol levels rose to normal, erythrocyte hemolysis *in vitro* decreased, and mean hemoglobin level rose from 7.6 to 9.8 gm/dl with the mean reticulocyte count falling from 8.2 to 3.9%. In a subsequent prospective trial, these workers found that 13 infants supplemented orally with tocopherol from 3 days of age showed less of a fall in hemoglobin and less prominent reticulocytosis in comparison to 12 vitamin E-deficient prematures. ^{51}Cr-RBC survival was measured in two infants with low serum tocopherol levels and found to be "shortened" to half-times of 11 and 15 days, although the survival time of erythrocytes of vitamin E-treated and control infants was not determined.

Subsequent to these findings, several groups obtained data supporting the relationship of vitamin E deficiency to falling hematological indices in premature infants. Chadd and Fraser (1970), for instance, reported that hemoglobin levels are significantly higher 8–10 weeks after birth in babies provided with vitamin E supplements. Additionally, Lo *et al.* (1973) reported a statistically significant rise in hemoglobin and fall in reticulocyte count in 6–8-week-old prematures after 2–3 weeks of oral treatment with 10 mg of α-tocopherol per day.

Perhaps the most extensive study of the hematological effects of vitamin E deficiency in premature infants has been conducted by Gross and Melhorn (1972). These investigators evaluated 234 prematures between 1968 and 1971 and showed that whereas infants of either 28–32 or 32–36 weeks of gestation on standard formula exhibited a 51% decline in hemoglobin level at 8 weeks of age, corresponding premature infants supplemented with 25 IU of water-miscible α-tocopheryl acetate per day showed decreases of 45% and 46%, respectively. Although the magnitude of improvement in terms of absolute hemoglobin level amounted to only 1 gm per deciliter of blood, the differences were highly significant ($p < 0.001$) in both groups of treated prematures, as were the lower reticulocyte counts. In addition, from studies on the interplay of tocopherol and dietary iron, it was clearly demonstrated that the administration of large amounts of medicinal iron exaggerates the "hemolytic process."

On the other hand, Panos *et al.* (1968) were unable to confirm the improvement in hemoglobin concentration and fall in reticulocyte count in vitamin E-supplemented premature infants, despite the demonstration that such therapy led to increased blood tocopherol. Their study, which focused on 47 infants at approximately 10 weeks of age, included measurement of ^{51}Cr-labeled RBC survival in 27 infants, before and after vitamin E supplementation in 14 of these. Perhaps the most significant finding by these investigators was that no improvement in the shortened ^{51}Cr-labeled RBC survival time was evident after vitamin E administration. Similarly negative results relative to hemoglobin levels were reported by

Goldbloom and Cameron (1963), who studied 14 premature infants for 6 months on either low-tocopherol diets or those fortified with the vitamin. In another negative trial, Sartain *et al.* (1967) found no improvement in various hematological indices of premature infants fed tocopherol-supplemented formulas. Additionally, Hashim and Asfour (1968), in a study of term infants receiving either diets inadequate in vitamin E as compared to PUFA or, alternatively, a tocopherol-fortified formula, reported that the group with vitamin E deficiency did not develop an exaggerated anemia. Instead, they showed spontaneous improvement in hemoglobin levels at a rate comparable to that of the control group.

Because hemolytic anemia may result in hyperbilirubinemia, especially in newborns, another approach to assessing the role of vitamin E has been to monitor serum bilirubin levels in neonates treated with tocopherol. Interestingly, neither Richards *et al.* (1957) nor Abrams *et al.* (1973) were able to show a significant effect of the vitamin on the degree of hyperbilirubinemia developed in infants given daily doses of α-tocopheryl acetate sufficiently large to raise serum tocopherol levels and reduce the hemolytic tendency *in vitro*.

Therefore, from a consideration of all studies bearing on the status of the erythrocyte in vitamin E-deficient premature infants which are recorded in the literature prior to 1976, it is clear that significant discrepancies are present and that further questions of a fundamental nature need to be asked. Those investigators who claim hematological improvement after supplementation with vitamin E can demonstrate statistically significant increases in blood hemoglobin concentrations at approximately 8–10 weeks of age accompanied by reduced reticulocytosis. Nonetheless, it should be noted that, even with tocopherol supplementation, reticulocytosis and anemia both become manifest, and thus tocopherol *does not fully correct* the hematological disturbances of prematurity.

In view of the fact that hemolytic anemia may be defined as a condition with shortened RBC survival associated with an inadequate acceleration of red cell production, establishing an unequivocal role for α-tocopherol in the anemia of prematurity will depend upon convincing demonstration that erythrocyte survival (a) is depressed in tocopherol-deficient infants and (b) is improved after treatment of deficient infants with vitamin E.

2. *Malabsorption States*

A second category of human subjects who manifest vitamin E deficiency are patients with various forms of intestinal malabsorption. This is a heterogeneous group in which the steatorrhea can be ascribed to a number of different disturbances in digestive or absorptive capability (see Tables V and VI). As discussed previously, the uptake and transfer of vitamin E

TABLE VI
BLOOD TOCOPHEROL LEVELS REPORTED IN HUMAN VITAMIN E
DEFICIENCY STATES (continued)

Condition	Mean plasma or serum tocopherol (mg/dl)	Range	Reference
C. Malabsorption syndromes other than cystic fibrosis			
Biliary atresia	0.11	—[a]	Gordon et al. (1958)
Biliary cirrhosis	0	—[b]	Woodruff (1956)
Biliary obstruction (cause unspecified)	0.08	0–0.14	Muller and Harris (1969)
Celiac disease	0.64	—[b]	Minot (1944)
Celiac disease	0.20	0–0.35	McWhirter (1975)
Celiac disease	0.39	—[a]	Muller et al. (1974)
Chronic pancreatitis	0.40	0.17–0.79	Binder et al. (1965)
Gastrectomy	0.34	0.1–0.80	Leonard et al. (1966)
Gastrectomy	0.37	0.1–0.77	Leonard et al. (1966)
Gastrectomy	0.58	0.41–0.74	Binder et al. (1965)
Intestinal lymphangectasia	0.28	—[a]	Muller et al. (1974)
Intestinal resection	0.31	—[b]	Binder et al. (1965)
Nontropical sprue	0.25	0.12–0.32	Darby et al. (1946)
Regional enteritis plus intestinal resection	0.27	0.15–0.39	Binder et al. (1965)
Tropical sprue	0.28	—[a]	Ramirez et al. (1973)
Ulcerative colitis	0.24	0.17–0.36	Binder et al. (1965)
Whipple's disease	0.30	0.14–0.45	Binder et al. (1965)
D. Protein-calorie malnutrition			
	0.43	0.33–0.65	Majaj et al. (1963)
	—[a]	0.09–0.55	Thanangkul et al. (1966)
	0.28	0–0.91	Sandstead et al. (1965)
	0.37	0.10–0.69	Baker et al. (1968)
	0.30	—[a]	Kulapongs (1975)
	0.83	—[a]	McLaren et al. (1969)
	0.49	—[a]	McLaren et al. (1969)

[a] Data not reported.
[b] Only one patient studied.

across the epithelial cell membrane of the small intestine is considered to be dependent on the coincidental absorption of lipids. Thus, whatever the cause of the steatorrhea, if it is of sufficient duration and magnitude, vitamin E deficiency would likely ensue as a consequence of tocopherol malabsorption.

Of those patients with enteropathies leading to chronic steatorrhea, subjects with pancreatic exocrine insufficiency, especially cystic fibrosis

(CF), have been of particular interest to investigators concerned with tocopherol deficiency in man (di Sant'Agnese and Talamo, 1967). There are a number of reasons why these patients are appropriate for extensive study and have been the focus of many investigators: (1) they appear to represent the largest group of human subjects in developed countries with severe, persistent steatorrhea; (2) they manifest a permanent digestive defect that cannot be corrected, but only ameliorated, by pancreatic replacement therapy; (3) cystic fibrosis patients are largely found in the pediatric age group that, by analogy to animal experimentation, appears to represent the ideal population for studies of tocopherol depletion in man.

To the authors' knowledge, the first report describing vitamin E deficiency in cystic fibrosis patients, as well as in other subjects with malabsorption, appeared in 1949 and resulted from a survey of 200 hospitalized patients by Darby et al. (1949). Subsequently, a number of investigators have confirmed the reduction in blood tocopherol concentrations in cystic fibrosis patients as well as the enhanced susceptibility of red cells to hydrogen peroxide originally noted by Gordon et al. (1955). From the results listed in Table V, it is evident that all surveys have disclosed vitamin E deficiency in cystic fibrosis and that reasonably good agreement exists with respect to the average concentration of circulating tocopherol in this form of pancreatogenous steatorrhea. It is equally apparent, however, that such patients display a wide range of blood vitamin E concentrations. Nonetheless, as illustrated in Fig. 2, reductions in plasma α-tocopherol are closely related to results obtained in assessing the degree of malabsorption by measurement of either dietary fat absorption or serum carotene level. In addition to plasma, Underwood and Denning (1972) measured tocopherol concentrations in red cells, liver, and skeletal muscle and reported that cystic fibrosis patients show substantial reductions in each of these tissues.

In comparison to the amount of attention directed toward vitamin E deficiency in cystic fibrosis, a relative paucity of information is available on vitamin E status in the other malabsorptive states presented in Table VI. From the list, it is evident that disturbances affecting nearly every component of the digestive or absorptive process may precipitate tocopherol depletion. In addition to being a heterogeneous group with regard to etiology, these disorders vary widely in regard to the type and age of the population afflicted and in the degree of vitamin E deficiency. Of considerable interest is the magnitude of tocopherol deficiency in hepatobiliary disturbances and the observation that blood vitamin E levels in these subjects are refractory to orally administered, water-miscible tocopherol preparations. Clinical investigations have not as yet defined the length

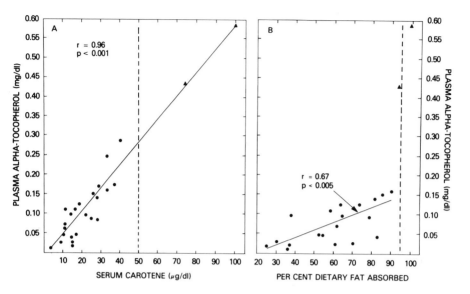

Fig. 2. The correlation between plasma α-tocopherol levels in cystic fibrosis (CF) patients and their degree of malabsorption. The latter was evaluated by measurement of serum carotene concentration and fecal fat excretion during balance studies. The lower limit of normal fat absorption, 95%, is indicated by the dashed line; normal carotene values range from 50 to 300 μg/dl. Triangles represent two CF patients with intact or nearly intact pancreatic function as demonstrated by assay of duodenal contents. (A) $r = 0.96$; $p < 0.001$. (B) $r = 0.67$, $p < 0.005$. Unpublished data of P. M. Farrell and P. A. diSant'Agnese.

of time necessary for development of tocopherol depletion in older children and adults, but this would ostensibly depend upon the amount of tissue storage in comparison to the degree of steatorrhea. Limited clinical studies (Binder *et al.*, 1965) suggest that several months are required to exhaust tissues in cases where intestinal uptake is severely compromised.

To elucidate the relationship between generalized steatorrhea and tocopherol malabsorption in patients with disorders other than cystic fibrosis, MacMahon and Neale (1970) administered tritiated α-tocopherol orally and studied its absorption. α-Tocopherol absorption was found to be most severely impaired in patients with biliary obstruction and somewhat less severely impaired in patients with pancreatic exocrine insufficiency. Most noteworthy was the observation that the degree of tocopherol malabsorption could be correlated statistically with the magnitude of fecal fat excretion.

Studies on the possible consequences of vitamin E deficiency in malabsorption states have focused on the neuromuscular system, erythrocyte stability, and the morphology of the intestinal tract. The neuromuscular system attracted the earliest attention owing in part to the recognition that the myopathy of vitamin E deficiency in animals (nutritional muscular dystrophy) can be readily produced under appropriate conditions in virtually every species that has come under study. Taking as their clue the prevailing clinical impression of the time that cystic fibrosis patients were characteristically weak with "flabby and atrophic muscles," Nitowsky et al. (1962) investigated 27 such subjects with vitamin E deficiency over a course of several years. Creatinuria was employed as the principal marker of muscle dysfunction, and it was observed that 69% of the patients excreted excessive creatine, which could be corrected in most of the patients by tocopherol supplementation. Excessive urinary creatine excretion, however, is not specific for muscle disease per se but may develop secondary to a number of conditions (Cantarow and Trumper, 1962). A more sensitive and specific index of skeletal muscle damage in man is release of sarcoplasmic enzymes into the blood stream. Creatine phosphokinase (CPK) and aldolase are especially useful in this regard since their activities are markedly and invariably elevated in progressive muscular dystrophy of genetic origin (Munsat et al., 1973). Farrell et al. (1975) measured serum CPK and aldolase activities in a series of 50 vitamin E-deficient cystic fibrosis patients and found only two with significant elevation in these enzymes. In addition, one 8-year-old boy with hepatic disease on cholestyramine therapy has been found to show a markedly elevated CPK activity in association with virtually undetectable plasma tocopherol (P. M. Farrell and L. Tomasi, unpublished data).

Unequivocal diagnosis of muscular degeneration depends upon morphological examination of biopsied tissue. Unfortunately, the lesions in vitamin E-deficient skeletal muscle, as described in over 20 different species of animals, tend to be focal and of varying severity, such that their demonstration in small muscle samples is difficult. Limited investigations of muscle structure have been carried out in cystic fibrosis patients. Oppenheimer (1956) in a restrospective review of necropsy tissue from 48 children found abnormalities in only one; these consisted of focal areas of muscle necrosis, hyalinization, and leukocytic infiltration—lesions not unlike those found in animal dystrophy. In addition, similar histopathological changes were found in one child with biliary atresia (Weinberg et al., 1958). More recently, muscle biopsies from the quadriceps femoris of four of our CF patients have been examined histologically and histochemically. All the patients were vitamin E deficient as disclosed by low plasma α-tocopherol levels and virtually undetectable concentrations in muscle specimens, and two displayed elevated plasma CPK and aldolase activities. Histologically, the architecture of muscle fibers was intact, but mild abnormalities were noted on histochemical evaluation. These consisted primarily of darkly staining type II fibers with the esterase procedure.

The question arises as to muscle strength in vitamin E-deficient cystic fibrosis patients and the effect of tocopherol supplementation on muscle function in these subjects. This issue has been carefully investigated by Levin et al. (1961) and by Darby and associates (1973). Both groups were unable to document objectively a significant degree of muscular weakness in these patients. The results of muscle testing following tocopherol treatment to normal plasma vitamin E levels were likewise unrevealing.

Erythrocyte stability represents a second area of research interest relative to the role of vitamin E deficiency in malabsorption. Although the results of *in vitro* studies with blood from cystic fibrosis patients have established the increased susceptibility of erythrocytes to oxidant damage, the most significant issue clinically is whether or not red cells function adequately *in vivo*. Farrell et al. (1975) have recently employed the ^{51}Cr-labeled RBC survival technique to assess erythrocyte stability in 19 vitamin E-deficient patients. As shown in Table VII, data from these measurements indicated that vitamin E-deficient red cells were statistically abnormal in terms of survival with a mean $t_{1/2}$ of 22 days. Three subjects were particularly low, with survivals of less than 18 days, but several manifested normal survivals. In what apparently represents the only other assessment of ^{51}Cr-labeled RBC survival in cystic fibrosis, Goldbloom (1960) reported that one patient with markedly diminished serum tocopherol showed a red cell half-life of 25 days. Six cystic fibrosis patients studied by Farrell et al. (1975) were available for repeat ^{51}Cr-labeled RBC survival measurements after supplementation with oral tocopherol. This group showed a significant increase in $t_{1/2}$ from 19 days to 27 days after treatment (Table VII).

Additionally, Leonard and Losowsky (1971) reported slightly lowered red cell survivals in a group of eight adults with malnutrition due to either steatorrhea (six subjects) or chronic alcoholism with poor diet. Seven of these patients showed abnormal ^{51}Cr-labeled RBC half-lives (less than 25 days) and the mean $t_{1/2}$ of the group was 19 days. Following oral plus intramuscular treatment with α-tocopherol and relabeling of red cells, it was observed that $t_{1/2}$ values increased to a normal range in five subjects and that the group as a whole showed a significantly greater post-treatment value of 25 days.

It should be noted that the average degree of shortening of RBC survival in tocopherol-deficient patients with malabsorption is not sufficient to produce a frank hemolytic anemia (^{51}Cr-labeled RBC half-lives in

TABLE VII

ERYTHROCYTE SURVIVAL IN VITAMIN E DEFICIENT CYSTIC FIBROSIS PATIENTS[a]

Group	Number	^{51}Cr-labeled RBC half-life (days) Mean ± S.E.	Range
Control	28	28.0 ± 0.5	25–35
Vitamin E deficiency	19	22.4 ± 0.9[b]	16–29
After vitamin E supplementation	6	27.6 ± 0.9[c]	25–31

[a] From Farrell et al. (1975) and unpublished data.
[b] As compared to the control subjects, $p < 0.001$.
[c] Mean ± S.E. survival of this group prior to treatment was 19 ± 1 days ($p < 0.001$).

hemolytic diseases approximate 5–15 days). Furthermore, it has been found that vitamin E-deficient patients show no clinical evidence of hemolysis and no change in hematological indices upon supplementation with vitamin E (Farrell et al., 1975; Leonard and Losowsky, 1971). This suggests that reduced red cell survival is adequately compensated for by erythropoietic mechanisms. Nonetheless, the demonstration of a shortened ^{51}Cr-labeled RBC half-life in unsupplemented patients and the finding that erythrocyte stability in vivo could be corrected upon adequate vitamin E therapy provides strong evidence that these subjects, and hence humans in general, require the vitamin for maintenance of normal red cell function.

The morphology of the intestinal tract and other smooth muscle-containing tissues has been of considerable interest to investigators concerned with aspects of vitamin E deficiency in human malabsorption. As mentioned earlier, an acid-fast pigment, referred to as ceroid or lipofuscin, accumulates in the smooth muscle and may become disseminated throughout the reticuloendothelial system after prolonged vitamin E deficiency in animals. Although factors responsible for the genesis of this pigment have not been identified precisely, ceroid appears to reflect the intracellular accumulation of peroxidized, highly unsaturated lipids as a manifestation of inadequate antioxidant protection. Examination of necropsy tissue from vitamin E-deficient cystic fibrosis patients of greater than 2 years of age has invariably revealed the presence of ceroid pigment. This was first noted by Blanc and associates (1958), who quantitated the extent of lipofuscin formation and correlated this with the presumed degree of antioxidant deficiency. Subsequently, Kerner and Goldbloom (1960) conducted an extensive retrospective survey of postmortem material and demonstrated ceroid deposition in esophagus, stomach, duodenum, jejunum, ileum, appendix, colon, urinary bladder, trachea, lungs, and liver.

3. A-betalipoproteinemia

First described by Bassen and Kornzweig (1950), a-betalipoproteinemia (ABL) or acanthocytosis has proved to be a fascinating disease, as recently reviewed by Kayden (1972). Because of its rarity (25 patients have been described to date), only limited data are available on the nature and effects of nutritional deficiencies occurring in this disorder. The steatorrhea and lipid transport abnormalities manifested by ABL patients have stimulated research on fat-soluble vitamins. Shortly after Simon and Ways (1964) reported that acanthocytes from their patients hemolyzed spontaneously *in vitro*, Kayden and Silber (1965) reported that four subjects, aged 8–11 years, with a-betalipoproteinemia had no measurable tocopherol in plasma as determined with techniques sensitive enough to detect 0.05 mg/dl. The apparent absence of circulating tocopherol in unsupplemented patients was confirmed by Bieri and Poukka (1970b) and also by Muller and Harries (1969). A total of seven patients have now been documented as showing a lack of plasma or serum tocopherol.

Erythrocyte tocopherol levels and fatty acid concentrations were also measured by Bieri and Poukka (1970b) on blood samples from ABL patients receiving a daily oral dose of 750 mg of α-tocopheryl succinate. They observed that although α-tocopherol concentrations remained low in plasma (mean = 0.20 mg/dl), red cells were able to develop and maintain normal levels (mean = 0.21 mg/dl packed cells). The ratio of RBC tocopherol to its concentration in plasma was approximately 4-fold greater in ABL patients compared to normal subjects. This level was found to be sufficient in terms of preventing the marked *in vitro* hemolytic tendency present in red cells from unsupplemented ABL patients. Thus, plasma α-tocopherol values cannot be considered a satisfactory index of tissue concentrations in a-betalipoproteinemia.

Studies exploring the possible effects of vitamin E deficiency in patients with a-betalipoproteinemia are hampered not only by the small number of subjects available, but also by the severity and complexity of the disorder. The lack of evidence for hemolytic anemia has been documented, and there have been no reports of myopathy (Kayden, 1972). At least one patient, a 9-year-old child, has been found to exhibit ceroid pigment deposition in the intestinal tract.

Although two children with ABL studied by Molenaar *et al.* (1968) must be regarded as atypical in terms of plasma vitamin E levels in the unsupplemented state (0.3 and 0.5 mg/dl), ultrastructural study of jejunal biopsies has formed the basis for a proposed subcellular, morphological disturbance in human vitamin E deficiency. Molenaar and co-workers reported that membranes of mitochondria and endoplasmic reticulum could not be visualized, i.e., were totally absent, upon routine preparation methods. Four months after tocopherol treatment, however, "a dramatic change" was evident with "a completely normal cellular ultrastructure." This cytological abnormality represents a striking finding, and the response claimed after tocopherol therapy raises exciting possibilities. Subcellular changes, however, could not be confirmed in cystic fibrosis patients with severe vitamin E deficiency (Farrell *et al.*, 1975).

4. *Protein-Calorie Malnutrition*

Infants and children with the severe form of protein-calorie malnutrition (PCM), i.e., kwashiorkor, and a limited number with less severe malnutrition, have been shown by numerous investigators to have depressed plasma vitamin E levels. Diminished tocopherol levels in these patients can be attributed to both poor vitamin intake, reduced blood lipids, and impaired intestinal absorption. Little need be said in this review about the general features and clinical consequences of protein-calorie malnutrition, for these have been described in detail by others (Olson, 1975). Nonetheless, a word about the anemia of protein-calorie malnutrition is in order since studies on the effects of vitamin E deficiency have largely focused on the erythropoietic system. In the absence of concomitant deficiencies of iron or the B vitamins, acute PCM typically leads to a normochromic, normocytic anemia with a generally normal or reduced reticulocyte count. There have been many reports of hypochromia and macrocytosis, however, and demonstrations of megaloblastic changes in the bone marrow in areas where folic acid deficiency is also present.

Although evaluation of the deficiency of a single nutrient, such as vitamin E, in patients with kwashiorkor presents obvious difficulties, children of 5 months to 4 years of age with protein-calorie malnutrition have come under intensive study in developing countries with respect to vitamin E status. Ever since 1957, when Scrimshaw and associates (1957) reported low blood tocopherol levels in patients with kwashiorkor, there has been little dispute regarding the occurrence of vitamin E depletion in these subjects. At least 6 other studies have verified this observation (Table VI), and McLaren *et al.* (1969) reported that depressed vitamin E levels correlate with the severity of the disease. Not unexpectedly, abnormal erythrocyte hemolysis in the presence of hydrogen peroxide has also been reported in these patients.

Investigations exploring the possible effects of vitamin E deficiency in protein-calorie malnutrition have, as mentioned previously, been directed toward hematological aspects of the syndrome. Majaj *et al.* (1963) first claimed that megaloblastic anemia in PCM responded favorably to vitamin E on the basis of data indicating that tocopherol therapy is associated with reticulocytosis and correction of low hemoglobin and hematocrit values. Review of their study, however, indicates that it was not adequately controlled, particularly with regard to administration of other nutrients. Whitaker and co-workers (1967) repeated the trial with 60 children hospitalized in Northern Thailand, but they too failed to control the investigation in terms of patient selection and various therapeutic measures. From the standpoint of validly assessing responses to tocopherol therapy, perhaps the most disconcerting aspect of the trial by Whitaker et al. (1967) is that the vitamin E-treated group entered the protocol with an apparently greater severity of malnutrition as evidenced by a lower mean initial hemoglobin value as compared to the control group. It was observed that those in the control group showed a progressive fall in mean hemoglobin concentration over 40 days from 9.5 to 8.3 gm/dl. In contrast, patients receiving 250 mg/day of vitamin E demonstrated a statistically significant hemoglobin increase from 7.8 to 9.6 gm/dl and also a rise in reticulocyte count.

These reports aroused considerable interest regarding a possible bone marrow-stimulating effect of vitamin E. More carefully controlled studies were thus conducted by a number of investigators, but none of these trials produced data indicating that hemoglobin synthesis responds to vitamin E. On the contrary, the subsequent investigations by Baker et al. (1968), Halstead et al. (1969), and Kulapongs (1975) have served to strengthen the hypothesis that protein deficiency, and at times iron deficiency, are the main factors relating to defective hematopoiesis in children with protein-calorie malnutrition. The study by Kulapongs is particularly noteworthy in that (1) the same population of Thai children were evaluated as in the trial of Whitaker et al. (1967), and (2) the experimental design was excellent, with proper use of controls. In contrast to tocopherol, reproducible responses can be elicited in the macrocytic anemia of PCM when folic acid is provided in pharmacological amounts. Accordingly, on the basis of the foregoing observations, it is reasonable to conclude that vitamin E cannot be incriminated as an important etiologic factor in the anemia of PCM, nor can it be advocated as a bone marrow stimulant.

5. Overview

From these considerations of vitamin E deficiency states in man, several generalizations and conclusions emerge as follows.

1. The infant, particularly the premature infant, is susceptible to vitamin E deficiency because of relatively poor transfer of the vitamin from placenta to fetus. It is important, therefore, to be certain that the vitamin

E intake, which frequently depends on foods other than mother's milk, be kept at adequate levels by careful planning of diets.

2. Growth in infants provides a further stress upon the vitamin E stores as the organism expands in size; this emphasizes the importance of proper diet intake.

3. In adult persons, the tocopherol stores are abundant and resistant to depletion. Thus, tissue vitamin E is not exhausted until dietary deprivation has continued for many months, possibly years. These large stores make the adult subject less than ideal for studying the effects of vitamin E deficiency.

4. Contrariwise, growing children with vitamin E deficiency represent a situation more analogous to tocopherol-deprived animals.

5. Intestinal malabsorption syndromes, if persistent and prolonged, will regularly lead to vitamin E depletion unless very large, oral tocopherol supplements are administered. The degree of deficiency appears to be proportional to the extent of malabsorption, as reflected by steatorrhea and other signs.

6. Biliary atresia and other hepatobiliary disturbances cause marked tocopherol deficiency and have been proved to be extremely difficult to treat with oral vitamin E supplements.

7. The most carefully studied group of patients with malabsorption are children with cystic fibrosis, and these have been shown to have severe vitamin E deficiency. Although the neuromuscular and hematological systems appear to be affected only minimally, subtle pathological changes and other chemical indicators of visceral disease, such as enzyme leakage, are present in a small percentage of these patients. The histological lesions are mild, and muscular performance is not affected.

8. Patients with a-betalipoproteinemia, a disorder resulting from a genetic absence of apoprotein for chylomicrons and low-density lipoproteins, are quite uniformly vitamin E deficient, show enhanced red blood cell hemolysis *in vitro* but, again, limited neuromuscular disease.

9. Infants with protein-calorie malnutrition show vitamin E depletion in proportion to the severity of their general protein-calorie lack, but do not respond dramatically to tocopherol supplementation. The vitamin E levels in their plasma are depressed, partially owing to tissue depletion and partially because of reduced lipoprotein (carrier) concentrations. There is no conclusive evidence that vitamin E supplementation to children with PCM enhances their hemopoietic capacity or specifically corrects their anemia. Protein, iron, folic acid, and other hematinic nutrients correct the anemia satisfactorily.

10. Enhanced peroxide susceptibility of tocopherol-deficient red cells *in vitro* and a slightly shortened erythrocyte survival time *in vivo* in

human subjects with tocopherol depletion provide evidence that vitamin E has an effect upon the red cell membrane. It is not yet established, however, that vitamin E deficiency, itself, causes hemolytic anemia.

11. Ceroid pigment accumulation has been detected in a number of organs from human subjects with vitamin E deficiency, particularly those containing smooth muscle. Although ceroid is associated with vitamin E lack, its contribution to organ pathology has not been determined.

B. Approaches to Therapy

Approaches to therapy will be discussed only in relation to deficient or potentially deficient patients (see Section IV, C for a discussion of vitamin E supplements in nondeficient individuals). The less than dramatic clinical and biochemical responses of patients to vitamin E supplementation has already been mentioned.

With regard to prematurely delivered infants, particularly those of early gestational ages, Barness et al. (1968) and subsequently Gross and Melhorn (1972) have shown that vitamin E is poorly absorbed for the first several weeks of life. Oral supplementation with relatively large doses of α-tocopheryl acetate, e.g., 5–25 IU/kg, has proved to be insufficient in newborns delivered 8–12 weeks prematurely. It is not until they attain full maturity *ex utero* that these infants respond favorably to oral supplementation. Thus, neither the diets provided for such patients nor the oral preparations of water-miscible tocopherol presently on the market, assure adequate blood and tissue vitamin E levels in infants with low birth weights. These results indicate a need for an approved, injectable preparation.

A second category of patients who are resistant, if not refractory, to the oral supplementation approach are those with biliary atresia and other severe hepato-biliary disturbances leading to reduced bile acid secretion. This group of patients provides a particularly difficult therapeutic challenge since in many instances they also receive cholestyramine resin in an attempt to lower bilirubin levels. The efforts of Gordon et al. (1958) to replete children with biliary atresia, as well as those of Woodruff (1956) in an adult patient with biliary cirrhosis, suggest that there is an absolute requirement for parenteral tocopherol in such subjects. Oral administration of tocopherol, in fact, has failed to raise vitamin E levels in every patient described in the literature to date fitting this category.

Patients with a-betalipoproteinemia are likewise difficult to supplement orally. Nonetheless, once it became recognized that plasma levels in these patients were not necessarily reflective of tissue concentrations, it was evident that massive doses of water-miscible tocopherol (e.g., 0.75–1.5

gm/day) suffice to increase erythrocyte vitamin E to normal levels and prevent hemolysis *in vitro*.

Cystic fibrosis patients with pancreatic insufficiency present less of a therapeutic challenge in regard to tocopherol supplementation. In our experience (P. M. Farrell and P. A. di Sant'Agnese, unpublished data), however, even these patients require the routine use of water-miscible vitamin E preparations rather than the unmodified, fat-soluble forms. This is in accordance with the findings of Harries and Muller (1971), who studied the absorption of both preparations in cystic fibrosis patients and demonstrated more efficient uptake of the water-miscible form. Absorption of nutrients in cystic fibrosis may be affected by many factors in addition to the lack of pancreatic enzymes (di Sant'Agnese and Talamo, 1967). In keeping with findings in patients with biliary atresia and cirrhosis, it has been observed in our clinic and also by Harries and Muller (1971) that cystic fibrosis patients with hepatic involvement, which may occur in up to 30% of cases (Kattwinkel *et al.*, 1973), may be more difficult to replete with oral vitamin E. Such patients poorly absorb tocopherol to such an extent that their plasma vitamin E concentrations cannot be raised even with 1 gm of a water-miscible preparation per day. Thus, a parenteral form of tocopherol is also required for these patients.

Recently, an injectable vitamin E preparation has been described in the literature by Bauernfeind *et al.* (1974) and Newmark *et al.* (1975). They reported that the free alcohol form, rather than the acetate form, of α-tocopherol is more efficiently absorbed from tissues used for intramuscular injections. Although further investigation of their parenteral vitamin E preparation is required, results of limited trials in premature infants by Johnson and associates (1974) have been encouraging and suggest that this agent may meet the requirements described above.

C. Possible Pharmacological Effects

1. *Doses Consumed and Blood Levels Achieved*

No aspect of vitamin E nutrition in man is currently more controversial, nor more popular among the lay public, than the possible pharmacological role of tocopherol when taken in large dietary supplements ("megavitamin E therapy"). Although the pharmacological use of vitamins in quantities far exceeding their daily nutritional requirements is not new, mechanisms are needed to explain the special physiological effect achieved. Experience in the past several years indicates that beneficial effects may accrue from the administration of selected nutrients in doses equivalent to 10–100 times their usual intake (Scriver, 1970).

The literature bearing on the pharmacological use of vitamin E is voluminous and replete with contradictory statements. Many case reports purporting to show evidence for therapeutic value do not represent controlled, scientific studies but rather are anecdotal comments. For a detailed discussion of the early clinical trials of α-tocopherol in large doses, the reader is referred to the comprehensive article by Marks (1962). In this review, the approach will be to focus on the most timely aspect of megavitamin E investigation, viz., tocopherol "therapy" for cardiovascular disease.

A number of tocopherol preparations for oral use are commercially available. These include capsules containing fat-soluble preparations and those providing water-miscible forms of vitamin E in the presence of a variety of emulsifying agents. Such capsules commonly contain 30, 50, 100, or 200 mg of α-tocopherol, although larger doses are available from some manufacturers. Tocopherol doses either self-prescribed or recommended by physicians vary widely but average approximately 400 IU/day (Farrell and Bieri, 1975). Curiously, little information is available on the blood or tissue levels of vitamin E achieved with supplementary ingestion by subjects with normal gastrointestinal function. In view of the limited capacity for tocopherol absorption from the alimentary canal, one might suspect that considerable amounts are lost through fecal excretion. Indeed, this appears to be the case as inferred from studies by Larsson and Haeger (1968) and by Farrell and Bieri (1975). The former investigators reported a mean plasma tocopherol concentration of 3.07 mg/dl in subjects receiving 300–600 IU/day (control mean = 1.13 mg/dl). Larsson and Haeger (1968) also determined the tocopherol content of *soleus* muscle in a limited number of supplemented patients and found a 3-fold greater level than that of unsupplemented patients or control subjects.

The group of subjects on supplementary vitamin E studied by Farrell and Bieri (1975) were consuming the vitamin for 2.9 years on the average with a dosage range of 100–800 IU/day. Plasma α-tocopherol was found to be significantly elevated in the group of megavitamin E consumers with a mean $\pm$ SD of 1.34 $\pm$ 0.10 mg/dl as compared with a control group of normal volunteers showing a corresponding figure of 0.65 $\pm$ 0.14. The levels varied widely, however, with one-fourth of the values falling within two standard deviations of the control mean. Plasma α-tocopherol concentrations did not correlate with total daily dose or duration of treatment, but did correlate with serum triglyceride and cholesterol values.

2. Ischemic Heart Disease

Ischemic heart disease due to coronary arterial occlusion, and manifested symptomatically as recurrent angina pectoris, has emerged as *the* major health problem of middle-aged adult males in the United States. Although the advent of cardiac surgical techniques in recent years using vascular grafts offers a possible alternative, therapy for ischemic heart disease has traditionally depended upon the use of vasodilators and anti-coagulants. In view of the serious nature of this disorder, it is not surprising that a number of agents, such as vitamin E, have come under study as "innovative" approaches to therapy.

The first claim that vitamin E could be useful in ischemic heart disease appeared in the brief report by Vogelsang and Shute (1946). They reported that tocopherol in doses of 200–600 mg/day diminished, or in some instances completely abolished, anginal pain. One year later, Shute *et al.* (1947) reported 84 case histories of patients, 90% of whom showed reduced symptomatic manifestations of coronary occlusion after 12 weeks on vitamin E therapy. These investigators have continued to be strong advocates of vitamin E treatment for cardiovascular disease.

The dramatic claim of Shute led to early investigations attempting to confirm the purported efficacy of vitamin E. Negative reports were published within two years of the original proposal and continue to appear at the time of this writing. At least 17 reports contrary to the claim of the Shute brothers may be found in the literature (cf. Ravin and Katz, 1949; Rinzler *et al.*, 1950; Anderson, 1972; Olson, 1973; Hodges, 1973). Some of the clinical trials were uncontrolled, just as was the study of Shute *et al.* (1947), whereas others represent carefully controlled and double-blind investigations with placebo capsules given randomly along with vitamin E. The common denominator of such investigations has been an unequivocal rejection of the proposal that vitamin E is effective in the therapy of ischemic heart disease.

Relative to tocopherol therapy for anginal symptoms, the recent reports of Anderson (1972) and Aanderson and Reid (1974) are particularly noteworthy since they describe a randomized, double-blind trial in a group of subjects in Toronto, Ontario, which was selected to correspond closely to the patients of the Shute Clinic in terms of epidemiological factors of importance in ischemic heart disease. In addition to assessing the course of angina objectively and carefully controlling the use of vitamin E versus placebo, Anderson (1972) employed an extremely high dose (3200 IU of vitamin E daily), as has been advocated by the Shutes in recent years. The criteria of Anderson included evaluation of (a) nitroglycerin consumption, (b) anginal status (by exercise testing and by severity of symptoms), (c) electrocardiograms, and (d) blood pressure. None of these indices showed significant improvement in the group receiving vitamin E, and no convincing evidence could be gathered in support of tocopherol ingestion for ischemic heart disease. A previous double-blind trial of vitamin E supplementation for angina by Rinzler *et al.* (1950) also yielded negative results, but may be criticized along with the Anderson trial because of the short duration of tocopherol supplementation.

In conclusion, there is abundant evidence against the claim that vitamin E is effective for ischemic heart disease.

3. *Peripheral Vascular Disease with Intermittent Claudication*

Closely allied to the claim that megavitamin E supplementation is beneficial in ischemic heart disease is the recommendation that tocopherol be prescribed for intermittent claudication. This symptomatic manifestation of arteriosclerotic, peripheral vascular disease may be as debilitating as recurrent angina pectoris. It afflicts the middle-aged and elderly population, particularly males, shows a variable course, and is typically treated in much the same fashion as arteriosclerotic heart disease (vasodilators, anticoagulants, and vascular surgery).

Vitamin E has been used by selective groups of physicians for intermittent claudication ever since Boyd *et al.* (1949) presented supporting evidence in a limited group of patients. Subsequently, a large number of studies have been conducted addressing this issue and leading to a nearly continuous stream of reports. In general, a review of the literature on the possible pharmacological role of vitamin E in intermittent claudication leaves one with a considerably more favorable impression than that gained from reviewing studies on tocopherol treatment for ischemic heart disease. Boyd *et al.* (1949) reported that 78% of 76 patients with moderately severe claudication were improved with vitamin E therapy over a 6-month period. In addition, an early controlled trial by Ratcliffe (1949), which included objective assessment with a walking test, indicated that patients with moderate claudication receiving 400 mg of tocopherol per day were improved in 34 of 41 cases, whereas only 5 of 25 untreated subjects showed improvement. This was followed by a study lasting 40 weeks in which Livingstone and Jones (1958) were able to document positive results in a double-blind study of 34 patients. More recently, Williams *et al.* (1971) reported improvement in 19 of 30 patients with femoral–popliteal occlusion after vitamin E therapy, whereas only 2 of 15 subjects on placebo showed improvement. Furthermore, Haeger (1973, 1974) has observed a significant increase in walking distance and arterial blood flow in patients with intermittent claudication receiving 300 mg of α-tocopheryl acetate per day for 2–5 years.

On the other hand, negative studies have also been published along with negative anecdotal comments by physicians who conducted small trials. Baer and Heine (1949) and Hamilton *et al.* (1953) failed to observe improvement in double-blind trials conducted over a 3-month period. The relatively short duration of treatment, however, precludes definitive interpretation of their data, since the nature of the disease is such that a lag period of several months often occurs before improvement is noted with any treatment. Indeed, even proponents of tocopherol treatment for intermittent claudication emphasize the long delay before significant responses are evident.

To summarize, it is clear that, although these studies favor the use of large doses of vitamin E in intermittent claudication, further clinical studies are needed.

4. *Vitamin E and Blood Coagulation*

Recent studies of platelets, which are known to contain a relatively high tocopherol content (Nordoy and Strom, 1975), offer a possible link between vitamin E and reduced blood coagulability. Machlin *et al.* (1975) have observed that vitamin E-deficient rats show increased platelet aggregation and an elevated platelet count. The latter finding is in agreement with that of Melhorn and Gross (1971), who reported that tocopherol-deficient infants tend to show high platelet counts, which are reduced to normal levels after administration of vitamin E. Regarding platelet aggregation, it has been observed by Steiner and Anastasi (1976) not only that this key step in coagulation is inhibited by tocopherol but that the apparent mechanism for the effect is in keeping with a known function of vitamin E—protection against lipid peroxide formation. The proposal that tocopherol is involved in platelet function is both provocative and attractive since decreased platelet aggregation could conceivably explain some of the positive clinical observations relative to amelioration of cardiovascular disease by vitamin E. Additional investigation, however, will be required to confirm these findings and assess their clinical implications.

5. *Other Proposed Pharmacological Uses*

The long-appreciated disturbances in fetal development noted in vitamin E-deficient pregnant animals led to an early exploration of a possible role of vitamin E in women with a history of habitual, spontaneous abortion (Marks, 1962). Although this proposed prophylactic use of tocopherol was apparently accepted by many obstetricians in the 1940s and 1950s, sound evidence supporting such treatment is lacking. One approach to assessing the possible role of tocopherol in spontaneous abortion has been the determination of circulating vitamin E levels in groups of pregnant women with normal or pathological outcomes. It has been established that blood tocopherol levels normally increase in a steady fashion from the first few weeks of pregnancy until delivery, in association with increased blood lipids. An extensive survey of 1611 pregnant women by Ferguson *et al.* (1955) revealed that patients with previous spontaneous abortions and other pathological conditions did not show significant abnormalities in blood tocopherol.

Chronic cystic mastitis is a relatively common, benign lesion of the female breast giving rise to symptoms of pain and tenderness that vary in severity and spontaneously regress in many instances. The intense discomfort of some women with this disease has led to a number of therapeutic adventures of questionable basis such as clinical trials with vitamin E. Although positive results with tocopherol therapy have been claimed (Abrams, 1965), the evidence is anecdotal at best and remains to be substantiated in a controlled trial.

Recent investigations in several countries have focused attention on the vitamin E status of patients with beta thalassemia major. In two series reported to date (Zannos-Mariolea *et al.*, 1974; Hyman *et al.*, 1974), statistically significant reductions in circulating tocopherol have been documented in children with this disease. Erythrocyte hemolysis in the presence of hydrogen peroxide was abnormal in each thalassemia patient tested, but a large number of subjects with normal serum tocopherol levels also demonstrated enhanced hemolysis *in vitro*. An important issue relative to vitamin E and thalassemia major concerns the question of whether or not such patients should be treated with supplementary doses of tocopherol. Although controlled trials of long-term vitamin E administration in pharmacological doses remain to be carried out, Hyman *et al.* (1974) comment that "vitamin E therapy did not affect transfusion requirements" in a short-term trial. In addition, Modell and associates (1974), after treatment of children for periods up to a year with large doses of vitamin E, reported that such treatment had little effect on either the hemoglobin pattern or on blood transfusion requirements. Thus, there is no sound basis at present for recommending tocopherol supplementation in thalassemia, but rather a need for further clinical research.

Several reports have appeared relating supplementary tocopherol to improved exercise tolerance in humans as well as animals (Cureton, 1954). The subjective nature of the evaluations in early studies, as well as the small doses utilized and the failure to allow for athletic training effects, make it impossible to attach credence to this claim. More recently, Sharman and associates (1971) conducted a double-blind trial using more objective techniques of evaluation and allowing for the effects of training on athletic ability. It was observed that a group receiving 400 mg of α-tocopheryl acetate daily showed no improvement in muscular performance, whereas training had a significant effect.

Nair and associates (1971) have reported that administration of supplementary vitamin E to a limited number of patients with porphyria resulted in a slightly reduced excretion of porphyrin and its precursors. Subsequently, Watson et al. (1973) and Mustajoki (1972) repeated the evaluation but were unable to confirm earlier findings. Therefore, the majority of the evidence supports the position that tocopherol is ineffective in porphyria.

REFERENCES

Abrams, A. A. (1965). N. Engl. J. Med. 272, 1080.
Abrams, B. A., Gutteridge, J. M. C., Stocks, J., Friedman, M., and Dormandy, T. L. (1973). Arch. Dis. Child. 48, 721.
Anderson, T. W. (1972). Can. Med. Assoc. J. 110, 401.
Anderson, T. W., and Reid, D. B. (1974). Am. J. Clin. Nutr. 27, 1174.
Armstrong, D., Dimmitt, S., Grider, L., Van Wormer, D., and Austin, J. (1973). Trans. Am. Neurol. Assoc. 98, 3.
Baer, S., and Heine, W. I. (1949). J. Am. Med. Assoc. 139, 733.
Baker, S. J., Pereira, S. M., and Begum, A. (1968). Blood 32, 717.
Barness, L. A., Oski, F. A., Williams, M. L., Morrow, G., and Annand, S. B. (1968). Am. J. Clin. Nutr. 21, 40.
Bassen, F, A., and Kornzweig, A. L. (1950). Blood 5, 381.
Bauernfeind, J. C., Newmark, H., and Brin, M. (1974). Am. J. Clin. Nutr. 27, 234.
Bieri, J. G. (1969). In "The Fat-Soluble Vitamins" (H. F. De Luca and J. W. Suttie, eds.), p. 307. Univ. of Wisconsin Press, Madison.
Bieri, J. G. (1972). Ann. N.Y. Acad. Sci. 203, 181.
Bieri, J. G., and Evarts, R. P. (1973). J. Am. Diet. Assoc. 62, 147.
Bieri, J. G., and Evarts, R. P. (1975a). Fed. Proc., Fed. Am. Soc. Exp. Biol. 34, 913.
Bieri, J. G., and Evarts, R. P. (1975b). Proc. Soc. Exp. Biol. Med. 149, 500.
Bieri, J. G., and Evarts, R. P. (1975c). J. Am. Diet. Assoc. 66, 134.
Bieri, J. G., and Poukka, R. K. H. (1970a). J. Nutr. 100, 557.
Bieri, J. G., and Poukka, R. K. H. (1970b). Int. J. Vitam. Res. 40, 344.
Bieri, J. G., and Prival, E. L. (1965). Proc. Soc. Exp. Biol. Med. 120, 554.
Bieri, J. G., Teets, L., Belavady, B., and Andrews, E. L. (1964). Proc. Soc. Exp. Biol. Med. 117, 131.
Bieri, J. G., Evarts, R. P., and Gart, J. J. (1976). J. Nutr. 106, 124.
Binder, H. J., Herting, D. C., Hurst, V., Finch, S. C., and Spiro, H. M. (1965). N. Engl. J. Med. 273, 1289.
Blanc, W. A., Reid, J. D., and Anderson, D. H. (1958). Pediatrics 22, 494.
Blomstrand, R., and Forsgren, L. (1968). Int. J. Vitam. Res. 38, 328.
Boyd, A. M., Ratcliffe, A. H., Jepson, R. P., and James, G. W. H. (1949). J. Bone Joint Surg., Br. Vol. 31, 325.
Brubacher, G., and Weiser, H. (1967). Wiss. Veroeff Dtsch. Ges. Ernaehr. 16, 50.
Bunnell, R. H., Keating, J., Quaresimo, A., and Parman, G. K. (1965). Am. J. Clin. Nutr. 17, 1.
Bunyan, J., Green, J., Edwin, E. E., and Diplock, A. T. (1960). Biochem. J. 77, 47.
Burk, R. F., and Seely, R. J. (1973). U.S. Army Med. Res. Nutr. Lab., Rep. 335.
Cantarow, A., and Trumper, M. (1962). "Clinical Biochemistry," 6th ed., pp. 180–181. Saunders, Philadelphia, Pennsylvania.
Catignani, G. L. (1975). Biochem. Biophys. Res. Commun. 67, 66.

Catignani, G. L. (1976) *In* "Vitamin E" (L. J. Machlin, ed.). Dekker, New York.

Catignani, G. L., Chytil, F., and Darby, W. J. (1974). *Proc. Natl. Acad. Sci. U.S.A.* **71**, 1966.

Chadd, M. A., and Fraser, A. J. (1970). *Int. J. Vitam. Res.* **40**, 610.

Cheeke, P. R., and Oldfield, J. E. (1969). *Can. J. Anim. Sci.* **49**, 169.

Cureton, T. K. (1954). *Am. J. Physiol.* **179**, 628.

Curran, J. S., Cantolino, S. J., Edwards, W. C., and Van Cader, T. C. (1975). *Pediatr. Res.* **9**, 364.

Dam, H. (1962). *Vitam. Horm. (N.Y.)* **20**, 527.

Darby, C. W., Davidson, A. G. F., and Desai, I. D. (1973). *Arch. Dis. Child.* **48**, 72.

Darby, W. J., Cherrington, M. E., and Ruffin, J. M. (1946). *Proc. Soc. Exp. Biol. Med.* **63**, 310.

Darby, W. J., Ferguson, M. E., Furman, R. H., Lemley, J. M., Ball, C. T., and Meneely, G. R. (1949). *Ann. N.Y. Acad. Sci.* **52**, 328.

Davies, T., Kelleher, J., and Losowsky, M. S. (1969). *Clin. Chim. Acta* **24**, 431.

Davis, K. C. (1972). *Am. J. Clin. Nutr.* **25**, 933.

De Leon, A. S., Elliott, J. H., and Jones, D. B. (1970). *Pediatr. Clin. North Am.* **17**, 309.

De Villers, A., Simard, P., and Srivastava, U. (1973). *Can. J. Biochem.* **51**, 450.

Dicks-Bushnell, M. W., and Davis, K. C. (1967). *Am. J. Clin. Nutr.* **20**, 262.

Dilley, R. A., and McConnell, D. G. (1970). *J. Membr. Biol.* **2**, 317.

Dinning, J. S. (1962). *Vitam. Horm. (N.Y.)* **20**, 511.

Diplock, A. T. (1974). *Am. J. Clin. Nutr.* **27**, 995.

di Sant'Agnese, P. A., and Talamo, R. C. (1967). *N. Engl. J. Med.* **277**, 1399.

Evarts, R. P., and Bieri, J. G. (1974). *Lipids* **9**, 860.

Farrell, P. M., and Bieri, J. G. (1975). *Am. J. Clin. Nutr.* **28**, 1381.

Farrell, P. M., Fratantoni, J. C., Bieri, J. G., and di Sant'Agnese, P. A. (1975). *Acta Paediatr. Scand.* **64**, 150.

Ferguson, M. E., Bridgforth, E., Quaife, M. L., Martin, M. P., Cannon, R. O., Mc-Ganity, W. J., Newbill, J., and Darby, W. J. (1955). *J. Nutr.* **55**, 305.

Filer, L. J. (1968). *Am. J. Clin. Nutr.* **21**, 3.

Filer, L. J., Wright, S. W., Manning, M. P., and Mason, K. E. (1951). *Pediatrics* **8**, 388.

Food and Nutrition Board. (1968). "Recommended Dietary Allowances." Natl. Acad. Sci.—Natl. Res. Counc., Washington, D.C.

Food and Nutrition Board (1974). "Recommended Dietary Allowances." Natl. Acad. Sci.—Natl. Res. Counc., Washington, D.C.

Fukuba, H. (1972). *In* "International Symposium on Vitamin E" (N. Shimazono and Y. Takagi, eds.), p. 63. Kyoritsu Shuppan Co., Ltd., Tokyo.

Fukuba, H. (1975). "Proceedings of the Symposium Sponsored by the Malnutrition Panels of the U.S.-Japan Cooperative Medical Sciences Program: Influence of Environmental and Human Factors on Nutritional Requirements, Tokyo."

Gallo-Torres, H. E. (1970). *Lipids* **5**, 379.

Gloor, U., Wursch, J., Schwieter, U., and Wiss, O. (1966). *Helv. Chim. Acta* **49**, 2303.

Goldbloom, R. B. (1960). *Can. Med. Assoc. J.* **82**, 1114.

Goldbloom, R. B., and Cameron, D. (1963). *Pediatrics* **32**, 36.

Gordon, H. H., and McNamara, H. (1940). *Am. J. Dis. Child.* **62**, 328.

Gordon, H. H., and Nitowsky, H. M. (1968). "Modern Nutrition in Health and Disease" (M. G. Wohl and R. S. Goodhart, eds.), 4th ed., pp. 238–246. Lea & Febiger, Philadelphia, Pennsylvania.

72 JOHN G. BIERI AND PHILIP M. FARRELL

Gordon, H. H., Nitowsky, H. M., and Cornblath, M. (1955). *Am. J. Dis. Child.* **90,** 669.
Gordon, H. H., Nitowsky, H. M., Tildon, J. T., and Levin, S. (1958). *Pediatrics* **21,** 673.
Gross, S., and Melhorn, D. K. (1972). *Ann. N.Y. Acad. Sci.* **203,** 141.
Haeger, K. (1973). *Vasa* **2,** 280.
Haeger, K. (1974). *Am. J. Clin. Nutr.* **27,** 1179.
Halstead, C. H., Sourial, N., Guindi, S., Mourad, K. A. H., Kattab, A. K., Carter, J. P., and Patwardhan, V. N. (1969). *Am. J. Clin. Nutr.* **22,** 1371.
Hamilton, M., Wilson, G. M., Armitage, P., and Boyd, J. T. (1953). *Lancet* **1,** 367.
Harries, J. T., and Muller, D. P. R. (1971). *Arch. Dis. Child.* **46,** 341.
Harris, P. L., Hardenbrook, E. G., Dean, F. R., Cusack, E. R., and Jansen, J. L. (1961). *Proc. Soc. Exp. Biol. Med.* **107,** 381.
Harris, R. S. (1962). *Vitam. Horm. (N.Y.)* **20,** 603.
Hashim, S. A., and Asfour, R. H. (1968). *Am. J. Clin. Nutr.* **21,** 7.
Hassan, H., Hashim, S. A., Van Itallie, T. B., and Sebrell, W. H. (1966). *Am. J. Clin. Nutr.* **19,** 147.
Herting, D. C., and Drury, E. E. (1969). *Am. J. Clin. Nutr.* **22,** 147.
Hodges, R. E. (1973). *J. Am. Diet. Assoc.* **62,** 638.
Hoekstra, W. G. (1975). *Fed. Proc., Fed. Am. Soc. Exp. Biol.* **34,** 2083.
Horwitt, M. K. (1960). *Am. J. Clin. Nutr.* **8,** 451.
Horwitt, M. K. (1962). *Vitam. Horm. (N.Y.)* **20,** 541.
Horwitt, M. K. (1974). *Am. J. Clin. Nutr.* **27,** 1182.
Horwitt, M. K., Harvey, C. C., and Harmon, E. M. (1968). *Vitam. Horm. (N.Y.)* **26,** 487.
Horwitt, M. K., Harvey, C. C., Dahm, C. H., Jr., and Searcy, M. T. (1972). *Ann. N.Y. Acad. Sci.* **203,** 223.
Hyman, C. B., Fanding, B., Alfin-Slater, R., Kozak, L., Weitzman, J., and Ortega, J. A. (1974). *Ann. N.Y. Acad. Sci.* **232,** 211.
Ikehata, H., Tanaka, H., and Kamishima, C. (1968). *Vitamins (Japan)* **38,** 253.
Jager, F. C. (1972). *Ann. N.Y. Acad. Sci.* **203,** 199.
Johnson, L., Schaffer, D., and Boggs, T. R. (1974). *Am. J. Clin. Nutr.* **27,** 1158.
Johnson, P., and Pover, W. F. R. (1962). *Life Sci.* **1,** 115.
Kanno, C., Hayashi, M., Yamauchi, K., and Tsugo, T. (1970). *Agric. Biol. Chem.* **34,** 878.
Kater, R. M. H., Unterecker, W. J., Kim, C. Y., and Davidson, C. S. (1970). *Am. J. Clin. Nutr.* **23,** 913.
Kattwinkel, J., Taussig, L. M., Statland, B. E., and Verter, J. I. (1973). *J. Pediatr.* **82,** 234.
Kayden, H. J. (1972). *Annu. Rev. Med.* **23,** 285.
Kayden, H. J., and Silber, R. (1965). *Trans. Am. Assoc. Physicians* **78,** 334.
Kelleher, J., and Losowsky, M. S. (1970). *Br. J. Nutr.* **24,** 1033.
Kerner, I., and Goldbloom, R. B. (1960). *AMA J. Dis. Child.* **99,** 597.
Kinsey, V. E. (1956). *Arch. Ophthalmol.* **56,** 481.
Kinsey, V. E., and Chisholm, J. F. (1951). *Am. J. Ophthalmol.* **34,** 1259.
Klatskin, G., and Molander, D. W. (1952). *J. Clin. Invest.* **31,** 159.
Kulapongs, P. (1975). *In* "Protein-Calorie Malnutrition" (R. E. Olson, ed.), pp. 263–273. Academic Press, New York.
Larsson, H., and Haeger, K. (1968). *Pharmacol. Clin.* **1,** 72.
Leonard, P. J., and Losowsky, M. S. (1967). *Am. J. Clin. Nutr.* **20,** 795.
Leonard, P. J., and Losowsky, M. S. (1971). *Am. J. Clin. Nutr.* **24,** 388.

Leonard, P. J., Losowsky, M. S., and Pulvertaft, C. N. (1966). *Gut* **7**, 578.
Levin, S., Gordon, M. H., Nitowsky, H. M., Goldman, C., di Sant'Agnese, P. A., and Gordon, H. H. (1961). *Pediatrics* **27**, 578.
Livingstone, P. D., and Jones, C. (1958). *Lancet* **2**, 602.
Lo, S. S., Frank, D., and Hitzig, W. H. (1973). *Arch. Dis. Child.* **48**, 360.
Losowsky, M. S., Kelleher, J., Walker, B. E., Davies, T., and Smith, C. L. (1972). *Ann. N.Y. Acad. Sci.* **203**, 212.
Lucy, J. A. (1972). *Ann. N.Y. Acad. Sci.* **203**, 4.
McCormick, E. C., Cornwell, D. G., and Brown, J. B. (1960). *Lipid Res.* **1**, 221.
Macdougall, L. G. (1972). *J. Pediatr.* **80**, 775.
Machlin, L. J., Filipski, R., Willis, A. L., Kuhn, D. C., and Brin, M. (1975). *Proc. Soc. Exp. Biol. Med.* **149**, 275.
Mackenzie, J. B. (1954). *Pediatrics* **13**, 346.
McLaren, D. S., Shirajian, E., Loshkajian, H., and Shadarevian, S. (1969). *Am. J. Clin. Nutr.* **22**, 863.
MacMahon, M. T., and Neale, G. (1970). *Clin. Sci.* **38**, 197.
MacMahon, M. T., and Thompson, G. R. (1970). *Eur. J. Clin. Invest.* **1**, 161.
MacMahon, M. T., Neale, G. and Thompson, G. R. (1970). *Eur. J. Clin. Invest.* **1**, 288.
McWhirter, W. R. (1975). *Acta Paediatr. Scand.* **64**, 446.
Majaj, A. S., Dinning, J. S., Azzam, S. A., and Darby, W. J. (1963). *Am. J. Clin. Nutr.* **12**, 374.
Marks, J. (1962). *Vitam. Horm.* (*N.Y.*) **20**, 573.
Mason, K. E., and Horwitt, M. K. (1972). *In* "The Vitamins" (W. H. Sebrell, Jr., and R. S. Harris, eds.), 2nd ed., Vol. 5, pp. 293–309. Academic Press, New York.
Melhorn, D. K., and Gross, S. (1969). *J. Lab. Clin. Med.* **74**, 798.
Melhorn, D. K., and Gross, S. (1971). *J. Pediatr.* **79**, 581.
Melhorn, D. K., Gross, S., Lake, G. A., and Leu, J. A. (1971). *Blood* **37**, 438.
Mellors, A., and Barnes, M. M. (1966). *Br. J. Nutr.* **20**, 69.
Mengel, C. F., Kann, H. E., Jr., and Meriwether, W. D. (1967). *J. Clin. Invest.* **46**, 1715.
Minot, A. S. (1944). *J. Lab. Clin. Med.* **29**, 772.
Modell, C. B., Stocks, J., and Dormandy, T. L. (1974). *Br. Med. J.* **3**, 259.
Molenaar, I., Hommes, F. A., Braams, W. G., and Polman, H. A. (1969). *Proc. Natl. Acad. Sci. U.S.A.* **61**, 982.
Molenaar, I., Vos, J., and Hommes, F. A. (1972). *Vitam. Horm.* (*N.Y.*) **30**, 45.
Moyer, W. T. (1950). *Pediatrics* **6**, 893.
Muller, D. P. R., and Harries, J. T. (1969). *Biochem. J.* **112**, 28P.
Muller, D. P. R., Harries, J. T., and Lloyd, J. K. (1974). *Gut* **15**, 966.
Munsat, T. L., Baloh, R., Pearson, C. M., and Fowler, W. (1973). *J. Am. Med. Assoc.* **226**, 1536.
Mustajoki, P. (1972). *J. Am. Med. Assoc.* **221**, 714.
Nair, P. P., Mezey, E., Murty, H. S., Quartner, J., and Mendeloff, A. I. (1971). *Arch. Intern. Med.* **128**, 411.
Newmark, H. L., Pool, W., Bauernfeind, J. C., and De Ritter, E. (1975). *J. Pharm. Sci.* **64**, 655.
Nitowsky, H. M., Cornblath, M., and Gordon, H. H. (1956). *AMA J. Dis. Child.* **92**, 164.
Nitowsky, H. M., Tildon, J. T., Levin, S., and Gordon, H. H. (1962). *Am. J. Clin. Nutr.* **10**, 368.
Nordoy, A., and Strom, E. (1975). *J. Lipid Res.* **16**, 386.

Nutrition Survey of East Pakistan. (1966). U.S. Department of Health, Education, and Welfare, Public Health Service, Bethesda, Maryland.

Olson, R. E. (1967). *Am. J. Clin. Nutr.* **20**, 604.

Olson, R. E. (1973). *Circulation* **48**, 179.

Olson, R. E. (1974). *Am. J. Clin. Nutr.* **27**, 1117.

Olson, R. E. (1975). In "Protein Calorie Malnutrition" (R. E. Olson, ed.), pp. 275–297. Academic Press, New York.

Oppenheimer, E. H. (1956). *Bull. Johns Hopkins Hosp.* **98**, 353.

Oski, F. A., and Barness, L. A. (1967). *J. Pediatr.* **70**, 211.

Oski, F. A., and Barness, L. A. (1968). *Am. J. Clin. Nutr.* **21**, 45.

Oski, F. A., and Naiman, J. L. (1972). "Hematologic Problems in the Newborn," 2nd ed., pp. 1–30. Saunders, Philadelphia, Pennsylvania.

Owens, W. C., and Owens, E. U. (1949). *Am. J. Ophthalmol.* **32**, 1.

Panos, T. C., Stinnett, B., Zapata, G., Eminians, J., Marasigan, B. V., and Beard, A. G. (1968). *Am. J. Clin. Nutr.* **21**, 15.

Patnaik, R. N., and Nair, P. P. (1975). *Experientia* **31**, 1021.

Peake, I. R., Windmueller, H. G., and Bieri, J. G. (1972). *Biochim. Biophys. Acta* **260**, 679.

Pearson, C. K., and Barnes, M. M. (1970). *Br. J. Nutr.* **24**, 581.

Poukka, R. K. H., and Bieri, J. G. (1970). *Lipids* **5**, 757.

Rajaram, O. V., Fatterpaker, P., and Sreenivasan, A. (1974). *Biochem. J.* **140**, 509.

Ramirez, I., Santini, R., Corcino, J., and Santiago, P. J. (1973). *Am. J. Clin. Nutr.* **26**, 1045.

Ratcliffe, A. H. (1949). *Lancet* **2**, 1128.

Ravin, I. S., and Katz, K. H. (1949). *N. Engl. J. Med.* **240**, 331.

Richards, J. E., Goldbloom, R. B., and Denton, R. L. (1957). *Pediatrics* **20**, 92.

Rinzler, S. H., Bakst, H., Benjamin, Z. H., Bobb, A. L., and Travell, J. (1950). *Circulation* **1**, 288.

Rose, C. S., and György, P. (1952). *Am. J. Physiol.* **168**, 414.

Rubinstein, H. M., Dietz, A. A., and Srinavasan, R. (1968). *Clin. Chim. Acta* **23**, 1.

Sandstead, H. H., Gabr, M. K., Azzam, S., Shuky, A. S., Weiler, R. J., Din, O. M. E., Mokhtar, N., Prassad, A. S., Hifney, A. E. and Darby, W. J. (1965). *Am. J. Clin. Nutr.* **17**, 27.

Sartain, P., Kay, J. L., and Dorn, P. M. (1967). *South. Med. J.* **60**, 1371.

Schmandke, H., and Proll, J. (1964). *Int. Z. Vitaminforsch.* **34**, 312.

Scrimshaw, N. S., Behar, M., Arroyave, G., Tejada, C., and Viteri, F. (1957). *J. Am. Med. Assoc.* **164**, 555.

Scriver, C. R. (1970). *Pediatrics* **46**, 493.

Sharman, I. M., Down, M. G., and Sen, R. N. (1971). *Br. J. Nutr.* **26**, 265.

Shute, W. E., Shute, E. V., and Vogelsang, A. (1947). *Med. Rec.* **160**, 91.

Silber, R., Winter, R., and Kayden, H. J. (1969). *J. Clin. Invest.* **48**, 2089.

Simon, E. R., and Ways, P. (1964). *J. Clin. Invest.* **43**, 1311.

Smith, C. L., Kelleher, J., Losowsky, M. S., and Morrish, N. (1971). *Br. J. Nutr.* **26**, 89.

Steiner, M., and Anastasi, J. (1976). *J. Clin. Invest.* **57**, 732.

Stockman, J. A. (1975). *Semin. Hematol.* **12**, 163.

Taylor, B. W., Watts, J. L., and Fosbrooke, A. S. (1973). *Arch. Dis. Child.* **48**, 657.

Thanangkul, O., Whitaker, J. A., and Fort, E. G. (1966). *Am. J. Clin. Nutr.* **18**, 379.

Thompson, J. N., Beare-Rogers, J. L., Erdody, P., and Smith, D. C. (1973). *Am. J. Clin. Nutr.* **26**, 1349.

Underwood, B. A., and Denning, C. R. (1972). *Pediatr. Res.* **6**, 26.

Vogelsang, A., and Shute, E. V. (1946). *Nature (London)* **157**, 772.

Vogtmann, H., and Prabucki, A. L. (1971). *Nutr. Metab.* **13,** 274.

Watson, C. J., Bossenmaier, I., and Cardinal, R. (1973). *Arch. Intern. Med.* **131,** 698.

Weber, F., and Wiss, O. (1966). *Nutr. Dieta* **8,** 54.

Weber, F., Weiser, H., and Wiss, O. (1964). *Z. Ernaehrungswiss.* **245,** 1.

Weinberg, T., Gordon, H. H., Oppenheimer, E. H., and Nitowsky, H. M. (1958). *Am. J. Pathol.* **34,** 565.

Weiss, P., and Bianchine, J. R. (1969). *Am. J. Med. Sci.* **258,** 275.

Whitaker, J. A., Fort, E. G., Vimokesant, S., and Dinning, J. S. (1967). *Am. J. Clin. Nutr.* **20,** 783.

Williams, H. T. G., Fenna, D., and Macbeth, R. A. (1971). *Surg., Gynecol. Obstet.* **132,** 662.

Witting, L. A. (1972). *Am. J. Clin. Nutr.* **25,** 257.

Witting, L. A., and Horwitt, M. K. (1964). *J. Nutr.* **82,** 19.

Witting, L. A., and Lee, L. (1975). *Am. J. Clin. Nutr.* **28,** 571.

Wo, C. K. W., and Draper, H. H. (1975). *Am. J. Clin. Nutr.* **28,** 808.

Woodruff, C. W. (1956). *Am. J. Clin. Nutr.* **4,** 597.

Wright, S. W., Filer, L. J., and Mason, K. E. (1951). *Pediatrics* **7,** 386.

Zannos-Mariolea, L., Tzortzaton, F., Dendaki-Svolaki, K., Katerellos, C., Kavallari, M., and Matsaniotis, N. (1974). *Br. J. Haematol.* **26,** 193.

The Biochemistry of Vitamin E in Plants

W. JANISZOWSKA*† AND J. F. PENNOCK

*Department of Biochemistry, University of Liverpool,
Liverpool, England*

I. INTRODUCTION

It is now over 50 years since Evans and Bishop (1922) described the condition of fetal resorption in pregnant female rats kept on certain diets. This paper initiated a search for a dietary factor that could alleviate the symptoms and resulted in the discovery of α-tocopherol, vitamin E in the late 1930s (Evans et al., 1936; Fernholz, 1937, 1938). In the ensuing years literally thousands of publications have described deficiency syndromes in a variety of animals, levels of vitamin E in diets and flora and fauna, chemical studies on vitamin E and its closely related family of compounds and its metabolism in animals, but to the frustration of an army of researchers vitamin E has refused to reveal its mode of action in animals. Theories come and go with regard to its function, but only the antioxidant theory survives, and even that not without many knocks. α-Tocopherol is easily oxidized, and in tissues it will act as an antioxidant to neighboring lipids—it has little option. Whether this role is sufficient to explain all the facts is much more debatable.

α-Tocopherol is a plant product. Although it can be found in meat, fish, eggs, etc., there is no evidence that it is synthesized in any tissue other than

---

* Present address: Department of Biochemistry, University of Warsaw, Warsaw, Poland.

† Unilever European Fellow.

a plant tissue. Perhaps if its function in plants were known, its role in animals could more easily be understood, but there is a paucity of evidence or even ideas on its function in plants. In this review we shall cover quite briefly the distribution and role of tocopherols in plants and describe new work carried out in our laboratory on tocopherol interconversions, which we believe has a major bearing on ideas of biosynthesis and chemistry of tocopherols.

A. CHEMISTRY OF THE TOCOPHEROLS AND TOCOTRIENOLS

As will become apparent in the section on biosynthesis, there is now reason to believe that some tocopherols not currently thought to have a natural occurrence in fact do occur, albeit in very small quantities, in plants. Paradoxically, these very tocopherols were a one time described as being present in seed oils and bran, but later their chemical identifications were shown to be erroneous. Thus it seems useful at this stage to revise the history of the discovery of the tocopherol family of compounds.

(I)   (II)

The isolation of α-tocopherol and its characterization as 5,7,8-trimethyltocol (I) was followed by the discovery over the next 20 years of six other methylated derivatives of tocol (II) in cereal brans and germ oils, and thus all seven possible methylated tocols had been found in nature (see Table I).

The chemistry seemed neat and tidy and logical until Green and his co-workers (1959) found that ϵ- and ζ-tocopherols were not identical with the synthetic 5- and 5,7-dimethyltocols, respectively, and finally showed that both compounds had an unsaturated side chain at position 2 (Green et al., 1960; McHale et al., 1963). ϵ-Tocopherol turned out to be related to β-tocopherol, but with three double bonds in the side chain, and ζ-tocopherol was similarly related to α-tocopherol. These new derivatives were called tocotrienols, and when Pennock et al. (1964) showed that η-tocopherol (found in rice and palm oil) was actually 7,8-dimethyltocotrienol and also described 8-methyltocotrienol, a component of palm oil, a new family of tocochromanols (tocochromanol is a term that can be used to describe both tocopherols and tocotrienols) was complete. This too seemed entirely

TABLE I
KNOWN TOCOPHEROLS FOUND IN PLANTS CA 1958

Compound	Structure	Reference
α-Tocopherol	5,7,8-Trimethyltocol	Fernholz (1937, 1938)
β-Tocopherol	5,8-Dimethyltocol	Emerson et al. (1936)
γ-Tocopherol	7,8-Dimethyltocol	Emerson et al. (1936)
δ-Tocopherol	8-Methyltocol	Stern et al. (1947)
ε-Tocopherol	5-Methyltocol	Eggitt and Ward (1953, 1955)
ζ-Tocopherol	5,7-Dimethyltocol	Green et al. (1955)
η-Tocopherol	7-Methyltocol	Green and Marcinkiewicz (1956)

logical. Instead of the seven possible methylated derivatives of tocol we have the eight possible tocopherols and tocotrienols that possess an 8-methyl group (Fig. 1).

As will be described later, Janiszowska and Pennock (1976) have now found small amounts of 7-methyltocol in leaves of *Phaseolus vulgaris* (French dwarf bean), and evidence from biosynthetic studies suggests that 5-methyltocol and 5,7-dimethyltocol may also be present in very small amounts. However, this is not to say that ε-, ζ-, and η-tocopherols are other than the tocotrienols mentioned above. It is tempting to suggest that, by analogy with the tocopherols in *P. vulgaris*, there may be in, say, *Hevea brasiliensis* latex very small amounts of 5- and 7-methyltocotrienols and 5,7-dimethyltocotrienol—but this is attempting to rely on logic once more, and such logic has caused too many problems so far.

B. DISTRIBUTION OF TOCOCHROMANOLS IN PLANTS

There are a great many papers describing tocopherols in various plants and parts of the plant, and Dicks (1965) has compiled a most compre-

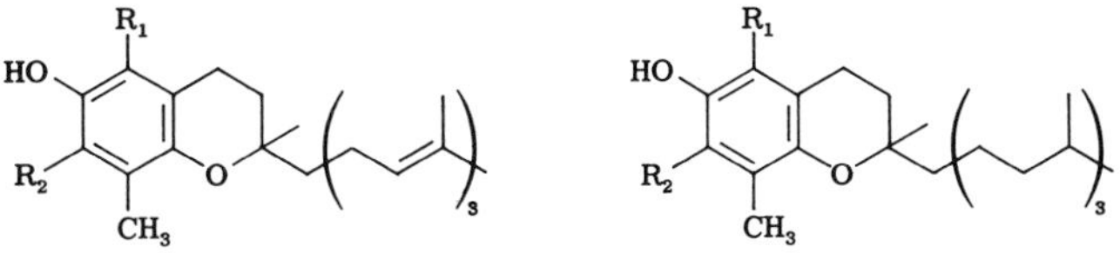

$R_1 = R_2 = CH_3$: α-Tocotrienol
$R_1 = CH_3, R_2 = H$: β-Tocotrienol
$R_1 = H, R_2 = CH_3$: γ-Tocotrienol
$R_1 = R_2 = H$: δ-Tocotrienol

$R_1 = R_2 = CH_3$: α-Tocopherol
$R_1 = CH_3, R_2 = H$: β-Tocopherol
$R_1 = H, R_2 = CH_3$: γ-Tocopherol
$R_1 = R_2 = H$: δ-Tocopnerol

FIG. 1. Naturally occurring tocopherols and tocotrienols.

hensive survey of the tocopherol content of foods and feedstuffs. All we should like to do is attempt to summarize the situation.

All higher plants that have been examined contain α-tocopherol, and this compound is found always in the leaves or wherever photosynthesis is taking place. Amounts vary, but as a general rule young fast-growing plants have very little α-tocopherol whereas slow-growing or evergreen plants contain quite large amounts. This has led both Booth and Hobson-Frohock (1961) to suggest that the α-tocopherol content of leaves is inversely proportional to growth rate. Presumably α-tocopherol is being used up rapidly in the fast growing plant since its synthesis is also proceeding quite rapidly. Older leaves also have a much higher content of chloroplasts, and so all chloroplastidic components are found at a high level.

The non-α-tocopherols, β-, γ-, and δ-, have not been reported as occurring in leaves to any great extent, but we agree with Threlfall (1971) that γ-tocopherol is often, if not always, found in the leaves of higher plants (Table II). It is usually present in smaller quantities than α-tocopherol. δ-Tocopherol is found in some leaves, but β-tocopherol is quite a rarity. Table III shows values for the tocopherol content of variegated tissues, and it is immediately clear that the α-tocopherol content is much lower in yellow tissue than in green. The γ-tocopherol level usually decreases in the yellow tissue, but to a much lesser extent than does the α-tocopherol level. These results largely confirm the data on intracellular distribution discussed in the next section. That is, α-tocopherol is located mainly in the

TABLE II

TocopHerol Content of Leaves of Some Higher Plants[a]

	Tocopherol (μg/gm fresh weight)			
Plant	α	β	γ	δ
Spinacea oleracea	24.3	ND[b]	4.2	Trace
Rumex sanguineus	16.9	Trace	6.9	2.9
Coleus blumei	32.3	ND	14.8	ND
Zea mays	2.4	ND	2.1	0.13
Polygonum cuspidatum	28.4	ND	12.2	2.7
Ligustrum vulgare	41.4	ND	10.3	ND
Tussilago farfara	12.1	ND	2.1	ND
Hevea brasiliensis	71.2	1.0	18.4	2.3
Hordeum vulgare	15.7	ND	8.3	ND
Phaseolus aureus	39.7	ND	29.4	8.1

[a] R. P. Newton and J. F. Pennock, unpublished observations.
[b] ND, not detected.

TABLE III
TOCOPHEROL CONTENT OF SOME VARIEGATED LEAF TISSUES[a]

| Plant[b] | Tocopherol (μg/gm fresh weight) | | | |
	α	β	γ	δ
Coleus hybridus schwartzei: G	19.8	ND[c]	9.4	ND
Y	6.9	ND	5.0	0.4
Peperomia americana: G	30.1	2.7	5.1	ND
Y	2.4	1.7	2.9	ND
Ficus elastica: G	34.7	ND	5.2	ND
Y	11.8	ND	9.5	ND
Abutilon sp.: G	43.5	ND	12.3	ND
Y	9.1	ND	7.4	ND
Ilex aquifolium: G	169	ND	43.0	6.1
Y	7.8	ND	4.6	7.1

[a] R. P. Newton, I. R. Peake, and J. F. Pennock, unpublished observations.
[b] G, green tissue; Y, yellow tissue.
[c] ND, not detected.

chloroplast whereas γ-tocopherol and δ-tocopherol are found mainly outside the chloroplast. The α-tocopherol in the yellow tissue may be in the supernatant fraction of the cell, but more likely it is contained in the few chloroplasts present and also in chromoplasts (see also Lichtenthaler, 1968). The fall in γ-tocopherol level from green to yellow tissue may suggest that some γ-tocopherol occurs in the chloroplast.

In other parts of the plant, such as stem, roots, fruits, seeds, α-tocopherol can be found, but often the predominating tocopherol present is γ-tocopherol (Dicks, 1965). The pea (*Pisum sativum*) seed is a good example in having up to 100% of the tocopherols present as γ-tocopherol (Green, 1958). Wheat germ oil is unusual in possessing quite large amounts of β-tocopherol accompanying the α-tocopherol (Green *et al.*, 1955). These distribution studies indicate that the non-α-tocopherols are not just biosynthetic intermediates in the formation of α-tocopherol, but probably function in their own right. Furthermore, the virtual absence of β-tocopherol in some tissues and its occurrence at a level of over 30% of the total tocopherols in wheat germ indicates that considerable variations in biosynthetic routes occur.

Tocopherols have been found in all brown, green, and red algae examined, and all but one of the blue-green algae have tocopherols. The exception, *Anacystis nidulans,* is currently unique in being the only green photosynthetic plant or alga not to contain α-tocopherol (Henninger *et al.*, 1965; Powls and Redfearn, 1967). No bacterium has been found unambiguously to contain tocopherols, and *Anacystis* is in many respects very similar to bacteria, as are other blue-green algae. Tocopherols have also been described in yeasts and mushrooms, i.e., nonphotosynthetic plants (Diplock *et al.*, 1961; Kubin and Fink, 1961), but Skinner and Sturm (1968) were unable to detect tocopherol in a variety of yeasts, and J. F. Pennock (unpublished observations) has failed to find tocopherols in fungi. Clearly another opinion is required.

Tocotrienols have a somewhat unusual distribution. They are not found in leaves or algae, but occur in some cereal seed oils and brans, palm oil, and the latex of *Hevea brasiliensis*. They are also unusual in being the only tocochromanols to have been found esterified (Dunphy *et al.*, 1965).

C. Intracellular Location of Tocopherols

There seems to be little doubt that in green leaves or algae most of the α-tocopherol occurs in the chloroplast (Booth, 1963; Bucke, 1968; Lichtenthaler and Tevini, 1970; Newton and Pennock, 1971a; Hughes *et al.*, 1971). In nonphotosynthetic tissues α-tocopherol occurs in the "plastid" fraction (e.g., the 3000 g sediment), and here it is presumably in the various plastids and chromoplasts (Lichtenthaler, 1968). Newton and Pennock (1971a), for instance, found over 90% of the α-tocopherol in the "plastid" fraction of parenchymatous tissue of a tangerine mutant of *Lycopersicon esculentum* (tomato). This fraction contained mostly chromoplasts and a few chloroplasts.

It is much more difficult to decide whether α-tocopherol is present in any cellular fraction other than chloroplast or a related plastid. In most studies on cell fractionation, some breakage of chloroplasts occurs and the fragments sediment with other factors. Furthermore, developing plastids are often small and do not sediment with the chloroplast fraction. Several workers have found that not all the α-tocopherol is present in the chloroplast fraction and suggest the mitochondria as a possible site in some cases (Threlfall and Goodwin, 1967; Dilley and Crane, 1963; Hughes *et al.*, 1971). Thomas and Stobart (1971), working with callus cultures of *Kalanchoë crenata* (these cultures produce chlorophyll in the light but cannot photosynthesize), found only 56% of the α-tocopherol in the plastid fraction in green cultures and 100% of the α-tocopherol in the 20,000 g sediment in dark grown cultures. When green cultures were treated with [^{14}C]-mevalonic acid, the α-tocopherol from the 20,000 g sediment had a specific activity three times that of the α-tocopherol in the plastid fraction. This not only indicates an extra chloroplastid site, but also synthesis outside the plastid fraction. However, another explanation may be that the 20,000 g fraction contains small immature plastids that are forming α-tocopherol quite rapidly.

Similar results were obtained by Botham and Pennock (1976). When *Phaseolus vulgaris* leaves were treated with [3,4-^{14}C]γ-tocopherol, there was conversion to α-tocopherol; although nearly all the α-tocopherol (weight) was in the chloroplast, most of the radioactivity was in the supernatant (after a 3000 g sediment was removed). The evidence seems to favor some α-tocopherol at least having an extrachloroplastidic site.

There have been fewer studies on the intracellular localization of the non-α-tocopherols, but Booth (1963) and Newton and Pennock (1971a) found that most of the γ- and δ-tocopherol was extrachloroplastidic. Newton and Pennock (1971a) later examined tocopherols in *Fucus spiralis* thallus tissue in particular. In *Fucus* species, in addition to α-tocopherol there are relatively large amounts of β- and γ-tocopherol and almost as much δ-tocopherol as α-tocopherol (Jensen, 1961). α-Tocopherol was found in the chloroplast fraction, β- and γ-tocopherol in the 30,000 and 100,000 g sediments, and δ-tocopherol in the 200,000 g sediment and supernatant. In a survey of subcellular fractions of the leaves of *Pisum sativum* (Hughes *et al.*, 1971), γ- and δ-tocopherol were found in each fraction, γ-tocopherol being mainly in the chloroplasts and microsomal fraction and δ-tocopherol mainly in the chloroplasts and supernatant. Dada (1968), too, found over half the γ-tocopherol in chloroplasts.

Non-α-tocopherols appear to be localized in the chloroplast to some extent and perhaps also on the endoplasmic reticulum. Newton and Pennock (1971b) found that γ-tocopherol was not a component of nuclei, cell walls, or mitochondria but was sedimented with the microsomal fraction at 25,000 g whereas δ-tocopherol was present in this fraction only after very gentle homogenization methods. Neither tocopherol was present in ribosomes. The two tocopherols seem to be components of the microsomal fraction but can be separated from one another to some extent by differential centrifugation of this fraction.

D. FUNCTION OF TOCOPHEROLS

The fact that large amounts of all four tocopherols can be found, not necessarily together, in various tissues suggests that all have a function. Perhaps there is one common function carried out in different parts of the cell by different tocopherols or several independent functions. At this stage three likely areas for possible tocopherol functioning can be recognized: (1) antioxidant role, (2) membrane stability, probably via (1), and (3) possible role in initiation of flowering.

1. *Antioxidant Role*

Chemically, tocopherols are easily oxidized to either quinones or dimers and trimers, and in animal tissues tocopherols are seen as preventing the spread of peroxidation through lipids, perhaps in a membrane (Tappell, 1974). Initially a fatty acid (unsaturated) is attacked by ozone or perhaps by a pollutant chemical or is irradiated to form a free radical. This reacts with oxygen and then attacks a neighboring fatty acid, removing a hydrogen and forming a new radical. The process goes on until α-tocopherol interrupts the spiral by reducing an offending radical.

$$RH \rightarrow R \cdot$$
$$R \cdot + O_2 \rightarrow R-O-O \cdot$$
$$R-O-O \cdot + R_1H \rightarrow R-O-O-H + R_1 \cdot$$
$$R_1 \cdot + O_2 \rightarrow R_1-O-O \cdot$$
$$\text{etc.}$$
$$ROO \cdot + \alpha\text{-tocopherol} \rightarrow ROOH + \text{oxidized } \alpha\text{-tocopherol}$$

Such a role for α-tocopherol (or other tocopherols) in plants is clearly feasible, particularly, for instance, in lipid stores. Large amounts of tocopherols are found in seed oils, and Hove and Harris (1951) suggested that there is a correlation between the highest tocopherol content and the highest degree of unsaturation in the component fatty acids. Furthermore γ- and δ-tocopherol, which *in vitro* are the most potent antioxidants of the tocopherol family (Lea and Ward, 1959), are found in those oils with the most unsaturated fatty acids.

In the chloroplast, α-tocopherol could protect vulnerable lipids from photooxidation by chlorophyll. Plastoquinone C, a series of hydroxylated derivatives of plastoquinone (Wallwork and Pennock, 1969), can be formed (on paper) by either epoxidation or hydroperoxidation of the double bonds of plastoquinone. α-Tocopherol could be present to keep this destruction of plastoquinone to a minimum.

2. *Membrane Stability*

Siegenthaler (1972) found that during aging chloroplasts lost linoleic and linolenic acids and developed some abnormalities of function. These acids are typical of those vulnerable to peroxidation. Baszynski (1974) has shown that α-tocopherol can restore photosystem I activity to heptane-extracted chloroplasts; since partial reconstitution can be achieved with either phytol or tocol, Baszynski suggested that α-tocopherol might have a structural role to play in thylakoid membranes. Bishop and Wong (1974) tentatively came to a similar conclusion. They isolated a tocopherol-deficient mutant of *Scenedesmus obliquus* that could not grow autotrophically but grew either heterotrophically or mixotrophically (heterotrophically with lights on). The mutant could photosynthesize to a reduced extent (20–60% of wild type), but high-intensity white light inhibited photosynthesis in the mutant but not the wild type. The mutant had normal levels of plastoquinone, but otherwise resembled the mutants of this organism blocked in photosystem II. Bishop and Wong found abnormalities in the stacking of the thylakoids in the mutant—an imperfection presumably in membrane structure.

There is little or no evidence for α-tocopherol functioning in chloroplasts on the electron transport chain as a redox couple with α-tocopherolquinone, although the latter compound is found in chloroplasts. α-Tocopherolquinone, but not α-tocopherol, undergoes changes in level in isolated chloroplasts illuminated in the presence of $NADP^+$, and α-tocopherolquinol is probably involved in these changes (Dilley and Crane, 1963).

3. Initiation of Flowering

α-Tocopherol has also been implicated in flower initiation in plants requiring thermal or photo induction. Baszynski (1967) showed that α-tocopherol could induce flowering in the "long-day" plant *Calendula officinalis* when grown "short-day" but control "short-day" plants without α-tocopherol did not blossom. Similar studies were carried out by Michniewicz and Kamienska (1964, 1965) on "long-day" plants and "cold-requiring" plants with identical results. It is not clear whether this is a direct effect of tocopherols or whether the action is through gibberellins. It is of interest in this area to mention the preliminary report of work by Battle *et al.* (1976), who find that there is a daily rhythm in the level of γ-tocopherol (but not α-tocopherol) in the leaves of *Xanthium strumarium* under vegetative photoperiods and that, when the leaves were switched to flowering photoperiods, there was a marked increase in γ-tocopherol only.

II. BIOSYNTHESIS OF TOCOCHROMANOLS

There are almost certainly two pathways at least leading to biosynthesis of α-tocopherol, namely, the tocotrienol route and the tocopherol route. In the *tocotrienol route* homogentisic acid (or a related derivative) condenses with geranylgeraniol (as the pyrophosphate), and a monomethyl tocotrienol results. Methylation yields first a dimethyl and then trimethyl tocotrienol (α-tocotrienol), and the side chain is then saturated to yield α-tocopherol. Such a pathway probably works in *Hevea latex*. The *tocopherol route* involves phytyl pyrophosphate, and thus the final saturation step is not needed. A prenyltoluquinol is a likely intermediate in both schemes.

When reviewed by Threlfall (1971), evidence from incorporation studies using [β-¹⁴C]tyrosine, [α-¹⁴C]homogentisic acid, [1,6-¹⁴C]shikimic acid, and [¹⁴CH₃]methionine favored the scheme shown in Fig. 2.

Although the tocopherol route has been studied in greater detail, the main evidence in favor of the above scheme is the same for both tocopherol and tocotrienol pathways. All tocochromanols have an 8-methyl group; α- and γ-tocochromanol, but not δ-tocochromanol, were labeled following incubations with [¹⁴CH₃]methionine, and homogentisate labeled in the α-carbon was incorporated into all tocochromanols (see Threlfall, 1971). Specific activity is useful in determining precursor product relationships, and on this basis the tracer studies indicated that γ-tocopherol was a precursor of α-tocopherol, but it seemed unlikely that δ-tocopherol was a precursor of γ-tocopherol (Whistance and Threlfall, 1968; Peake *et al.*, 1970). However, specific activities can be misleading, especially when,

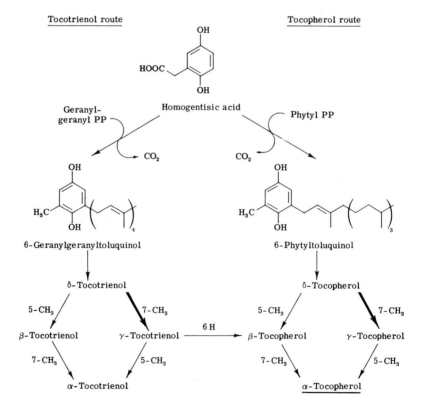

FIG. 2. Possible biosynthetic routes to α-tocopherol. 7-CH₃, 7-methylation; 5-CH₃, 5-methylation.

as is likely with γ- and δ-tocopherol, there are two pools present in the cell, one concerned in biosynthesis and the other functional.

A. TOCOPHEROL PATHWAY

1. *Methyltocols as Precursors of Dimethyltocols and α-Tocopherol*

To study the possible involvement of δ-tocopherol and other methyltocols in tocopherol biosynthesis, Janiszowska *et al.* (1976) prepared samples of [3,4-³H]5-, 7-, and 8-methyltocol (the latter is δ-tocopherol) from toluquinol and [1,2-³H]isophytol. The chemical synthesis favored formation of 7-methyltocol, that is, introduction of the side chain in the para position to the ring methyl and the ratio of 5-:7-:8-methyltocol in the reaction product was 2:5:3.

In the initial experiment, an ethereal solution of 25 μCi of [3,4-³H] δ-tocopherol was applied to the leaf of *Hevea brasiliensis* and the incubation was continued for 24 hours. Considerable incorporation of radioactivity into γ-tocopherol (specific activity 87,594 dpm/mg) and α-tocopherol (specific activity 2202 dpm/mg) occurred and confirmed that δ-tocopherol could be a precursor of γ-tocopherol and α-tocopherol.

Janiszowska *et al.* (1976) then examined the possible incorporation of 5-, 7-, and 8-methyltocol into other tocopherols in 4-week-old plants of *Phaseolus vulgaris*. In a series of experiments, 50 μCi of each tritiated methyltocol isomer was incubated in turn for 24 hours with leaves of *P. vulgaris;* the results are shown in Table IV.

TABLE IV

THE INCORPORATION OF RADIOACTIVITY FROM TRITIATED METHYLTOCOLS INTO TOCOPHEROLS BY LEAVES OF *Phaseolus vulgaris*[a]

Compound	[3,4-³H]5-Methyltocol, 50 μCi (dpm)	[3,4-³H]7-Methyltocol, 50 μCi (dpm)	[3,4-³H]8-Methyltocol, 50 μCi (dpm)
α-Tocopherol (5,7,8)[b]	11,640	43,500	17,500
β-Tocopherol (5,8)	13,790	ND[c]	9,750
γ-Tocopherol (7,8)	ND	137,070	25,000
5,7-Dimethyltocol	7,390	4,315	ND

[a] 3,4-³H-labeled methyltocol (50 μCi) was applied to the leaf surface of 4-week-old *P. vulgaris* plants, and the plants were left in a greenhouse for 24 hours. The leaves were extracted, and 1-mg quantities of the three dimethyl tocols and α-tocopherol were added as carrier. The tocopherols were separated and purified.

[b] Figures in parentheses refer to methyl groups present in tocopherol.

[c] ND, not detected.

Although the total incorporation of label from the tritiated methyltocols into tocopherols was low mainly because a large proportion of each compound applied to the leaf surface did not penetrate the leaf cells, the results show that all three methyltocols can act as precursors of tocopherols in *P. vulgaris*. Not only are the two "unnatural" tocopherols, 5- and 7-methyltocols, converted into β- and γ-tocopherol, respectively, but both compounds also yield to some extent another "unnatural" compound, 5,7-dimethyltocol. Each methyltocol isomer is methylated to yield two dimethyltocols and α-tocopherol. It is not clear whether all the dimethyltocols can act as precursors of α-tocopherol, but it seems likely.

7-Methyltocol appears to be the best precursor of γ-tocopherol and eventually α-tocopherol, but the 8-methyltocol is also quite a good precursor of γ-tocopherol. The problem is then to determine whether there are several possible pathways in the plant or merely that its methyltransferases are nonspecific. From knowledge of the distribution of tocopherols, it is clear that some specificity occurs. It seems unlikely that there is only one methylating enzyme, but the total number needed to introduce methyl groups into the 5, 7, and 8 positions on the various substrates is not known. It is perhaps not unreasonable to assume that there is present a 5-methyltransferase, a 7-methyltransferase, and an 8-methyltransferase, each exerting some specificity of reaction on particular substrates. If this is the case, does the 8-methyltransferase use both 7-methyltocol and 5,7-dimethyltocol as substrates? Thus there is still much to learn in this area. However, the results in Table IV clearly demonstrate that there is a very active 8-methyltransferase working, and this would not be required in the biosynthetic scheme shown in Fig. 2.

2. Incubation of P. vulgaris Leaves with Tritiated Tocol

In an effort to investigate the specificity—or perhaps lack of specificity —of the methyltransferases, Janiszowska and Pennock (1976) synthesized a sample of [3,4-^{3}H]tocol and applied it to leaves of *P. vulgaris*. After the incubation period, carrier amounts of each of the monomethyl and dimethyltocols and α-tocopherol were then added to the lipid extract from the leaves. These compounds, together with any labeled endogenous counterparts that might be formed, were reisolated and purified.

No radioactivity was detected in any tocopherol after rigorous purification. Therefore tocol cannot act as a substrate for any of the methyltransferases, and clearly there is a requirement for the presence in the molecule of at least one nuclear methyl group before the methyltransferases can act. This is very good supporting evidence for the idea that one nuclear methyl group comes from the α-carbon of homogentisic acid and also adds credibility to the view that the incorporation of 5- and 7-methyltocols into tocopherols by *P. vulgaris* leaves results from the action of key functional enzymes, and is not due merely to coincidental nonspecific methylations.

3. Further Experiments as to the Role of 7-Methyltocol in the Biosynthesis of Tocopherols

DL-[β-^{14}C]Tyrosine can be used as a precursor of tocopherols (Whistance and Threlfall, 1967) in higher plants, and Janiszowska and Pennock (1976) attempted to "dilute out" radioactivity from this precursor by the preadministration of 7-methyltocol or δ-tocopherol to the plants. In these experiments, 7-methyltocol or δ-tocopherol (1 mg) was applied in ether to the leaf surface of *P. vulgaris* plants. After 24 hours, another 1 mg of tocopherol was added, and after a further 4 hours 5 μCi of DL-[β-^{14}C]tyrosine was also applied to the leaf surface. Control plants were treated with ether only and the labeled tyrosine. The results of the experiments are shown in Table V.

Both 7-methyltocol and δ-tocopherol were able to "dilute out" incorporation of label from radioactive tyrosine into γ- and α-tocopherol. On the face of it, 7-methyltocol appears to be a better diluent than δ-tocopherol, incorporation of label into γ-tocopherol being reduced to 68% of the control with 7-methyltocol present and only 80% with δ-tocopherol present. In the case of α-tocopherol, incorporation was reduced to 40% with 7-methyltocol and 88% with δ-tocopherol. One might argue that the tocopherol coated on the leaf surface reduces uptake of tyrosine, but

TABLE V

INCORPORATION OF RADIOACTIVE TYROSINE INTO TOCOPHEROLS BY LEAVES OF
Phaseolus vulgaris PREVIOUSLY TREATED WITH 7-METHYLTOCOL OR δ-TOCOPHEROL[a]

Compound	+δ-Tocopherol (dpm)	Control (dpm)	+7-Methyltocol (dpm)	Control (dpm)
α-Tocopherol	759	866	1,318	3,226
γ-Tocopherol	4,873	6,107	7,358	10,839
δ-Tocopherol	456	452	2,150	909
7-Methyltocol	NE[b]	NE	228	151
Plastoquinone	1,014	1,008	1,878	1,828

[a] 7-Methyltocol (1 mg) or δ-tocopherol (1 mg) was applied to *P. vulgaris* leaves at zero time and after 24 hours as an ethereal solution. After a further 4 hours, 5 μCi of DL-[β-^{14}C]tyrosine was applied to the leaf surface of these plants and controls which had only received ether. Tocopherols (1 mg) were added to the leaf extract to aid isolation and purification.

[b] NE, not examined.

incorporation into the internal control in plastoquinone is identical in the experimental and control.

The presence of 7-methyltocol caused an increased incorporation into δ-tocopherol, a fact confirmed quite clearly on autoradiograms. One could argue that the presence of 7-methyltocol in the system inhibited its own synthesis, perhaps by feedback inhibition, and this block resulted in increased synthesis of δ-tocopherol. Radioactivity was detected in 7-methyltocol when it had been applied to the leaf surface, but the amounts were very small. The tocopherol was purified on two absorption—thin-layer chromatography systems and one reversed-phase system, and a nitroso derivative was prepared and purified and finally counted for radioactivity and amount of material present estimated. Certainly no sign of 7-methyltocol was detected on autoradiograms.

Perhaps the main result of the experiment was that 7-methyltocol could "dilute out" radioactivity from [^{14}C]tyrosine and further supported the view that 7-methyltocol is a real and important precursor of γ- and α-tocopherol.

4. Isolation of 7-Methyltocol

Leaves of P. vulgaris were removed from young plants; 920 gm of tissue was extracted, and the lipid was chromatographed on a Brockmann Grade 3 alumina column. The fraction eluted by 12% diethyl ether in light petroleum was further examined by thin-layer chromatography with 20% diethyl ether in light petroleum and chloroform as solvents, and in each case the material between 7-methyltocol markers was eluted. The fraction was then purified on a reversed-phase system, and the UV spectrum of the fraction was determined. The spectrum agreed with that of 7-methyltocol; allowing for some losses, it was estimated at 0.045 μg/gm wet weight of leaf. The material was then nitrosated and the nitroso derivative migrated with 5-nitroso-7-methyltocol on thin-layer chromatography.

5. Incubations with Radioactive Dimethyltocols

a. γ-Tocopherol. Botham and Pennock (1976) incubated [3,4-^{14}C] γ-tocopherol with nasturtium (Tropaeolus majus) leaves and P. vulgaris leaves by applying the tocopherol in ether to the surface of the leaves. About 4.7 μCi of radioactive γ-tocopherol (4.64 μCi/mg) was applied to about 20 gm of either T. majus or P. vulgaris leaves, and the tissue was extracted after a 24-hour incubation. In two experiments with T. majus, total incorporations into α-tocopherol were 28,100 and 18,730 dpm, amounting to about 0.27% and 0.18% conversion from γ-tocopherol, respectively. These incorporations are not very high, but the method of application of γ-tocopherol is not very successful, and probably little of the applied material actually enters the leaf.

When γ-tocopherol was incubated with *P. vulgaris* leaves incorporation into α-tocopherol was 5640 dpm and considerable radioactivity (6680 dpm) was found in α-tocopherolquinone. It is clear from these experiments that γ-tocopherol can be a precursor of α-tocopherol in these two higher plants.

b. 5,7-Dimethyltocol. Condensation of [1,2-³H]isophytol with 3,5-dimethylquinol gave [3,4-³H]5,7-dimethyltocol, which was applied to the surface of *P. vulgaris* leaves. After a 24-hour incubation, the leaves were extracted to yield α-tocopherol (164,000 dpm) from 25 μCi of [³H] 5,7-dimethyltocol. This represents quite a high percentage conversion to α-tocopherol (0.30%), but it is impossible to compare with the conversions using γ-tocopherol because of differences in specific activity of precursors. The [¹⁴C]γ-tocopherol was 4.64 μCi/mg, and the [³H]5,7-dimethyltocol was 220 μCi/mg.

Nevertheless, 5,7-dimethyltocol is formed in *P. vulgaris* after application of 5- or 7-methyltocol to leaves and is itself converted to α-tocopherol. Whether we are observing the activity of a biosynthetic route that plays an important role in the plant or whether the results are due to nonspecific enzymes working on artificial precursors is more difficult to assess. Although the conversion of 5,7-methyltocol to α-tocopherol looks quite high, it must be remembered that formation of 5,7-dimethyltocol from 5- or 7-methyltocol was quite small compared with, say, the formation of γ-tocopherol from 7-methyltocol (Table IV). Therefore, in the overall scheme production of α-tocopherol from γ-tocopherol would greatly exceed that from 5,7-dimethyltocol because of the differences in rates of formation of these precursors. The findings really indicate the probable presence of a relatively nonspecific 8-methyltransferase that can utilize several substrates: 7-methyltocol (to form γ-tocopherol), 5-methyltocol (to form β-tocopherol), or 5,7-dimethyltocol (to form α-tocopherol). Some specificity must, however, be exercised by the enzyme, as it will not methylate tocol itself (see Section II, A, 2).

No experiments have as yet been carried out with β-tocopherol as a precursor for α-tocopherol.

6. *Phytyltoluquinones* (PTQ)

If phytyl pyrophosphate or geranylgeranyl pyrophosphate condenses with homogentisic acid with the loss of CO_2 and pyrophosphate, a toluquinol with a terpenoid side chain will be formed. Pennock *et al.* (1964) suggested 6-geranylgeranyltoluquinol as a possible precursor of the tocopherols, and Threlfall (1971) preferred 6-PTQ. If tissues are extracted to look for such a quinol, it is highly unlikely that it would survive the extraction procedure and much more likely that the related quinone would appear in extracts.

In 1971 Threlfall *et al.* isolated a PTQ from a streptomycin-bleached strain of *Euglena gracilis* strain Z, which was characterized as 6-phytyl-toluquinone [described by Threlfall *et al.* as 2-demethylphytylplasto-quinone (III)]. This compound (as the quinol) could be a precursor of δ-tocopherol. Three years earlier, Burnett and Thomson had described the

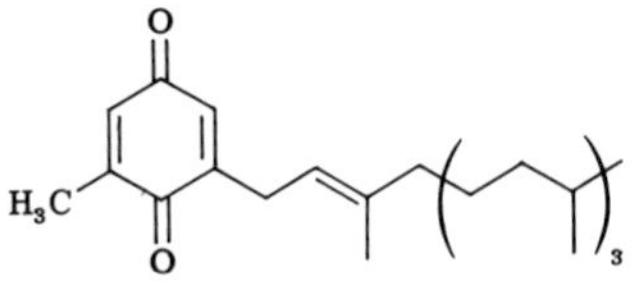

(III)

isolation of a quinonoid constituent of the leaves of *Pyrola media*, which was identified as 5-geranyl-2-methyl-1,4-benzoquinone (5-geranyltolu-quinone IV). The structure was confirmed by synthesis from toluquinol and geraniol. A homologous quinone (with only one isoprenoid unit in the side chain) was also found in *P. media*. Although this compound could

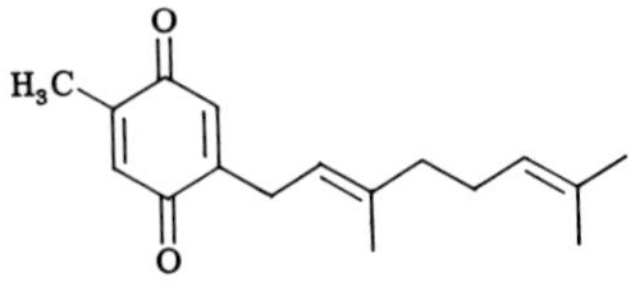

(IV)

not be a precursor of the tocopherols or tocotrienols, the presence of such a compound in nature with the methyl group para to the side chain was extremely interesting since cyclization of such a compound would yield a 7-methylchromanol (V). In view of the relatively high activity of 7-meth-yltocol as a tocopherol precursor in *P. vulgaris* leaves, Janiszowska and Pennock (1976) examined this plant for PTQ content.

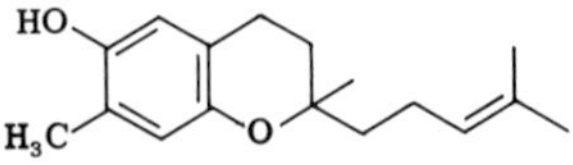

(V)

Before examination of the plant tissue, synthesis of 5-PTQ was carried out according to the method of Burnett and Thomson (1968). Phytol (or isophytol) was condensed with toluquinol in dioxane in the presence of boron trifluoride etherate. When Burnett and Thomson condensed geraniol and toluquinol, only one product (5-geranyltoluquinone) appeared to be

3-Phytyltoluquinone (3-PTQ)
(VI)

5-Phytyltoluquinone (5-PTQ)
(VII)

6-Phytyltoluquinone (6-PTQ)
(VIII)

formed. However, we obtained three products, (VI)–(VIII), which were identified as the three isomeric PTQs. The three compounds had almost identical UV absorption properties (λ_{max}. 252 nm in cyclohexane, E 17,700). The compounds were examined by infrared analysis, nuclear magnetic resonance, and mass spectrum; in each case the three compounds behaved quite similarly, and final structural identification was only confirmed by cyclization of the quinol with $KHSO_4$ in acetic acid (Hoffman et al., 1960) to yield the related methylated tocol, i.e., 5- and 7-methyltocol and δ-tocopherol.

When isophytol was used (isophytol appeared to give a higher yield than phytol), the situation was complicated by the formation of both 2'-cis and 2'-trans-quinones. On thin-layer chromatography it is possible to separate the cis- and trans-quinones, as usually the 2'-cis-quinone runs ahead of the 2'-trans. However, on thin layers of silica gel G with 8% diethyl ether in light petroleum as solvent, the three PTQs migrated quite closely with R_f values as follows: 3-PTQ, 0.46; 5-PTQ, 0.41; 6-PTQ, 0.37. Therefore there is some overlap of the 2'-cis-6-PTQ with the 2'-trans-5-PTQ and of the 2'-cis-5-PTQ with 2'-trans-3-PTQ. The best separation could be achieved using 8% ether in light petroleum as solvent with precoated thin-layer plates, silica gel 60 (Merck). The percentage composition of the PTQ reaction product was estimated by spectrophotometry of the separated PTQs or by conversion to tocopherols and then estimation of the tocopherols by Emmerie–Engel reaction. The results were very similar by both methods: 3-PTQ, 14%; 5-PTQ, 48%; and 6-PTQ, 38%.

About 1 kg of leaves from 4-week-old P. vulgaris plants was extracted with organic solvents, and, after column and thin-layer chromatography of the lipid extract, a small amount of PTQ was isolated. This material was a mixture of 3-PTQ (11% of total), 5-PTQ (61%) and 6-PTQ (28%), and the total concentration was about 0.45 μg per gram of leaf (fresh weight). On reductive cyclization, only two products were identified: δ-tocopherol and 7-methyltocol arising from 6-PTQ and 5-PTQ, respectively. Unfortunately not sufficient material was available for another cyclization. Reductive cyclization of small amounts of phytyltoluquinone does not always proceed smoothly; on occasion, with synthetic material we have obtained no readily identifiable product. A further difficulty is that the best way of identifying the monomethyltocols is to treat them with diazotized o-dianisidine reagent after thin-layer chromatography. 7-Methyltocol gives a slate gray color, δ-tocopherol a deep purple, but 5-methyltocol, which apparently does not couple, gives only a weak brown color (Green and Marcinkiewicz, 1959). Therefore, not only is 5-methyltocol likely to be present in the cyclization product to a small extent, but it gives a very weak stain. Thus the final confirmation of the presence of 3-PTQ in *P. vulgaris* is required, but for now it is assumed that the PTQ from the extract migrating with the same R_f value as synthetic 3-PTQ is in fact 3-PTQ.

The finding of the three isomers of PTQ is highly significant in view of the earlier work with tritiated 5- and 7-methyltocol and δ-tocopherol, which indicated that the latter compounds could be precursors of dimethyltocols and α-tocopherol. Preliminary surveys with other tissues show that the PTQs are present in *Scenedesmus obliquus* (R. Powls and J. F. Pennock, unpublished observations), but could not be detected in mature leaves of grape ivy (*Rhoicissus rhomboidea*). In the examination of the extract from *R. rhomboidea*, one problem became apparent that may explain why PTQs have not been identified on many occasions. On thin-layer chromatograms (silica gel G/ether-light petroleum solvent) the phytylplastoquinones migrate just behind plastoquinone in a position where plastoquinone B (Griffiths, 1966) appears when present. Plastoquinone B is a common component of mature leaves in amounts much higher than those of phytylplastoquinones found in *P. vulgaris*, and so it is expected that the latter compounds would be masked. It is also possible that in the dark green leaves of *R. rhomboidea* (which have very large amounts of tocopherols present) tocopherol biosynthesis may be switched off and so intermediates in biosynthesis may not be present.

7. Incorporation of Tritiated Phytyltoluquinones into Tocopherols

Condensation of [1,2-³H]isophytol with toluquinone in the presence of boron trifluoride etherate gave the three 1',2-³H-labeled PTQs. Because of the formation of 2'-*cis*- and 2'-*trans*-quinones (see Section II, A, 6) it was not possible to prepare pure 2'-*trans*-quinones. After isolation by thin-layer chromatography, the 2'-*trans*-6-PTQ appeared to be pure, but 2'-*trans*-5-PTQ was contaminated with some 2'-*cis*-6-PTQ, and 2'-*trans*-3-PTQ was contaminated with 2'-*cis*-5-PTQ. However, the *cis* quinones always isomerize to a large extent to the *trans*-quinones (the stable mixture for other terpenoid quinones, e.g., vitamin K_1, is 70% *trans*, 30% *cis*). Light appears to initiate this isomerization. Therefore, having isolated, say, 2'-*trans*-5-PTQ with some 2'-*cis*-6-PTQ, the fraction could be left for some time in the laboratory and then rechromatographed to remove the 2'-*trans*-6-PTQ (and 2'-*cis*-5-PTQ) formed during standing. Nevertheless some contamination always remained.

Samples (10 μCi) of [1',2'-^{3}H]5- and 6-phytyltoluquinone were applied to young *P. vulgaris* plants in the usual manner. Carrier tocopherols were added to the extracted lipids and reisolated. The results are shown in Table VI. *Phaseolus vulgaris* leaves are clearly capable of converting the two phytyltoluquinones used in the experiments into the respective methyltocol. Conversion of 5-PTQ to 7-methyltocol proceeds much more efficiently than formation of δ-tocopherol from 6-PTQ. The reaction proceeds presumably by conversion to the quinol and then cyclization to the chromanol (see Threlfall, 1971).

The other products of the incubations, i.e., the dimethyltocols and α-tocopherol, show that the PTQs can act as precursors for the various tocopherols. In these experiments more α-tocopherol has been formed from 6-PTQ than from 5-PTQ, and it is possible that the incorporation

TABLE VI
INCORPORATION OF RADIOACTIVITY FROM [1',2'-^{3}H]5- AND 6-PTQ INTO
TOCOPHEROLS IN LEAVES OF *Phaseolus vulgaris*[a]

Compound	[1',2'-^{3}H]5-PTQ[b] (dpm)	[1',2'-^{3}H]6-PTQ (dpm)
α-Tocopherol	3,220	12,880
β-Tocopherol	NE[c]	9,272
γ-Tocopherol	74,270	3,680
δ-Tocopherol	5,280	55,900
7-Methyltocol	399,000	NE

[a] To leaves of 4-week-old *P. vulgaris* plants, 10 μCi of either [1',2'-^{3}H]5-PTQ or [1',2'-^{3}H]6-PTQ were applied and left for 24 hours. Carrier tocopherols (1 mg of each) were added to the extracted lipids to aid isolation and purification. Values are in total disintegrations per minute (dpm). PTQ = phytyltoluquinone.

[b] Contaminated with a little 2'-*cis*- and 2'-*trans*-[1',2'-^{3}H]6-PTQ.

[c] NE, not examined.

of radiolabeled 6-PTQ into the leaf proceeded faster than with 5-PTQ, and thus the reaction has proceeded further. Also the higher activity in β-tocopherol than in γ-tocopherol when 6-PTQ is the precursor is unusual in view of the results shown in Table IV. Clearly there can be big variations between different plants and experiments.

No quantitative data could be obtained for incorporation of tritiated 3-PTQ. The relatively small amount of 2'-trans-3-PTQ made in the radioactive synthesis was heavily contaminated with 2'-cis-5-PTQ. However, application of such a fraction to leaves indicated that 3-PTQ could in fact be cyclized by the leaf to 5-methyltocol.

8. Phytylplastoquinone (PPQ)

In 1970, Whistance and Threlfall isolated from *Euglena gracilis* a compound they identified as phytylplastoquinone (IX). It was suggested that PPQ could be a precursor of γ-tocopherol in *Euglena*. In the experiments just described involving incubation of *P. vulgaris* leaves with [1',2'-³H]5-PTQ, synthetic PPQ was added to the quinone fraction and reisolated by absorption and reversed-phase thin-layer chromatography. The PPQ had 86,250 dpm associated with it, a considerable incorporation and comparable with the amount of incorporation into γ-tocopherol (74,270). PPQ was also formed when 6-PTQ was incubated with *P. vulgaris* leaves, but we have no quantitative data about this conversion.

(IX)

Clearly this suggests another pathway for biosynthesis of γ-tocopherol (Fig. 3). From the data available, we cannot decide whether PPQ is a precursor of γ-tocopherol or not, but it is certainly plausible. One could also imagine PPQ being formed in tissues as a result of a small side reaction—the methylating enzyme normally involved in plastoquinone biosynthesis working nonspecifically to form PPQ. If the reaction were to be regarded only as a small side reaction, then it would be difficult to explain such a high conversion of 5-PTQ to PPQ in *P. vulgaris* leaves. It is probable that, whereas 5-phytyltolu*quinone* was applied to the leaf surface, 5-phytyltolu*quinol* is the likely intermediate formed within the plant cell. The 5-PTQ is perhaps easily methylated to PPQ whereas the

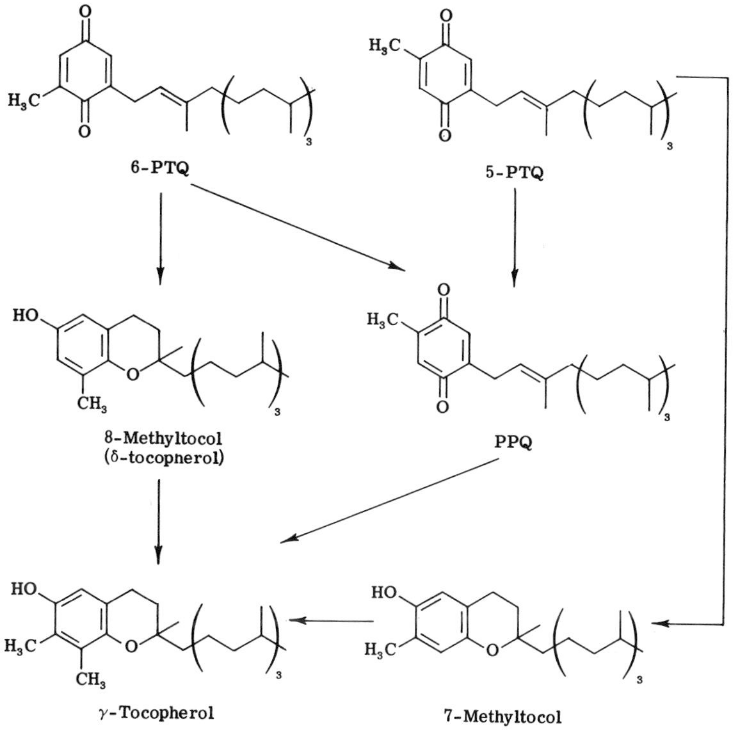

FIG. 3. Possible involvement of phytylplastoquinone (PPQ) in γ-tocopherol biosynthesis. PTQ, phytyltoluquinone.

5-PTQH$_2$ is cyclized to 7-methyltocol according to the scheme shown in Fig. 4.

9. Consideration of the Possible Pathways of Tocopherol Biosynthesis

Figure 5 shows the possible interconversions that have been shown to be possible or plausible in the leaves of *P. vulgaris* as a result of studies with precursors prepared from tritiated isophytol. The figure is restricted to the *tocopherol pathway*—no consideration is given in this representation to the *tocotrienol pathway*. As can be seen, every route tested works to some degree. The previously accepted route involving condensation of phytyl pyrophosphate with homogentisic acid eventually yielding 6-PTQ; cyclization to 8-methyltocol (δ-tocopherol); methylation at the 7-position to γ-tocopherol and further methylation at the 5-position to give α-tocopherol is confirmed. However, this is by no means the only pathway or, on the basis of our results, the major one.

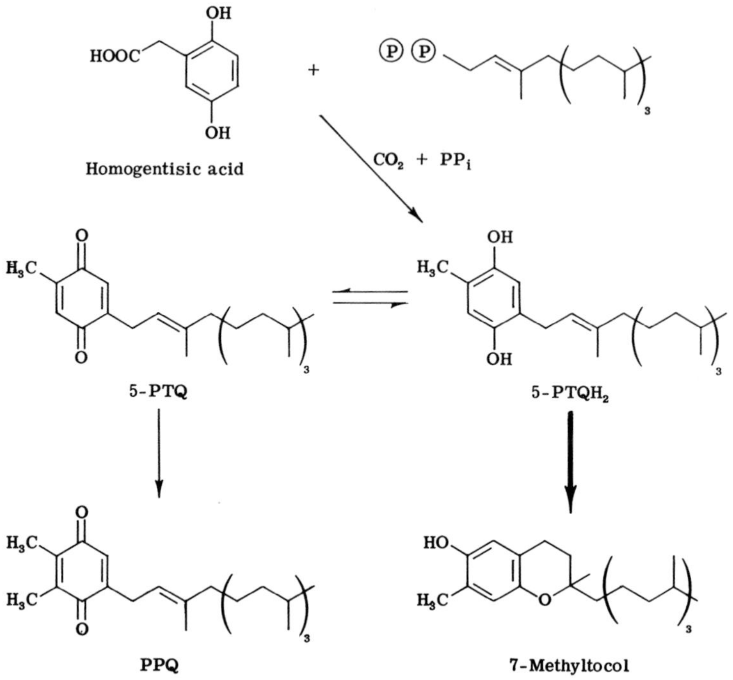

FIG. 4. Interconversions of phytyltoluquinone (PTQ) and phytylplastoquinone (PPQ). PTQH₂, phytyltoluquinol.

How do the above observations fit in with earlier work using water-soluble precursors, e.g., tyrosine, homogentisic acid, or mevalonic acid? It must be admitted that the only compounds ever found to be produced from the radiolabeled precursors mentioned above are α-, β-, γ-, and δ-tocopherols—never previously have 7- or 5-methyltocol been detected. This may mean that involvement of 7- or 5-methyltocol (or related quinones) occurs only when the plants are supplied exogenously with these tocols, and only by virtue of nonspecific enzymes. Certainly evidence in favor of 6-PTQ and δ-tocopherol as the sole route to tocopherols comes from the work of Whistance and Threlfall (1971) on the incorporation of shikimate into quinones and chromanols by maize shoots. DL[1,2-¹⁴C] shikimate was incorporated into α- and γ-tocopherol by maize shoots, and, by an ingenious degradation process based on the Kuhn–Roth oxidation to yield acetic acid from all C-methyl groups, it was deduced that the α-carbon of homogentisate gives rise to the methyl *meta* to the side chain in α- and γ-tocopherol; i.e., δ-tocopherol is the only precursor of these tocopherols. Had 7-methyltocol or 5-methyltocol been involved, then the

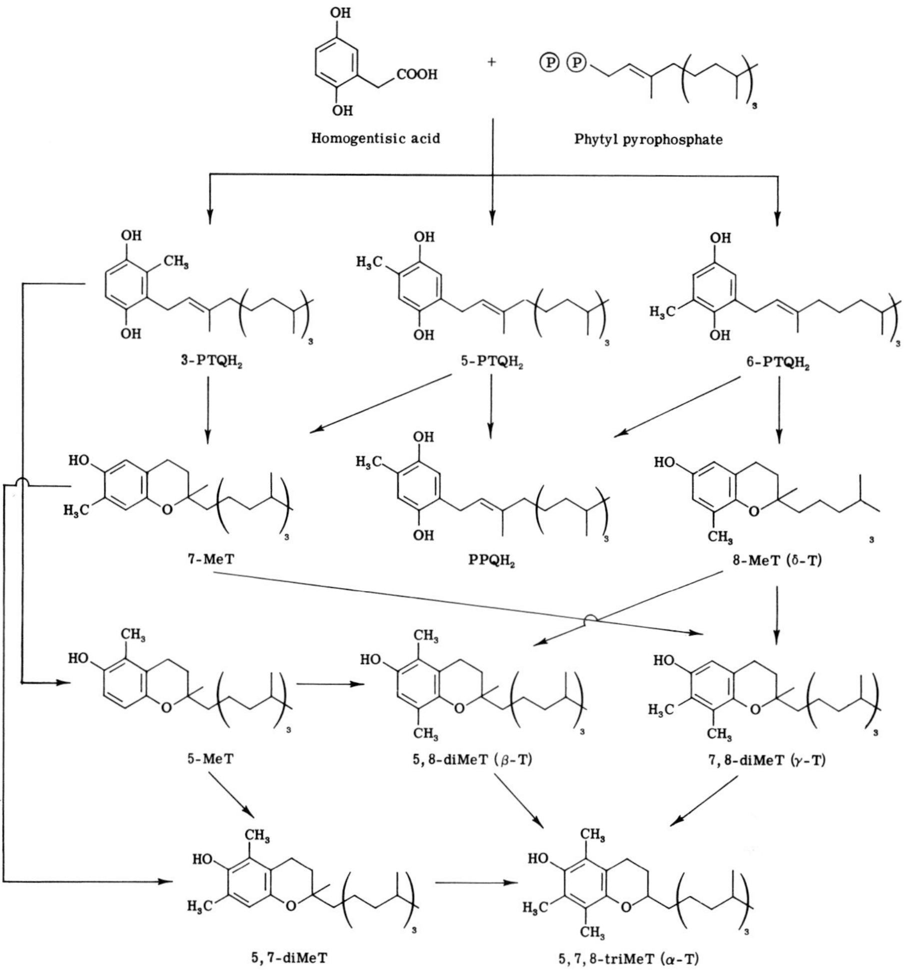

FIG. 5. Possible pathways of tocopherol biosynthesis in *Phaseolus vulgaris*. PTQH₂, phytyltoluquinol; PPQH₂, phytylplastoquinone; MeT, methyltocol; diMeT, dimethyltocol; triMeT, trimethyltocol; α-T, β-T, α- or β-tocopherol.

results would have been different. How can these facts be reconciled? Degradative evidence indicates that δ-tocopherol is the only precursor of the tocopherols whereas mainly 5-PTQ is found in *P. vulgaris* leaves and can be converted to γ- and α-tocopherol via 7-methyltocol at a high rate. Only one thing is clear—one must be wary of implicating compounds in a biosynthetic route simply because they are present in the tissue. In *P. vulgaris* leaves we find both 5-PTQ and δ-tocopherol, and if one biosynthetic route predominates, then one or other of these compounds is a "red herring." Certainly the absence of possible intermediates, or rather the inability to detect them, should not deter us from investigating schemes implicating them. There are clearly many intermediates in the biosynthesis of ubiquinone, but none have been detected in the higher plant; yet one still assumes that they participate in ubiquinone biosynthesis in these plants.

Perhaps there is a species difference between tocopherol biosynthesis in maize and that in *P. vulgaris*. This could possibly be the case, but is not regarded as very likely. A more likely explanation could be that there are different sites of tocopherol biosynthesis within the leaf and the pathway in one site is not necessarily the same as that in the other. For instance it is quite likely that there is a chloroplastidic biosynthesis of tocopherol quite distinct from an extrachloroplastidic pathway. The main pathway to α-tocopherol in the chloroplast may involve 6-PTQ and δ-tocopherol whereas the extrachloroplastidic route may involve 5-PTQ and 7-methyltocol. Different precursors may be transported to one or other of the biosynthetic routes and thus highlight different pathways. Shikimic acid taken up via the stem may be transported to the chloroplast and "label" the chloroplastidic (δ-tocopherol) route whereas lipid precursors applied to the leaf surface enter the extrachloroplastidic route (mainly proceeding via 7-methyltocol).

Clearly more work is required before it can be said whether there are several biosynthetic routes functioning normally in the higher plant or whether only one (the δ-tocopherol route) is present and the others are artifactual just from the plant tissues ability to deal with different potential basic precursors presented to them.

B. Tocotrienol Pathway

Studies on tocotrienols in *Hevea latex* suggest that δ-tocotrienol is formed from homogentisate and geranylgeranyl pyrophosphate, presumably with 6-geranylgeranyltoluquinol as an intermediate. Results with radioactive homogentisate indicate that δ-tocotrienol can be the precursor of γ-tocotrienol and α-tocotrienol, and the latter conversion is confirmed by studies with [$^{14}CH_3$]methionine (Whittle *et al.*, 1967; Peake *et al.*, 1970). Latex contains α-, β-, γ-, and δ-tocotrienol and a small amount of α-tocopherol, and it has usually been assumed that α-tocotrienol can be hydrogenated to α-tocopherol. Studies on *P. vulgaris* and *Avena sativa* using "A"-tritio NADPH (4*R*-diastereoisomer) indicates that this is the reducing coenzyme for production of phytol from geranylgeraniol and for formation of the reduced side chain of α-tocopherol (Wellburn, 1968). In another experiment (Wellburn, 1970) with [$^{14}CH_3$]methionine and tritiated "A" NADPH incubated with *Ficus elasticus* leaves in the presence of δ-tocotrienol, ^{14}C radiolabel appeared in γ- and α-tocotrienol formed during the incubation (i.e., no tocotrienols were present without added δ-tocotrienol). Tritium appeared in α-, β-, γ-, and δ-tocopherol and this was taken as evidence in favor of formation of tocopherols from tocotrienols. However, *Ficus elasticus* leaves contain latex, and it has to be considered that two distinct biogenetic pathways were operating, one in latex resulting in the formation of tocotrienols and the other in the leaf-forming tocopherols as suggested by Wellburn.

C. INTRACELLULAR SITES OF BIOSYNTHESIS

As described in Section C the main intracellular site for α-tocopherol is the chloroplast, while the main site for γ- and δ-tocopherol is extrachloroplastidic. However, some α-tocopherol is found outside the chloroplast and some γ- and δ-tocopherol is found inside the chloroplast. Have we then one biogenetic site followed by transport to other perhaps functional sites, or are there at least two distinct biogenetic sites?

Evidence has been found in two ways. Threlfall (1967) described experiments where either radioactively labeled mevalonic acid (MVA) or CO_2 was incubated with etiolated maize shoots in the light for 24 hours. The rationale behind these experiments was that during this "greening up" period there would be a great demand for CO_2 fixed in the chloroplast to be used for synthesis of chloroplastidic components while MVA taken up the stem would be chiefly used outside the chloroplast. Indeed, the chloroplast membrane was thought to be relatively impermeable to MVA. Consequently compounds found inside the chloroplast such as plastoquinone, β-carotene, and phylloquinone were heavily labeled from $^{14}CO_2$ but relatively poorly labeled from [2-^{14}C]MVA, whereas compounds found extrachloroplastidically, such as 3β-hydroxysterols and ubiquinone, were heavily labeled with [2-^{14}C]MVA as precursor and relatively poorly labeled from $^{14}CO_2$. α-Tocopherol (and α-tocopherolquinone) fitted into neither of these two patterns, being equally well labeled from either $^{14}CO_2$ or [2-^{14}C]MVA and if two pathways of biosynthesis occurred, one inside and one outside the chloroplast, this is the expected result.

Further evidence for two distinct sites of synthesis was obtained in fractionation studies with *P. vulgaris* leaves (I. R. Peake and J. F. Pennock, unpublished observation). *P. vulgaris* plants (20 days old) were excised and dipped in a solution containing 10 μCi of DL-[β-^{14}C]tyrosine, and after 24 hours the leaves were removed, homogenized, filtered through muslin cloth, and centrifuged at 2000 g for 10 minutes. Cell debris was trapped by the muslin; most of the chloroplasts precipitated at 2000 g, and the supernatant contained mitochondria, endoplasmic reticulum, cell sap, etc. The various fractions were extracted, and the tocopherols were estimated and radioactivity was determined. Table VII shows the results.

The cell debris contains some unbroken cells, but mainly small veins; relatively large amounts of γ-tocopherol are found in this fraction presumably in the vascular tissue. As expected, most of the α-tocopherol was in the chloroplast fraction, and most of the γ-tocopherol was in the supernatant. Radioactivity broadly followed the same pattern; most of that found in α-tocopherol was in the chloroplast, and most of that found in γ-tocopherol was in the supernatant. However, some α-tocopherol (chemically and radioactively detected) was in the supernatant, and some γ-tocopherol (chemically and radioactively detected) was in the chloroplast. The highest specific activity for α-tocopherol was in the supernatant whereas the highest specific activity for γ-tocopherol was in the chloroplast.

The most logical idea seems to be that there are biogenetic pathways for γ- and α-tocopherol in the chloroplast and in an organelle found in the supernatant fraction. Thus the α-tocopherol formed outside the chloroplast, where there is only a small pool of α-tocopherol, has a high specific activity whereas inside the chloroplast there is a large pool of α-tocopherol and the specific activity is relatively low. Exactly the reverse occurs with γ-tocopherol. The highest specific activity for γ-tocopherol occurs in the chloroplast, where there is only a small pool of this tocopherol.

P. vulgaris leaves were also fractionated after treatment with [3,4-^{14}C]γ-tocopherol (Botham and Pennock, 1976). The [3,4-^{14}C]γ-tocopherol was applied to the leaf surface, and after incubation for 24 hours the leaves were homogenized and fractionated to give cell debris, chloroplasts, and supernatant as before. α-Tocopherol was found in the cell debris (3.5 μg, 389 dpm, specific activity 110.8, chloroplasts 103.1 μg, 214 dpm, specific

TABLE VII

DETERMINATION OF α- AND γ-TOCOPHEROL IN CELLULAR FRACTIONS OF *Phaseolus vulgaris* LEAVES AFTER INCUBATION WITH DL-[β-^{14}C]TYROSINE

| Fraction | α-Tocopherol | | | γ-Tocopherol | | |
	μg	Dpm	Specific activity (dpm/μg)	μg	Dpm	Specific activity (dpm/μg)
Cell debris	17	547	32.2	66	3477	52.7
Chloroplasts	58	1558	26.9	10	829	82.9
Supernatant	22	1329	60.4	71	3577	50.4

activity 2.31) and supernatant (6.4 μg, 1164 dpm, specific activity 181.0). Clearly the conversion of γ-tocopherol to α-tocopherol has taken place outside the chloroplast.

III. SUMMARY

There are certainly two pathways of tocochromanol biosynthesis which we can term the "tocotrienol pathway" and the "tocopherol pathway." The work described in this review questions whether the tocopherol pathway is in fact one main biosynthetic route (as suggested by natural occurence of tocopherols and studies with [14C]homogentisic acid) or is a maze of pathways involving three isomeric phytyltoluquinols, three isomeric methyltocols, three isomeric dimethyltocols, and α-tocopherol (as suggested by studies with tritiated phytyluquinones and methyltocols). The latter studies suggest a major biogenetic route for α-tocopherol being 5-phytyltoluquinol $\longrightarrow$ 7-methyltocol $\longrightarrow$ 7,8-dimethyltocol (γ-tocopherol) $\longrightarrow$ 5,7,8-dimethyltocol (α-tocopherol).

It is also suggested that within the cell there are two distinct sites of tocopherol biosynthesis: one inside the chloroplast, resulting mainly in the formation of α-tocopherol, and one outside the chloroplast, resulting mainly in the formation of δ- and γ-tocopherol. It is not impossible that the chloroplastidic pathway differs in intermediates involved compared with those of the extrachloroplastidic pathway. The tocotrienol pathway is not present in leaf cells and has a very limited distribution.

ACKNOWLEDGMENTS

We would like to thank Drs. O. Isler and U. Würsch of F. Hoffmann-La Roche for very generous gifts of [1,2-³H]isophytol.

REFERENCES

Baszynski, T. (1967). *Naturwissenschaften* **54**, 339.
Baszynski, T. (1974). *Biochim. Biophys. Acta* **347**, 31.
Battle, R. W., Gaunt, J. K., and Laidman, D. L. (1976). *Biochem. Soc. Trans.* **4**, 484.
Bishop, N. I., and Wong, J. (1974). *Ber. Dtsch. Bot. Ges.* **87**, 359.
Booth, V. H. (1963). *Phytochemistry* **2**, 421.
Booth, V. H., and Hobson-Frohock, A. (1961). *J. Sci. Food Agric.* **12**, 251.
Botham, K. M., and Pennock, J. F. (1976). Submitted for publication.
Bucke, C. (1968). *Phytochemistry* **7**, 693.
Burnett, A. R., and Thomson, R. H. (1968). *J. Chem. Soc. C*, p. 857.
Dada, O. A. (1968). Cited by Threlfall (1971).
Dicks, M. W. (1965). *Wyo. Agric. Exp. St. Bull.* **435**.
Dilley, R. A., and Crane, F. L. (1963). *Plant Physiol.* **38**, 452.
Diplock, A. T., Green, J., Edwin, E. E., and Bunyan, J. (1961). *Nature (London)* **189**, 749.

Dunphy, P. J., Whittle, K. J., Pennock, J. F., and Morton, R. A. (1965). *Nature (London)* **207**, 521.

Eggitt, P. W. R., and Ward, L. D. (1953). *J. Sci. Food Agric.* **4**, 176.

Eggitt, P. W. R., and Ward, L. D. (1955). *J. Sci. Food Agric.* **6**, 329.

Emerson, O. H., Emerson, G. A., and Evans, H. M. (1936). *Science* **83**, 421.

Evans, H. M., and Bishop, K. S. (1922). *J. Metab. Res.* **1**, 319.

Evans, H. M., Emerson, O. H., and Emerson, G. A. (1936). *J. Biol. Chem.* **113**, 319.

Fernholz, E. (1937). *J. Am. Chem. Soc.* **59**, 1154.

Fernholz, E. (1938). *J. Am. Chem. Soc.* **60**, 700.

Green, J. (1958). *J. Sci. Food Agric.* **9**, 801.

Green, J., and Marcinkiewicz, S. (1956). *Nature (London)* **176**, 86.

Green, J., and Marcinkiewicz, S. (1959). *Analyst* **84**, 297.

Green, J., Marcinkiewicz, S., and Watt, P. R. (1955). *J. Sci. Food Agric.* **6**, 274.

Green, J., McHale, D., Marcinkiewicz, S., Mamalis, P., and Watt, P. D. (1959). *J. Chem. Soc.,* p. 3362.

Green, J., Mamalis, P., Marcinkiewicz, S., and McHale, D. (1960). *Chem. Ind. (London)*, p. 73.

Griffiths, W. T. (1966). *Biochem. Biophys. Res. Commun.* **25**, 596.

Henninger, M. D., Bhagavan, H. N., and Crane, F. L. (1965). *Arch. Biochem. Biophys.* **110**, 69.

Hoffman, C. H., Trenner, N. R., Wolf, D. E., and Folkers, K. (1960). *J. Am. Chem. Soc.* **82**, 4744.

Hove, E. L., and Harris, P. L. (1951). *J. Am. Oil Chem. Soc.* **38**, 405.

Hughes, C. T., Gaunt, J. K., and Laidman, D. L. (1971). *Biochem. J.* **124**, 9P.

Janiszowska, W., and Pennock, J. F. (1976). Submitted for publication.

Janiszowska, W., Botham, K. M., and Pennock, J. F. (1976). Submitted for publication.

Jensen, A. (1961). *J. Sci. Food Agric.* **20**, 449.

Kubin, H., and Fink, H. (1961). *Fette, Seifen, Anstrichm.* **63**, 280.

Lea, C. H., and Ward, R. J. (1959). *J. Sci. Food Agric.* **10**, 537.

Lichtenthaler, H. K. (1968). *Z. Pflanzenphysiol.* **59**, 195.

Lichtenthaler, H. K., and Tevini, M. (1970). *Z. Pflanzenphysiol.* **62**, 33.

McHale, D., Green, J., Marcinkiewicz, S., Feeney, J., and Sutcliffe, L. H. (1963). *J. Chem. Soc.,* p. 784.

Michniewicz, M., and Kamienska, A. (1964). *Naturwissenschaften* **51**, 295.

Michniewicz, M., and Kamienska, A. (1965). *Naturwissenschaften* **52**, 623.

Newton, R. P., and Pennock, J. F. (1971a). *Phytochemistry* **10**, 2323.

Newton, R. P., and Pennock, J. F. (1971b). *Biochem. J.* **124**, 21P.

Peake, I. R., Audley, B. G., and Pennock, J. F. (1970). *Biochem. J.* **119**, 58P.

Pennock, J. F., Hemming, F. W., and Kerr, J. D. (1964). *Biochem. Biophys. Res. Commun.* **17**, 542.

Powls, R., and Redfearn, E. R. (1967). *Biochem. J.* **104**, 24C.

Siegenthaler, P. A. (1972). *Biochim. Biophys. Acta* **275**, 182.

Skinner, W. A., and Sturm, P. A. (1968). *Phytochemistry* **7**, 1893.

Stern, M. H., Robeson, C. D., Weisler, L., and Baxter, J. G. (1947). *J. Am. Chem. Soc.* **69**, 869.

Tappell, A. L. (1974). *Am. J. Clin. Nutr.* **27**, 960.

Thomas, D. R., and Stobart, A. K. (1971). *New Phytol.* **70**, 163.

Threlfall, D. R. (1967). *In* "Terpenoids in Plants" (J. B. Pridham, ed.), p. 191. Academic Press, New York.

Threlfall, D. R. (1971). *Vitam. Horm. (N.Y.)* **29**, 153.

Threlfall, D. R., and Goodwin, T. W. (1967). *Biochem. J.* **103**, 573.
Threlfall, D. R., Law, A. L., and White, W. A. (1971). *Biochem. J.* **124**, 23P.
Wallwork, J. C., and Pennock, J. F. (1969). *Prog. Photosynth. Res., Proc. Int. Congr.* [*1st*], *1968,* p. 315.
Wellburn, A. R. (1968). *Phytochemistry* **7**, 1523.
Wellburn, A. R. (1970). *Phytochemistry* **9**, 743.
Whistance, G. R., and Threlfall, D. R. (1967). *Biochem. Biophys. Res. Commun.* **28**, 295.
Whistance, G. R., and Threlfall, D. R. (1968). *Biochem. J.* **109**, 577.
Whistance, G. R., and Threlfall, D. R. (1970). *Phytochemistry* **9**, 213.
Whistance, G. R., and Threlfall, D. R. (1971). *Phytochemistry* **10**, 1533.
Whittle, K. J., Audley, B. G., and Pennock, J. F. (1967). *Biochem. J.* **103**, 21C.

The Role of Prolactin in Carcinogenesis[*]

UNTAE KIM AND JACOB FURTH

Department of Pathology, Roswell Park Memorial Institute, New York State Department of Health, Buffalo, New York, and Institute of Cancer Research and Department of Pathology, Columbia University College of Physicians and Surgeons, New York, New York

I. INTRODUCTION

Of the 11 pituitary hormones of mammals (Li, 1972), mammotropic hormone (prolactin) may be functionally the most versatile (Nicoll and Bern, 1972). As many as 80 direct or indirect functions have been attributed to it in vertebrates, ranging from osmotic regulation in the hagfish to growth and function of the mammary gland in mammals. Included are stimulation of the sebaceous glands, hair follicles, lipid metabolism, erythropoiesis, sugar metabolism, sodium retention, promotion of fertility, androgen binding in the prostate, and stimulation of vaginal mucification (Nicoll and Bern, 1972). In the course of vertebrate phylogeny, the single outstanding function of this hormone in mammals emerged—stimulation

[*] Supported in part by USPHS Grant CA-02332 and Contract NO1-CB-23864 from the Breast Cancer Program Coordinating Branch, National Cancer Institute, U.S. Public Health Service.

of the growth and function of the mammary gland. This discourse is confined to the role of prolactin in mammary carcinogenesis based on observations of our own and those reported by others.

II. Historical Aspects. Overview of Recent Developments*

Atrophy of the mammary gland following hypophysectomy (Smith, 1927) and restoration of this deficiency by extracts of the anterior hypophysis (Stricker and Grüter, 1928) indicated the existence of mammogenic hormone(s) in the pituitary. Subsequent analytical studies (cf. Lyons, 1958) led to the conclusion that all of the 6 "classical" anterior pituitary hormones play some role in the physiology of the mammary gland. It was postulated that the two gonadotropins act via gonadal hormones, while prolactin can act both directly and indirectly via the ovary.

The pioneering observations related to mammary carcinogenesis followed two independent routes: one, the intuitive introduction of ovariectomy for control of human breast cancer (Beatson, 1896), which, in turn, led to mammary tumor induction in rodents by administration of estrogen; the other, an equally perceptive study of extrasellar pituitary grafts (Loeb and Kirtz, 1939), which led to induction of mammary tumors in mice, followed by the discovery of hypothalamic control of prolactin release. The isografting of pituitaries beneath the kidney capsule became a commonly used procedure to induce sustained elevation of circulating prolactin levels. Remarkably, both procedures—chronic estrogenic stimulation and extrasellar pituitary isografting—led to the induction of functional prolactin-secreting pituitary tumors (cf. Furth and Clifton, 1958; Mühlbock and Boot, 1959). It deserves emphasis that estrogens are the primary inducers of prolactin.

The term "prolactin" was first used by Riddle and associates (1932a,b), who introduced "cropmilk" stimulation in pigeons for its assay. Mammotropin (or mammotrophin, MtH) is a more correct term for this hormone, since its primary action in mammals is mammary gland stimulation; milk secretion calls for supplementary hormones, notably, glucocorticoids.

* Nomenclature and abbreviations: Mt = mammotrope, the pituitary cell secreting MtH; MtH = prolactin = lactogenic hormone = mammotropic hormone (P); h.P = human prolactin; o.P = ovine prolactin; MtT = mammotropic tumor; MT = mammary tumor; StH = somatotropic hormone; GH = growth hormone; St = somatotrope, the cell-secreting StH; P.RH (= P.RF) = prolactin (MtH) releasing hormone (or factor); P.IH (= P.IF) = prolactin (MtH) inhibiting hormone (or factor); TtH = thyrotropin; T.RH = thyrotropin-releasing hormone (or factor); RIA = radioimmunoassay; RRA = radioreceptor assay; IHCS = immunohistochemical staining; DES = diethylstilbestrol.

The term LtH (luteotropic hormone) used as a synonym for MtH is not advisable. There is an inverse relation between MtH and LH (luteinizing hormone) release. The effect of MtH on the ovary is manifested by persistence of large corpora lutea, (which are normally produced by LH), with failure to release progesterone. This luteotropic change is invariably associated with MtT in rodents. The *in vitro* studies of McNatty *et al.* (1974) suggest that MtH plays some role in the control of steroid secretion by the Graafian follicles of the human ovary. Maintenance of human granulosa cells *in vitro* are said to require physiological concentrations of MtH, whereas high concentrations of MtH are inhibitory. The pathogenesis of luteotropic effects in man as well as in animals requires further study.

The isolation of human prolactin in 1971 was followed by a flood of publications and conferences on prolactin in general and its role in mammary carcinogenesis, thereby terminating a long era during which the hormonal control of human mammary tumors was linked almost exclusively to gonadal steroids.

The first comprehensive symposium on "Lactogenic Hormones" was sponsored by the Ciba Foundation in London (Wolstenholme and Knight, 1972). It was dedicated to the memory of Sidney J. Folley, the English pioneer in research on milk secretion.

It was followed by a workshop on "Prolactin and Carcinogenesis" in Cardiff (Boyns and Griffiths, 1972), with sessions on prolactin, the pituitary, and breast cancer.

The proceedings of an international symposium on "Human Prolactin" edited by Pasteels *et al.* (1973) discussed the chemistry, morphology, receptors, assay methods, pathophysiology, control of prolactin secretion, and related pharmacological factors. This symposium also had a brief session on prolactin and mammary carcinogenesis.

In the same year, two reviews appeared on the same subject. In one, Friesen and Hwang (1973) considered the cell of origin of prolactin, its purification and chemistry, assays for prolactin, its concentration in serum, control of its secretion, effect of drugs, and its physiological role. In the other review, entitled "Prolactin: Physiology and Clinical Significance," Horrobin (1973) reviewed the relationship of prolactin to various human diseases not considered in the aforementioned publications (such as the nephrotic syndrome, hypertension, adrenal and thyroid disease, and diabetes). Its relation to cancer was only briefly discussed.

The proceedings of the most recent "Workshop on Human Prolactin" held in Amsterdam (edited by Kwa *et al.*, 1975) reached us as this paper went to press.

With advancement of knowledge, it has become clear that prolactin does not operate alone, nor is breast cancer a neoplasm related to only one hormone. References pertinent to the topic of this review can be found in books on hormones as well as on cancer. Examples are: *Recent Progress in Hormone Research* (annual proceedings of the Laurentian Hormone Conferences, edited by R. O. Greep); "Hormonal Proteins and Peptides" (edited by C. H. Li); "The Anterior Pituitary" (Tixier-Vidal and Farquhar, 1975), an excellent review of the ultrastructure of this gland; "Cancer: A Comprehensive Treatise," Vol. I (Becker, 1975), containing a comprehensive chapter on hormones and neoplasia; *Advances in Cancer Research* (series edited by G. Klein, S. Weinhouse, and A. Haddow); and *Methods in Cancer Research* (series edited by H. Busch).

III. ANATOMICAL AND PHYSIOLOGICAL CONSIDERATIONS

A. THE PROLACTIN CELL (MAMMOTROPE, MT)

The mammotrope is the most abundant cell of the anterior pituitary in adult female rodents. It is present at birth in relatively small numbers. A study of the histogenesis of the various pituitary cell types during embryonal life utilizing immunohistochemical or radioimmunoassay (RIA) techniques is yet to be done. In young adult virgin animals, Mts number about 40% of all anterior pituitary cells (Baker, 1970). They are not well visualized by conventional staining, in which they appear roughly spherical or slightly ovoid with centrally located nuclei, resembling the growth hormone cells (somatotrope, St), which are also "acidophilic."

The Mt granules are reliably visualized by fluorescent antibody staining (Emmart *et al.*, 1965) and immunohistochemical staining (IHCS) (Nakane and Pierce, 1967; cf. Nakane, 1975; Baker, 1970; cf. Furth *et al.*, 1973). A modification of the Nakane–Pierce procedure, which is also known as immunoglobulin-peroxidase bridge technique, was developed by Mason *et al.* (1969) and improved by Phifer *et al.* (1972). IHCS can distinguish between cells on the basis of size and location of hormone granules.

The St granules are scattered throughout the cytoplasm, while the Mt granules tend to form a "cap"-shaped clump in one part of the cytoplasm. The Mt granules measure 600–900 nm; the St granules, 350–400 nm.

The prolactin cells with their organelles and hormone granules are best visualized by electron microscopy (cf. Farquhar *et al.*, 1975; Herlant, 1975; Tixier-Vidal, 1975). Farquhar, with associates, has been correlating the physiological function with fine structure of all the anterior pituitary cells. Improved formulas for fixation and processing, such as that of Shiino *et al.* (1974), provide excellent preservation of subcellular details, e.g., visualization of microtubules in Mts, their association with mitochondria, secretory granules, ribosomes, nuclear envelopes, and plasma membranes. The Mt cells can be separated from other cells of the pituitary by 1 *g* velocity sedimentation (Hymer *et al.*, 1974; Hymer, 1975). The structure and function of dispersed cells, their synthesis, transport and release of granules in *in vitro* systems has been reported by Farquhar *et al.* (1975). A stereotopographic analysis of the organelles of the Mt cells in relation to secretion was reported by Warchol *et al.* (1974).

B. The Lactogenic Hormone (Prolactin, MtH)

In mammals there are three sources of lactogenic hormone: the chorion, the placenta, and the pituitary. Only the latter has been shown to be related to mammary tumorigenesis. In lower species, lactogenic hormones also have numerous other functions, which are not conspicuous in mammals and are not known to be related to carcinogenesis.

Preparation of a purified MtH was first reported by W. R. Lyons (1937). C. H. Li and others soon joined him (cf. Li, 1973) by extracting MtH from the pituitaries of various animal species.

The amino acid sequence of ovine prolactin was characterized by Li *et al.* (1969), and that of human prolactin by Lewis *et al.* (1971a,b) and Hwang *et al.* (1972). The complete covalent sequence of h.P was presented by Li (1972).

Although in lower animals MtH is readily distinguished from StH, in man it could not be separated from StH until 1971. All earlier preparations described as h.StH or human placental lactogen (HPL) had strong overlapping activities. The similarity of human and ovine MtH, HPL, and h.StH is indicated by amino acid sequence homology (cf. Li, 1972; Wolstenholme and Knight, 1972; Friesen and Hwang, 1973). Presently, all available preparations of these hormones have some overlapping biological and immunological activities, owing to their structural relationships. They have been well illustrated by Niall *et al.* (1973). A milligram of h.P possesses 25 IU of lactogenic and 0.4 USP units of StH activity, whereas h.StH has 2 IU of lactogenic and 2 USP units of StH activity, respectively. Computer techniques have also indicated the homology of these preparations. The structural similarity between StH and MtH may explain the overlapping immunological and biological activities encountered when the amount of hormones used is high, as with the overlapping mammosomatotropic effect seen in MtT-bearing animals. On the basis of polyacrylamide gel electrophoresis and isoelectric focusing, Rodbard and Bertino (1973) indicated the similarities between the various h.P preparations.

By a combination of procedures, Robertson and Friesen (1975) obtained 1300-fold purification of rat placental lactogen employing a specific radio-receptor assay (RRA). Utilizing this assay technique, Kelly *et al.* (1975) also purified and characterized chorionic MtH.

The RIA is the most sensitive technique for detection and quantitation of MtH. Those of various mammalian species exhibit a fair degree of group reactivity. The sensitivity of anti-o.P sera for h.P was comparable to the result of assays in homologous system (Aubert *et al.*, 1974a). In a collaborative study, Aubert *et al.* (1974b) compared various preparations of h.P, and the most sensitive preparations were those of Lewis *et al.* (1971a) and Hwang *et al.* (1972). Similar results were obtained in homologous and heterologous systems. The presence of P in unextracted urine of mouse and man was demonstrated by RIA (Sinha *et al.*, 1973).

The RRA for P and other hormones with lactogenic activity (chorionic MtH, StH), developed by Shiu *et al.* (1973), has a sensitivity of 5 ng/ml. "Cold" P preparations inhibited the binding of ^{125}I-labeled P to receptors in direct proportion to their biological potency.

The heterogeneity of pituitary hormones was reported by Yalow (1974). That of immunoreactive h.P in the plasma has been described by Rogol and Rosen (1974) and Suh and Frantz (1974) and confirmed by Aubert *et al.* (1975) by both RIA and RRA.

Disc electrophoresis on acrylamide gel can be used for both identification and quantitation of hormones. It gives sharp bands for the various pituitary hormones in characteristic locations (Jones *et al.*, 1965). The intensity of the bands, quantitated by densitometry, gives a fair estimation of the quantity of the respective hormones and also indicates impurities that may be present (Furth and Moy, 1967). This technique can detect hormones only in excess of ∼1 μg, whereas RIA can detect less than 1 ng. There is an inverse relation between serum and pituitary MtH levels. Administration of a large dose of MtH to rats (Yanai and Nagasawa, 1969) markedly decreases the optical density of the MtH band of the normal pituitary in the acrylamide gel, as does the MtT graft (MacLeod *et al.*, 1966).

Bioassays are less sensitive than RIA for detection of P, and the procedures do not always give concordant results. They can be done *in vivo* or *in vitro*. The *in vitro* morphological effects of P on human mammary gland kept for 3–5 days in organotypic culture are beautifully illustrated by Dilley and Kister (1976). The greatest growth of mammary gland occurred after adding insulin, h.MtH, and estradiol to the media. Ovine MtH was not mitogenic, and corticoids inhibited growth. These authors reviewed earlier studies on the effects of hormones on the mammary gland *in vitro*. Most of these studies were carried out with the aim of predicting the hormone sensitivity of mammary tumors. Noteworthy among the similar earlier studies are those of Lagios (1974) and of Ceriani et al. (1972) on hormone requirements of the human mammary gland for growth and differentiation in organ culture. In similar studies, Flaxman and Lasfargues (1973) found that additions of insulin and bovine P caused an increase in the number of human mammary ductal cells synthesizing DNA. Organ culture studies led Oka and Topper (1972) to conclude that MtH is not directly mitogenic on the mammary epithelium but acts indirectly on it after insulin sensitization. The morphological and mitogenic effects of MtH in organ cultures of rat mammary gland epithelium, but not of stromal fibroblasts, were described by Dilley (1971a).

Stoudemire et al. (1975) have studied the synergism between MtH and ovarian hormones on DNA synthesis in rat mammary gland. The effect of MtH and progesterone on specific binding of estradiol to mammary tissue in vitro was studied by Leung and Sasaki (1973). MtH secretion is enhanced in cocultures of Mt with mammary cells (Wilfinger et al., 1975).

By improving techniques of dissociation, viable single cell suspensions of all pituitary tropic cells, including Mt were obtained by Hopkins and Farquhar (1973). Throughout a period of 20 hours after dissociation, the cells incorporated [³H]leucine linearly for up to 4 hours at a rate 90% greater than did solid masses of hemipituitaries. The authors described synthesis, intracellular transport, and release of both StH and MtH. There is a transient inhibition of the cells' synthetic activity to secretogogues, but after 6–12 hours in culture, they seem to recover. The process of incorporation of [³H]leucine into StH and release of StH has been well worked out, but that of MtH is still fragmentary. Hopkins and Farquhar also reviewed earlier studies on secretory functions of undissociated and dissociated pituitary cells.

With respect to MtH, noteworthy are the studies of Tixier-Vidal and Picart (1967) on utilization of dl[³H]leucine in organ cultures and of Meldolesi et al. (1972) on in vitro synthesis of MtH and StH and pulse labeling of these hormones with radioactive leucine. Stumpf (1970) called attention to the technical errors in utilization of autoradiography, comparing it with fluorescent microscopy and histochemistry in visualization of hormones.

Polypeptide hormones generally act on the plasma membrane, and with the adenyl cyclase system being part of the receptor site, cyclic 3',5'-adenosine monophosphate (cAMP) works as the transmitter. Chomczynski and Topper (1974) suggest that MtH may perform some of its functions on the nuclei of the mammary epithelium. Like other polypeptide and glycoprotein hormones, MtH exerts its effects on target cells through interaction with receptors on the plasma membrane. However, according to Turkington (1972), unlike other pituitary hormones, the MtH effects are not mediated by adenyl cyclase.

C. Regulation of MtH Secretion

The prime inducers of MtH production are ovarian steroids, notably estrogens. MtH levels reach their height at the end of pregnancy. During pregnancy, extrapituitary hormones with MtH activity, the so-called "chorionic" and placental lactogens, assist in the buildup of the mammary epithelium. After delivery, MtH levels drop and reach low-normal levels subject to diurnal fluctuations. During nursing, MtH levels are relatively low, and milk production is promoted by glucocorticoids, the major lactogen for the adult mammary gland. It has long been known that forced pregnancies enhance mammary gland (and mammary tumor) development in the mouse, while prolonged and frequent nursing inhibits the tumor development.

The problem of whether estrogen renders cells of the mammary gland more receptive to prolactin stimulation was studied by Talwalker and Meites (1961) by inducing mammary lobuloalveolar growth with prolactin and growth hormone in adreno–ovariectomized and adreno–ovariectomized–hypophysectomized rats. Their results indicate that estrogen is not essential for the growth and function of the mammary gland. However, several investigators found that a prior priming of the mammary gland in vivo with estrogen or estrogen and progesterone permits fuller structural and functional development of mammary explants in vitro (Ichinose and Nandi, 1966; Stockdale et al., 1966; Ben-David, 1968; Nagasawa and Yanai, 1971). This effect was variously called "augmentation" and "sensitization."

Nicoll and Meites (1962) demonstrated a direct stimulatory effect of estrogen on the secretion of prolactin in vitro.

Systemic administration of prolactin in normal rodents causes an increase of RNA synthesis in the mammary gland, followed by DNA synthesis and cellular proliferation (Pelc, 1968; Denamur, 1969; Simpson and Schmidt, 1971). When prolactin (without estrogen) is directly added to in vitro explants of immature rat mammary glands in standard media containing insulin, DNA synthesis, mitotic activity, and alveolar development are stimulated (Dilley, 1971a,b), indicating the direct effect of prolactin on the mammary gland prior to lactation, confirming the findings of Stockdale and Topper (1966).

The existence of P.IH was first described by Pasteels in 1962 and by Talwalker et al. in 1963. The role of estrogen in the hypothalamic control of prolactin has been demonstrated by Kanematsu and Sawyer (1963) and

Ramirez and McCann (1964), who found that a minute estrogen pellet, implanted in the posterior tuberal hypothalamus of rabbits and rats, markedly stimulated synthesis and storage of prolactin in the pituitary without releasing it. When such a pellet was implanted in the pituitary, prolactin was released. The secretion of MtH was thought to be regulated by the interaction of the hypothalamic P.IH (Meites and Nicoll, 1966) and the P.RH (Tindal et al., 1967; cf. McCann et al., 1968).

The hypothalamic hormones are, in turn, influenced by hormonelike substances originating in or acting via the cerebral and limbic centers. By influencing P.RH and P.IH activity, the growth and function of mammary gland and its tumors may be affected.

Most of the classical studies on hypothalamic hormones were made independently by Guillemin and Schally with their associates. In 1973 both reviewed the hypothalamic control of adenohypophysial secretion (Blackwell and Guillemin, 1973; Schally et al., 1973). Stimulation of prolactin release by the thyrotropin releasing hormone (T.RH) was reported by Smith and Convey (1975), who used bovine pituitary cells. Machlin et al. (1974) found that addition of 1 ng or more of T.RH per milliliter increased release of MtH and thyrotropin (TtH), and subsequent addition of 10 ng/ml also increased release of StH. However, Frohman and Szabo (1975) reported that P.RH is distinct from T.RH.

A priming effect of T.RH on MtH secretion was reported by Rivier and Vale (1974), who noted that in vivo T.RH injection led to a greater rise of TtH and MtH in estrogen-progesterone-pretreated male rats than in untreated controls. The effect of MtH was found to be enhanced by thyroidectomy (Mittra, 1974).

The direct action of dopamine and norepinephrine on hypothalamic P.RH was found in the in vitro studies of Shaar and Clemens (1974). T.RH blockade of ergocryptine and apomorphine inhibition of MtH release in vitro was reported by Hill-Samli and MacLeod (1975).

The involvement of several neurotransmitters (adrenergic, dopaminergic, cholinergic, and serotoninergic drugs) on plasma MtH levels in ovariectomized, estrogen-treated rats was reported by Lawson and Gala (1975). It is suggested by studies of Gala and Boss (1975) that while CB-154 (2-Br-ergocryptine) prevents release of MtH, estrogen stimulates MtH synthesis despite the blocking of its release. MacLeod and Lehmeyer (1972) indicated that the sympathicometic catecholamines, acting on a discrete area of the hypothalamus or perhaps via P.IH, have an inhibitory effect on MtH release. Perphenazine stimulates MtH secretion and blocks the inhibitory effect of dopamine.

These investigations are the foundations of subsequent research efforts aimed at controlling breast cancer by chemicals, thereby eliminating drastic surgical intervention, and placing the control of prolactin secretion on an equal footing with the control of estrogen secretion. In light of these developments, there is even a possibility that psychoendocrine factors can also influence breast cancer growth, although thus far only anecdotal evidence supports this possibility (Stoll, 1974b, p. 401).

There is much yet to be learned about the homeostasis of MtH. Lloyd et al. (1975) suggested the existence of a simple intracellular negative feedback between the intracellular concentration of MtH and DNA synthesis. DNA synthesis is triggered when the stored MtH is depleted. Voogt and Ganong (1974) presented suggestive evidence against the anterior pituitary being the site of negative feedback of prolactin.

Recently, two new substances have been reported to have either direct or indirect effect on MtH. One is *somatostatin*, a hypothalamic hormone discovered by Guillemin and associates (cf. Vale et al., 1974). It not only regulates nonpituitary-mediated growth-promoting action, but also controls the spontaneous release of MtH from pituitary cells *in vitro* (Vale et al., 1974). The other substance, *somatomedin*, was isolated earlier by Salmon and Daughaday (1957). It is a secondary mediator of growth hormone for skeletal growth. However, MtH can also stimulate the production of somatomedin in the absence of StH (Francis and Hill, 1975).

Several recent books, such as those edited by Meites (1970) and Ganong and Martini (1973), review research on the hypothalamus. The very title of the excellent book edited by Stoll (1974), "Mammary Cancer and Neuroendocrine Therapy," indicates the practical significance of the relationship between the central nervous system and mammary tumorigenesis.

IV. Hyperplasia of Prolactin Cells and Mammotropic Tumors (MtT)

The historical aspects of MtT are thoroughly reviewed in "The Pathophysiology of Pituitaries and Their Tumors; Methodological Advances" (Furth et al., 1973). Here, we shall merely summarize the present state of basic knowledge concerning primary and transplanted MtT, with references to the more recent literature.

Although there are views to the contrary (cf. Olivier et al., 1975), it is our considered opinion that hyperplasia and neoplasia of Mt cells, as of all pituitary cells, result from multiplication of cells of the same type preexisting at birth. The existence of pluripotent reserve cells in postnatal life is conceivable, but requires better evidence than has thus far been presented.

The invariable development of pituitary tumors in rodents that had been treated with estrogenic hormones over long periods of time was recorded independently by several investigators, including Lacassagne, Aschheim and Zondek, Selye, and Gardner (cf. Gardner et al., 1959; Furth and Clifton, 1966), before the various pituitary cells and their specific hormones were identified. Transplantation studies of such tumors in isologous hosts clearly indicated that they were prolactin-secreting and therefore were named mammotropic tumors (MtT) (Furth, 1955). The first generation grafts of such tumors are usually dependent on the presence of estrogen in the host (i.e., intact ovaries) and fail to grow in ovariectomized females or in males (Furth et al., 1956).

Soon after the initial transplantation, 2 major changes are noted. The tumors lose complete dependency on ovarian estrogens, but remain hormone-responsive (i.e., stimulated by estrogens), and acquire the ability to secrete StH. Therefore, they were renamed mammosomatotropic tumors (MStT) (Furth and Clifton, 1966). At first puzzling, this phenomenon may now be explained by the structural homology between MtH and StH. Neoplasia is often associated with derepression of the genetic code. During the course of successive transplant generations of MStTs, MtH secretion tends to decrease, while StH secretion persists and usually increases. This change occurs regularly. Therefore, only by reisolation or preservation of highly functional specific tumor cell lines in a tumor bank can one obtain a "well defined" MtT or MStT.

The simplest method of MtT induction is the subcutaneous implantation of diethylstilbestrol (DES) pellets. A single pellet of 1 mg of DES fused in 9 mg of cholesterol, replaced once every 3 months for 9 months, is adequate; larger doses shorten the induction time but also increase mortality. Large doses of estrogens inhibit mammary gland growth and function but enhance MtT induction. The growth of such estrogen-induced MtTs is initially dependent on sustained high level of estrogen. Therefore, repeated DES pelletings of the host animals for several transplantation generations may be required until the MtT becomes autonomous.

In studies in which mice and rats were kept alive until natural death, it was noted that MtTs are the most common neoplasm, especially in old rats (Kim et al., 1960). A much higher incidence of spontaneous MtT was reported by Ito et al. (1972). Of 54 rats that were exsanguinated in extremis when older than 640 days, 38 had pituitary tumors. Hyperplasia of the mammary gland and RIA indicated that most, if not all, of these tumors were mammotropic. The 54 exsanguinated rats were a sample of 1040 rats autopsied after natural death in "life-span" nutritional studies of Kaunitz. The postmortem examinations of these male rats disclosed that at 400 days 38% of 316 rats had pituitary tumors, and at 640 days 48% [27% microscopic and 21% macroscopic (cf. Ito et al., 1972)]. The hormonal factors responsible for the high incidence of spontaneous MtTs in male rats are yet to be analyzed. In mice, the available data indicate marked strain differences. In studies of Upton *et al.* (1960), in which virgin LAF$_1$ mice were kept until natural death and the pituitaries were systematically examined, the spontaneous incidence of pituitary adenomas was less than 1% in males and more than 4% in females.

In women, MtTs masquerade under various syndromes such as gynecomastia, galactorrhea, and Forbes–Albright syndrome. RIA have clearly indicated that these patients had a prolactin-secreting pituitary adenoma. However, little is known about the pathophysiology of these tumors. Most, if not all, minute "chromophobe adenomas" of the human and rat pituitary, when tested for hormonal function, were found to be mammotropic.

The ultramicroscopic appearance of human MtTs, including those associated with amenorrhea and galactorrhea syndromes of women, is beautifully illustrated by Olivier *et al.* (1975). They also described and illustrated our trihormonal mutant of an MtT rat (strain F4), which has high ACTH, moderate MtH, and low StH activity (Furth and Clifton, 1966).

Most spontaneous pituitary tumors in man and rodents appear to be benign adenomas. Pleomorphic areas are not uncommon, but this alone does not indicate malignancy. Since intracranial tumors rarely metastasize, it will remain doubtful which, if any, of the human adenomas is truly malignant. Adenomatoid hyperplasias cannot be distinguished from true adenomas except by transplantation analyses. Most transplanted spontaneous pituitary adenomas tested were found to be functional. They appear to be "chromophobic" because they either produce very little hormone or rapidly discharge the hormones they produce, probably owing to hyperstimulation or an impaired mechanism for storage of hormones. Their function is best determined by the highly sensitive immunohistochemical staining of the tumor cells and radioimmunoassay of the host's plasma and the tumor.

McCormick and Halmi (1971) studied 1600 consecutive autopsies, classifying the pituitaries on the basis of histochemical staining. They found none to be unequivocally chromophobic: 59% were classified as "acidophilic," but only 3% of this type produced acromegaly, and MtTs were not recognized among them. However, it is possible that some, if not all, of the "nonacromegalic acidophilic" tumors were MtTs. A moderate degree of mammary gland hyperplasia is likely to be undetected unless it is highly secretory or the entire gland is studied microscopically.

The following are mostly abstracted from our general review article on tumors of the pituitary (Furth *et al.*, 1973).

Hwang *et al.* (1971a) identified MtH in 3 human tumors by incubating them in organ cultures, utilizing media containing [^{3}H]leucine, and tested the culture fluid and cells by precipitation with anti-StH and anti-MtH sera. The latter cross-reacts with h.MtH, but not with StH. Others used antisera against primate hormones with similar properties. From pooled culture fluids of human pituitaries with suggestive of Mt hyperplasia or neoplasia (including those with Forbes–Albright syndrome), relatively pure MtH was isolated, and its antisera were prepared. In tissue cultures MtH seemed to be more rapidly released from the pituitary cells than other pituitary hormones.

Finn and Mount (1971) studied 2 patients with Forbes–Albright tumor. One of them, a 32-year-old woman with gynecomastia, had 14 mU of MtH per milliliter and a normal level of StH in the serum. The other, an 18-year-old boy, had gynecomastia with galactorrhea.

Friesen et al. (1972), who pioneered in the isolation of human MtH and the preparation of antihuman MtH antisera, also documented the character of Forbes–Albright syndrome by RIA and demonstrated differences between human MtH and human StH.

Hwang et al. (1971b) found elevated MtH levels in 20 of 24 patients with galactorrhea. They quantitated the plasma MtH levels in various physiological states. The MtH levels were less than 30 ng/ml in normal children and adults of both sexes, less than 500 in newborns, owing probably to maternal contribution, and 30–1500 in patients with galactorrhea. During pregnancy, the plasma MtH level rose to 200 ng at term and fell to normal in 1–2 weeks post-partum. The suckling stimulus causes a 10- to 20-fold increase of MtH levels. Similarly, Turkington (1972) found high MtH serum values in 9 patients with Forbes–Albright adenoma, and elevated MtH levels in only 1 of 9 acromegalics. Of 11 patients with hypothalamic lesions, he observed abnormal MtH secretion in 2. He estimated the half-life of MtH to be about 15 minutes on the basis of plasma MtH assays following surgical removal of the Forbes–Albright tumor.

Ten human MtTs were studied by Racadot et al. (1971). In 6, the pathological findings correlated well with the clinical observations. Ultrastructural studies of the tumors disclosed active secretion. Four patients had "chromophobe adenomas" in which distinct Mts were recognized in small numbers.

Earlier, Peake et al. (1969) studied a Forbes–Albright tumor by electron microscopy and also found that while the granules of normal Sts ranged from 350 to 400 nm, those of the tumor cells ranged from 500–600 nm, the size of normal MtH granules.

The first clinical report on attempts to make use of the recent discoveries on pharmacological agents affecting MtH secretion was made by Malarkey et al. (1971). They measured serum MtH by RIA in 3 patients with Forbes–Albright syndrome and found that administration of 0.5 gm of L-DOPA produced a profound, but transient, fall in serum MtH in all 3.

If L-DOPA exerts its effects on the pituitary gland only via the hypothalamus, their observations suggest that the pituitary tumors responding to L-DOPA are autonomous though functional. (This is true for most experimental MtTs, which acquire autonomy but still maintain MtH activity.) Ergocryptine terminated galactorrhea in a patient with Forbes–Albright tumor (Lutterbeck *et al.*, 1971) and in a male patient with MtT (Copinschi *et al.*, 1973). For the latter and other references on inhibition of MtH with ergot alkaloids in advanced breast cancer, see Stoll (1974a, pp. 357–362).

V. The Role of Prolactin in Development of Mammary Tumors (MT)

Beatson (1896) was the first to link mammary cancer of women with the ovary. In the decades that followed, virtually all studies of MT revolved around the ovary and its hormones. The discoveries made by Bittner and his colleagues (cf. Bittner, 1946–1947) at the Jackson Laboratories represent the foundation of current knowledge and formed the basis for further research on MT. They recognized the triad of factors in the development of mammary tumors in mice: genetics, hormones, and a filterable agent named by them "mammary tumor agent" (MTA), now correctly named "mammary tumor virus" (MTV). All 3 factors have been proved to hold true for most mammals. In man, the existence of tumor viruses rests on indirect evidence. The limitation on experimentation in man with neoplastic diseases makes it difficult to bring solid proof for the existence of human MTV.

It has been well established that certain polycyclic aromatic hydrocarbons can readily induce MT in rodents (cf. Huggins and Yang, 1962). However, solid evidence for chemicals or radiations playing a causal role in human mammary cancer is still lacking.

The relative role played by these 3 major and several minor factors in the development of MT varies greatly not only with species, but also with strains within species. We shall review these factors with emphasis on the role of hormones, notably MtH. It may enable readers to form hypotheses of their own on the *modus operandi* of the various factors in the genesis of MT and on the fundamental nature of the neoplastic change, different from those to which we adhere presently.

We believe that carcinogenic agents change the genetic code, while hormones are mere homeostatic regulators of the number and function of cells. Although carcinogens alone can modify the differentiated (repressed) as well as undifferentiated genetic code in the absence of hormones (and thus produce a neoplasm), in nature, this type of carcinogenesis appears to be a rare event. It seems that in "spontaneous" carcinogenesis occurring in nature, hormones, which promote cell proliferation, can become a determining factor in the development of neoplasia. Furthermore, it may be possible that if the hormonal proliferative stimulus is unrestrained, this alone may lead to a neoplastic change.

A. Genetic Susceptibility: Strain and Species Factors

The widely varying incidence of MT in various close-bred species and strains suggested a genetic susceptibility. Leo Loeb and C. C. Little recognized the necessity of developing highly inbred, relatively homozygous animals through successive brother–sister mating. This resulted in the formulation of Bittner's *triad of factors* in mice. It now appears doubtful that any strain of mice is free from *virus*. Among them the strain with the greatest hereditary liability to the development of spontaneous MT is C3H of Bittner. Hybridization and other studies attribute this susceptibility to both a high genetic liability and to the presence of a virulent virus. Some inbred strains have a low incidence of MT, even if the virus is introduced in large quantities. Viruses with low virulence have also been isolated (cf. Bern and Nandi, 1961).

For a few decades, the MTV was the only virus capable of producing a malignant, organ-specific epithelial tumor in a mammal. Its mode of action remained unknown until the discovery of the reverse transcriptase (cf. Temin, 1974; Baltimore, 1976; Spiegelman, 1974a). This enzyme prepares a DNA copy of the RNA viruses, which becomes integrated with the cell's DNA, thereby explaining the mechanisms by which the genetic code of RNA viruses is inherited.

In some strains of mice the *incidence* of MT is high in both virgin and breeding females, but in others, only in breeders (cf. Bern and Nandi, 1961). This observation, the inhibitory effect of ovariectomy and other findings related to the MT incidence point to hormonal influences. Differences in susceptibility among strains have been attributed to the difference in sensitivity of the mammary gland to MT-promoting effects of progesterone and growth hormone, to the priming effect of estrogen and progesterone on mammary glands *in vivo* and *in vitro* (Nandi and Bern, 1960; Rivera, 1966; Singh *et al.*, 1970; Boot, 1970), and to the level of pituitary prolactin (Yanai and Nagasawa, 1970; Sinha *et al.*, 1974). Similar differences have been found in the course of experimental chemical carcinogenesis.

Epidemiological studies of mammary cancer in different races also suggest the existence of genetic differences in man, but they are often obscured by demographic differences (MacMahon *et al.*, 1973; Henderson *et al.*, 1974). Some have postulated differences in estrogen or androgen metabolism (Lemon, 1969; MacMahon *et al.*, 1974; Bulbrook, 1972), others, presumed high "risk factors" because plasma MtH is elevated in near relatives of breast cancer patients (Anderson, 1973; Kwa *et al.*, 1974; Henderson *et al.*, 1975).

A recent study of the inbred Parsee women in India, who are known to have extremely high incidence of breast cancer, disclosed an elevated level of the reverse transcriptase and other biochemical markers which are considered to be an indication of the presence of an RNA virus homologous to the mouse MTV (cf. Spiegelman, 1974b). The electron microscopic observation of B-type RNA virus particles in these women is of borderline significance (Moore *et al.*, 1969).

B. AGE FACTOR

The susceptibility of mice to MTV is highest at birth (cf. Bittner, 1946–1947) and during the nursing period (Moore *et al.*, 1970) and decreases with age.

In female rats receiving 400 r of whole-body irradiation at 3 days of age, the MT incidence was 18%. It slightly decreased at 21 days, and increased to a peak of 30% at 52 days of age (late puberty), and declined thereafter (Huggins and Fukunishi, 1963). Feedings of methylcholanthrene to 23-day-old and up to 50-day-old rats rapidly produced MT in all rats. Susceptibility to the chemicals, however, decreased with age, and no tumors were produced in rats older than 100 days (Huggins *et al.*, 1961).

The high susceptibility of newborn rats to radiation and newborn mice to infection with MTV may be attributed to high levels of lactogenic hormones. In humans, the serum prolactin levels of the newborn are reported to be nearly 17-fold that of normal adults, as high as the maternal levels at term (Hwang *et al.*, 1971b). However, there is no evidence linking h.MT to levels of serum prolactin at birth.

The peak susceptibility of the mammary gland to chemical carcinogenesis of young adult rats (40–65 days old) by either chemicals or radiation coincides with the eruptive maturation of the rudimentary mammary gland, with a vast number of mitotic figures in each mammary pad (Furth, 1973). This corresponds to the period of biochemical maturation of the human mammary pad into a breast tissue (Smithline *et al.*, 1975). The rapid decline of MT incidence in response to chemical carcinogens in virgin rats older than 70 days of age is puzzling. These age changes could not be correlated with plasma estrogen and prolactin levels. (H. J. Esber, unpublished data).

In women, a higher incidence of breast cancer has been found among those who had menarche at a younger age, birth of the first child at older age, and delayed menopause (MacMahon et al., 1973; Henderson et al., 1974). Pregnancy (Dao et al., 1960; Shellabarger et al., 1962), grafts of a functional MtT (U. Kim, unpublished data), or administration of a combination of progesterone and estradiol-17β (Huggins et al., 1962), which bring about the full growth and function of mammary glands prior to carcinogenic exposures, were found to suppress mammary tumor development. This suggests that cells are susceptible to carcinogens only while they grow and that they become resistant after they are fully matured and functioning.

C. Dietary Factors

After life insurance statistics linking overweight to early death and neoplosia, numerous experimental studies analyzed and confirmed this relationship; first among them was that of Tannenbaum (1959).

Carroll and Khor (1970) and Hui et al. (1971) found that high dietary fat increases MT incidence in rats given chemical carcinogens. This was attributed to elevated serum prolactin levels (Cohen et al., 1974; Chan et al., 1975). Similarly, high dietary fat consumption in women increases the risk of breast cancer (MacMahon et al., 1973; Drasar and Irving, 1973). In rats, lowering the serum prolactin levels with an ergot alkaloid was found to abolish such effects of dietary fat (Chan and Cohen, 1974).

Epidemiological reports indicate a higher incidence of breast cancer in the areas of endemic goiter (Eskin, 1970). In Japan, where the dietary intake of iodine is high, the breast cancer incidence is low (Wynder et al., 1960; Nagataki et al., 1967). As already mentioned, T.RH not only stimulates the synthesis and release of TtH, but also acts as a prolactin releaser (Jacobs et al., 1971; Bowers et al., 1971; Kelly et al., 1973). This may explain why goitrous patients with elevated prolactin levels have an increased risk of developing breast cancer (Mittra et al., 1974). Thus, all mammary cancer risk factors in man and animals reviewed point to the critical role of prolactin in mammary carcinogenesis.

D. Pathogenesis of Mammary Tumors

The basic physiological role of estrogen and prolactin (as of all hormones) is to regulate cell growth and function. Estrogen and prolactin are interrelated in that estrogen is an inducer of P. Both are aided by several other hormones and are subject to influences of hormones of higher centers, notably, of the hypothalamus. The development of neoplastic transformation of their major target organ, the mammary gland, is an accident in which these two hormones can play a dominant role.

The mechanism of action of estrogen via its cytosol receptors is well established, although the translation of the estrogen–cytosol–DNA complex is not yet fully understood. Nevertheless, evidence for the direct carcinogenic action of *estrogen* has been presented in several reviews by Jensen (cf. 1974).

The structural homology of estrogen and of potent chemical mammary carcinogens is intriguing, as discussed in Yang *et al.* (1961). Estrogen is inevitably linked to Mt.

Under estrogenic stimulation, the mammotropes promptly undergo hyperplasia, with increased secretion of prolactin. This is a reversible process. Regression of hypersecretion of prolactin follows cessation of estrogenic stimulation. But if the estrogenic stimulation is uninterrupted, some prolactin cells can undergo neoplastic transformation followed by formation of prolactin-secreting adenomas as discussed above.

Receptors for both estrogens and prolactin are present not only in the mammary gland, but also in their controlling centers and in cells of numerous organs in which the acceptance of these hormones is not followed by neoplastic transformation, e.g., liver cells have receptors for both of these hormones (Posner *et al.*, 1974; Kelly *et al.*, 1974), but neither is known to produce neoplasia in liver cells. The molecular biology of receptors and translation of their messages is beyond the scope of this review. However, it deserves emphasis that following neoplastic transformation of the mammary gland, the tumor cells often retain the receptor sites for estrogen and prolactin, albeit inadequately (Costlow *et al.*, 1974; McGuire *et al.*, 1974). The presence of *receptors for estrogens* in the mammary gland is required for its stimulation by estrogens, but mere acceptance of them does not imply that the message is translated into mammary gland stimulation. Notwithstanding, the estrogen receptor assay is widely used for assessing hormone responsiveness of MT in man and animals (McGuire *et al.*, 1974).

Prolactin binding sites in rat MT have also been demonstrated (Costlow *et al.*, 1974; Kelly *et al.*, 1974; Turkington, 1974). Costlow *et al.* (1975a) found that the activity of prolactin receptors was high in a transplanted prolactin-dependent mammary adenocarcinoma of the rat (strain MT-W9). The binding sites on the cell surface decreased as the tumor became less hormone-dependent or autonomous. Thus, some MTs can have both estrogen and prolactin receptors.

Vignon and Rochefort (1974) and Sasaki and Leung (1975) found that estrogen receptors in rat MT are dependent on or modulated by prolactin.

Posner *et al.* (1974) and Kelly *et al.* (1974) found prolactin receptors in the liver of female, but not of male, rats. Pregnancy and long-term administration of estrogen increased the activity (or concentration) of receptors in females and males (Posner *et al.*, 1974; Chamness *et al.*, 1975). Activity decreased after hypophysectomy (Posner *et al.*, 1975). Recent observations suggested that prolactin seems to induce its own receptor (Posner *et al.*, 1975; Costlow *et al.*, 1975b).

Estrogen is a unique hormone in that it produces cancer in various organs of seemingly "virus-free" rodents without the aid of any known carcinogen, e.g., in endocrine-related organs, such as the pituitary, mammary gland, uterus, cervix, and adrenal, and also in the kidney and hematopoietic tissue whose endocrine relation is slight (Burrows and Horning, 1952; Gardner, 1957). The growth of these tumors is usually dependent upon the continued supply of estrogens, at least in the original host and in the first few transplantation generations. It is generally believed that estrogens can both initiate and promote cancerous growth, either alone or through induction of prolactin. This view was challenged by Lacassagne, who reviewed the available evidence in 1961 and concluded that estrogens exert this influence via stimulation of prolactin.

The molecular configuration of estrogens is similar to carcinogenic polycyclic hydrocarbons (Yang *et al.*, 1961; Huggins and Yang, 1962), some of which as Jull (1958) demonstrated, have estrogenic properties. DES is not a hydrocarbon, but it is estrogenic and carcinogenic.

In general, when the force of any of the three classes of carcinogens (chemical, viral, or radiation) is weak, added prolactin is required to induce MT. Similar prolactin dependence of MT, induced by chronic estrogen treatment, had been reported by Cutts and Noble (1964).

When the neoplastic transformation induced by carcinogens is mild, the resultant neoplasm can remain latent. Expression of the neoplastic transformation may require sustained hormonal stimulation (Kim and Furth, 1960c). Analogous situations exist in the pregnancy-dependent mammary cancers of mice (Foulds, 1947, 1949); in suckling stimulus-dependent mammary carcinomas induced by DMBA in lactating rats (McCormick and Moon, 1965); and in estrone pellet-induced rat MT (Noble and Collip, 1941; Cutts and Noble, 1964; Cutts, 1964). Many carcinogen-induced MTs can regress after ovariectomy or hypophysectomy and be "resuscitated" by large concentrations of prolactin (Kim and Furth, 1960a).

There are numerous studies on the physiological and histological effects or prolactin on the prostate (cf. Boynes and Griffith, 1972). With respect to the role of prolactin in the induction and growth of prostatic carcinoma, Farnsworth concludes that it probably increases the gland's affinity for steroids, and therefore may exacerbate the growth of androgen-responsive tumors (cf. Boynes and Griffith, 1972).

E. Prolactin as a Carcinogenic Agent

There are four procedures to raise circulating prolactin levels which may lead to carcinogenesis. All require long-continued uninterrupted administration of P: (a) repeated (about daily) injections of homologous P (impractical because it calls for large quantities of homologous hormone); (b) administration of P.RH or other prolactin-releasing agents (also impractical until a long-acting preparation is developed); (c) grafts of isologous MtT, which secrete large quantities of MtH; and (d) ectopic pituitary grafts. Only the last two procedures have been well-explored.

Induction of MT by injections of homologous or heterologous prolactin was reported by Boot et al. (1962), Haran-Ghera (1963), Brock and Sutcliffe (1972), and Lorber et al. (1973). Induction of MT by grafts of syngeneic MtT was noted by us (Kim and Furth, 1960a; Yokoro and Furth, 1961, 1962). Ectopic pituitary grafts were introduced by Loeb and Kirtz (1939) for production of MT. The pathophysiological mechanism of this procedure was explained following the discovery of Everett (1954) that extrasellar grafts of the pituitary continuously secrete MtH, the latter procedure has subsequently been used by numerous investigators (Mühlbock, 1956; Mühlbock and Boot, 1959; Bruni and Montemurro, 1971a; and others). Welsch et al. (1970a) reported that stimulation of the *rat* mammary gland by multiple ectopic pituitary grafts produces a high incidence of fibroadenomas, but no carcinomas. A similar increase of fibroadenomas was produced by specific hypothalamic lesions which are known to produce increased prolactin secretion (Welsch et al., 1970b).

The studies reviewed indicate that prolactin can induce MT without estrogens and that it can resuscitate tumors that were induced by estrogens and regressed after ovariectomy or hypophysectomy and activate latent cancers. Neither the mammary gland nor hormone-responsive MT can be stimulated by estrogens in hypophysectomized animals (Kim et al., 1963). Correspondingly, Welsch and Rivera (1972) demonstrated that estrogen did not stimulate DNA synthesis in explants of a DMBA-induced mammary adenocarcinoma in media containing insulin and cortisone.

The discovery of the hypothalamic hormones and agents acting by way of the hypothalamus emphasized the role of MtH in mammary carcinogenesis. These studies were initiated by induction of hypothalamic lesions (Liebelt, 1959; Clemens et al., 1968; Klaiber et al., 1969; Bruni and Montemurro, 1971b). They were followed by administration of reserpine in animals and man (Lacassagne and Duplan, 1959; Welsch and Meites, 1969; Boston Collaborative Drug Program, 1974; Armstrong *et al.*, 1974; Heinonen *et al.*, 1974). It may be concluded that the procedures and agents discussed above play a determining role in the growth of established MT (Dunning, 1960; Kim and Furth, 1960a; Sterental *et al.*, 1964).

The interaction of pituitary MtH and ovarian hormones and their relationship to the central nervous and endocrine systems are well covered in the book edited by Stoll (1974a).

Mowles *et al.* (1971) noted that after injecting 50 μCi of [6,7-^{3}H] estradiol-17β into ovariectomized rats, the cytosolic uptake in the anterior hypothalamus and pituitary reached its peak promptly within 5 minutes and then decreased, while uptake in the uterine horn (probably also in the mammary gland) was maximal at 1 hour and declined gradually over a period of 6 hours (Leavitt *et al.*, 1969). The nuclear uptake in the hypothalamus and pituitary was not maximal until after 30 minutes, and the major part of the pituitary cytosol receptor protein was bound to form a 4.5 S complex, as compared to an 8–9.5 S uterine cytosol receptor. The pituitary and hypothalamic nuclear extracts contained 7 S complexes, which were also clearly separable from the 4.5 S uterine nuclear receptor. They concluded that differences in the concentrating and binding mechanisms of different but closely related target tissues may indicate the sequence of events in the differentiative expression of estrogenic activity.

Meites (1970, 1973) noted that a single injection of various drugs that act by way of the central nervous system can lower or raise MtH levels and thereby promote or inhibit mammary tumorigenesis. For example, methyl DOPA is promammary carcinogenic, whereas L-DOPA has the opposite effect. Yanai and Nagasawa (1971) reported that ergocryptine or ergocornine reduced the incidence of MT. Thus, the triggering mechanism of mammary tumorigenesis can lie in the central nervous system. MtH appears to be the key hormone, although estrogens also are often involved.

F. PROGRESSION

The progression of cancer from "bad to worse" was first reported by Rous and Beard (1935) during the course of their studies of viral Shope papillomas and extended by Rous and Kidd (1941) in their demonstration of subthreshold neoplastic states in the course of studies on induction of tumors with tar.

Our studies initiated the discovery that the estrogen-induced pituitary tumors were prolactin-secreting (Meyer and Clifton, 1956). Grafts of these tumors yielded large concentrations of isologous prolactin, enabling us to study the phenomenon of progression in chemically induced mammary adenocarcinomas (Kim and Furth, 1960b). Figure 1 illustrates the natural history of the MtH-dependent adenocarcinoma.

The MT-W9 strain was studied through 27 successive syngeneic transplantations (Kim et al., 1960, 1963). During the first two transplantation generations, the tumor grew only in MtH-enriched male and female hosts. Such tumors were designated *hormone-dependent*. In its third passage, it also grew in 2 of 13 (about 15%) intact female rats that did not receive MtH. When one of the tumors was transplanted into normal rats, it grew only in the female. This subline was designated as MT-W9A and as *hormone-responsive*. This tumor regressed promptly upon bilateral ovariectomy or hypophysectomy, indicating its dependence on physiological levels of ovarian or pituitary hormones. Its responsiveness to pituitary MtH was indicated by restoration of tumor growth in hypophysectomized rats by MtH, but not by estrogen (Kim et al., 1963). It maintained its hormone responsiveness with regularity, but in its fourth passage the tumor grew in 1 of 8 intact males and 2 of 8 ovariectomized females. One of the latter tumors grew equally well in both female and male rats. This subline was designated as MT-W9B and termed *fully autonomous*. It

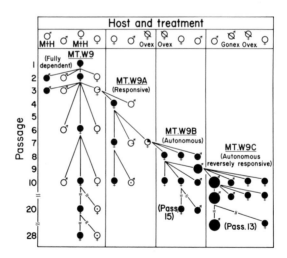

Fig. 1. Natural history of prolactin-dependent MT-W9. The shadowed area of the circles indicates the percentage of takes, and the size of the circle indicates the relative tumor size. Prolactin (MtH) was administered by a cograft of a mammotropic tumor (MtT) in the back of neck. Ovex, oophorectomy; Gonex, orchiectomy.

continued to grow well even in hypophysectomized rats. It maintained its autonomous character in subsequent transplantations, but again in its second passage it showed a change by growing in 2 of 6 intact males faster than in the other males or in females. When one of this new type was transplanted into normal rats, it grew faster in the males than in the females. This third subline, MT-W9C, was designated *androgen-responsive* or *reversely responsive*. The growth of this tumor could be stimulated by an injection of testosterone propionate and retarded by bilateral orchiectomy.

The growth of minimally deviated tumors such as MT-W9 (Kim and Furth, 1960c) requires stimulation by high (pharmacological) levels of exogenous MtH. These tumors regress promptly upon removal of the ovary or pituitary, but grow back rapidly at the original site when prolactin is replenished. It does so even 3 months after the tumor regression following ovariectomy or hypophysectomy. This indicates that the deprivation of stimulatory hormone does not eliminate all "dependent" cells, and a small number of transformed cells remain dormant. The neoplastic cells, unlike normal cells, are individualistic.

These four types of neoplastic MTs encompass almost the entire spectrum of breast cancers in man and animals with respect to their hormone sensitivity (Kim and Depowski, 1975). It is the characteristic concentration of carcinogens, their mode of administration, and random events that determine the character of transformation and the number of cells transformed. With a highly active dose, the resultant transformed cells are likely to be numerous and heterogeneous in character. Random isolation of tumors of the above types was reported (Lee, 1971); Mineshita and Yamaguchi (1965) reported on an autonomous spontaneous MT in an aging female mouse and an androgen-dependent variant isolated from an autonomous subline of an estrogen-dependent rat mammary carcinoma (Cutts, 1969).

Spontaneous or induced tumors may have features of any of these types at the time of their discovery or may acquire them by secondary mutations. The successive development of irreversible newer types proceeds via sequential clonal selection of the "fittest" in a given milieu. Chromosomal analysis may serve to characterize certain types (Kim and Depowski, 1975). Spontaneous mouse tumors tend to be autonomous and nonresponsive when discovered, and rat tumors are likely to be hormone-responsive; about 40% of human tumors are variously hormone-responsive at the time of their discovery. They are also subject to "progression." Since small tumors are completely removed only *in vitro*, studies can disclose the existence of fully hormone-dependent clones. To date, no h.MT proved to be curable by hormonal therapy alone.

VI. Harderian Gland Tumors and Prolactin

A remarkable recent finding of Fry *et al.* (1976) is that the induction and growth of tumors of the Harderian gland of mice are promoted by prolactin. As a source of prolactin, isologous pituitary grafts were used as well as DES. The inducers of this (and of mammary tumors) were ionizing radiations of various types. The maximum incidence was in the 80-rad fast-neutron group. The tumors ranged from benign functional adenomas to transplantable and metastasizing carcinomas. The maximum MT incidence by radiation was 3.8%; that of the Harderian gland was up to 37%.

VII. Concluding Comments

This review indicates that prolactin plays a major role in mammary carcinogenesis on a par with its natural inducer, estrogen. There are still numerous dark areas concerning carcinogenesis by both of these hormones. Their role is regulation of growth and function of the mammary gland, aided by several other hormones. Estrogens can be directly carcinogenic, i.e., capable of changing the genetic code. Natural estrogens have a structural homology with carcinogenic polycyclic hydrocarbons and are physiologically led to the nucleus complexed with their cytoplasmic receptors. However, the nonsteroidal estrogenic DES seems to be also carcinogenic. Thus, why the estrogen–cytosol–DNA complex, the physiological stimulant of the mammary gland, sometimes brings about a neoplastic transformation of the differentiated DNA, albeit very rarely, calls for an explanation. Prolactin, in contrast, acts on the plasma membrane, where its instructions for growth and function of the mammary epithelium are carried out by the "second messenger," cAMP. The latter understands the genetically defined language of various cells.

Estrogen is a "cosmopolitan" hormone in that it has receptor sites in many cells, in addition to the mammotrope of the pituitary. The fact that mammary tumors cannot be induced in hypophysectomized animals by estrogen, i.e., in the absence of prolactin, while prolactin can do so in the absence of steroids, calls for reconsideration of the commonly held view that the major direct mammary carcinogens are ovarian steroids.

REFERENCES

Anderson, I. E. (1973). *Cancer Bull. (M. D. Anderson)* **25**, 23.
Armstrong, B., Stevens, N., and Doll, R. (1974). *Lancet* **2**, 675.
Aubert, M. L., Grumbach, M. M., and Kaplan, S. L. (1974a). *Acta Endocrinol. (Copenhagen)* **77**, 460.

Aubert, M. L., Becker, R. L., Saxena, B. B., and Raiti, S. (1974b). *J. Clin. Endocrinol. Metab.* **35,** 1115.

Aubert, M. L., Garnier, P. E., Kaplan, S. L., and Grumback, M. M. (1975). *Proc. Endocrine Soc.* Abstract No. 59.

Baker, B. L. (1970). *J. Histochem. Cytochem.* **18,** 1.

Baltimore, D. (1976). *Harvey Lect. Ser.* **70,** 57.

Beatson, G. T. (1896). *Lancet* **2,** 104.

Becker, F. F. (1975). "Cancer: A Comprehensive Treatise," Vol. 1. Plenum, New York.

Ben-David, M. (1968). *J. Endocrinol.* **41,** 377.

Bern, H. A., and Nandi, S. (1961). *Prog. Exp. Tumor Res.* **2,** 90.

Bittner, J. J. (1946-1947). *Harvey Lect. Ser.* **42,** 221.

Blackwell, R. E., and Guillemin, R. (1973). *Annu. Rev. Physiol.* **35,** 357.

Boot, L. M. (1970). *Int. J. Cancer* **5,** 167.

Boot, L. M., Mühlbock, O., Ropcke, G., and Van Ebbenhorts Tengbergen, W. (1962). *Cancer Res.* **22,** 713.

Boston Collaborative Drug Program. (1974). *Lancet* **2,** 669.

Bowers, C. Y., Friesen, H. G., Hwang, P., Guyda, H. J., and Folkers, K. (1971). *Biochem. Biophys. Res. Commun.* **45,** 1033.

Boyns, A. R., and Griffiths, K. (1972). "Fourth Tenovus Workshop on Prolactin and Carcinogenesis." Alpha Omega Alpha Publ., Cardiff, Wales.

Brock, D. J. H., and Sutcliffe, R. G. (1972). *Lancet* **2,** 197.

Bruni, J. E., and Montemurro, D. G. (1971a). *Cancer Res.* **31,** 854.

Bruni, J. E., and Montemurro, D. G. (1971b). *Cancer Res.* **31,** 1903.

Bulbrook, R. D. (1972). *Proc. R. Soc. Med.* **65,** 646.

Burrows, H., and Horning, E. S. (1952). "Oestrogens and Neoplasia." Blackwell, Oxford.

Carroll, K. K., and Khor, H. T. (1970). *Cancer Res.* **30,** 2260.

Ceriani, R. L., Contesso, G. P., and Nataf, B. M. (1972). *Cancer Res.* **32,** 2190.

Chamness, G. C., Costlow, M. E., and McGuire, W. L. (1975). *Steroids* **26,** 363.

Chan, P. C., Didato, F., and Cohen, L. A. (1975). *Proc. Soc. Exp. Biol. Med.* **149,** 133.

Chan, P. C., and Cohen, L. A. (1974). *J. Natl. Cancer Inst.* **52,** 25.

Chomczynski, P., and Topper, Y. J. (1974). *Biochem. Biophys. Res. Commun.* **60,** 56.

Clemens, J. A., Welsch, C. W., and Meites, J. (1968). *Proc. Soc. Exp. Biol. Med.* **127,** 969.

Cohen, L. A., Didato, F., and Chan, P. C. (1974). *Fed. Proc., Fed. Am. Soc. Exp. Biol.* **33,** 601.

Costlow, M. E., Buschow, R. A., and McGuire, W. L. (1974). *Science* **184,** 85.

Costlow, M. E., Buschow, R. A., Richert, N. J., and McGuire, W. L. (1975a). *Cancer Res.* **35,** 970.

Costlow, M. E., Buschow, R. A., and McGuire, W. L. (1975b). *Life Sci.* **17,** 1457.

Cutts, J. H. (1964). *Cancer Res.* **24,** 1124.

Cutts, J. H. (1969). *J. Natl. Cancer Inst.* **42,** 485.

Cutts, J. H., and Noble, R. L. (1964). *Cancer Res.* **24,** 1116.

Dao, T. L., Bock, F. G., and Greiner, M. J. (1960). *J. Natl. Cancer Inst.* **25,** 991.

Denamur, R. (1969). *In* "Lactogenesis" (M. Reynolds and S. J. Folley, eds.), pp. 53–64. Univ. of Pennsylvania Press, Philadelphia.

Dilley, W. G. (1971a). *Endocrinology* **88,** 514.

Dilley, W. G. (1971b). *J. Endocrinol.* **50,** 501.

Dilley, W. G., and Kister, S. J. (1976). *J. Natl. Cancer Inst.* (in press).

Drasar, B. S., and Irving, D. (1973). *Br. J. Cancer* **27,** 167.

Dunning, W. F. (1960). *In* "Biological Activities of Steroids in Relation to Cancer" (G. Pincus and E. P. Vollmer, eds.), pp. 225–255. Academic Press, New York.

Emmart, E. W., Bates, R. W., and Turner, W. A. (1965). *J. Histochem. Cytochem.* **13**, 182.

Eskin, B. A. (1970). *Trans. N.Y. Acad. Sci.* [2] **32**, 911.

Everett, J. W. (1954). *Endocrinology* **54**, 685.

Farquhar, M. G., Skutelsky, E. H., and Kopkins, C. R. (1975). *In* "The Anterior Pituitary" (A. Tixier-Vidal and M. G. Farquhar, eds.), pp. 83–135. Academic Press, New York.

Finn, J. E., and Mount, L. A. (1971). *J. Neurosurg.* **35**, 723.

Flaxman, B. A., and Lasfargues, E. Y. (1973). *Proc. Soc. Exp. Biol. Med.* **143**, 371.

Foulds, L. (1947). *Br. J. Cancer* **1**, 362.

Foulds, L. (1949). *Br. J. Cancer* **3**, 230.

Francis, M. J. O., and Hill, D. J. (1975). *Nature (London)* **255**, 167.

Friesen, H., and Hwang, P. (1973). *Annu. Rev. Med.* **24**, 251.

Friesen, H., Webster, B. R., Hwang, P., Guyda, H., Munro, R. E., and Read, L. (1972). *J. Clin. Endocrinol. Metab.* **31**, 192.

Frohman, L. A., and Szabo, M. (1975). *Proc. Endocrine Soc.* Abstract No. 86, p. 93.

Fry, R. J. M., Garcian, A. G., Allen, K. H., Sallese, A., Staffeldt, E., Tahmisian, T. H., Devine, R. L., Lombard, L. S., and Ainsworth, E. J. (1976). *I.A.E.A.* **SM202** (in press).

Furth, J. (1955). *Recent Prog. Horm. Res.* **11**, 221–225.

Furth, J. (1973). *In* "Human Prolactin" (J. L. Pasteels and C. Robyn, eds.), pp. 232–248. Excerpta Med. Found., Amsterdam.

Furth, J., and Clifton, K. H. (1958). *Ciba Found. Colloq. Endocrinol. [Proc.]* **12**, 3.

Furth, J., and Clifton, K. H. (1966). *In* "The Pituitary Gland" (G. W. Harris and B. T. Donovan, eds.), pp. 460–497. Butterworth, London.

Furth, J., and Moy, P. (1967). *Endocrinology* **80**, 435.

Furth, J., Clifton, K. H., Gadsden, E. L., and Buffett, R. F. (1956). *Cancer Res.* **16**, 608.

Furth, J., Ueda, G., and Clifton, K. H. (1973). *Methods Cancer Res.* **10**, 201–277.

Gala, R. R., and Boss, R. S. (1975). *Proc. Soc. Exp. Biol. Med.* **149**, 330.

Ganong, W. F., and Martini, L. (1973). "Frontiers in Neuroendocrinology." Oxford Univ. Press, London and New York.

Gardner, W. U. (1957). *Proc. Can. Cancer Res. Conf.* **2**, 207.

Gardner, W. U., Pfeiffer, G. A., and Trentin, J. J. (1959). *In* "The Physiopathology of Cancer" (F. Homburger, ed.), pp. 152–237. Harper (Hoeber), New York.

Haran-Ghera, N. (1963). *Acta Unio Int. Cancrum* **19**, 765.

Heinonen, O. P., Shapiro, S., Tuominen, L., and Turunen, M. I. (1974). *Lancet* **2**, 675.

Henderson, B. E., Powell, D., and Rosario, I. (1974). *J. Natl. Cancer Inst.* **53**, 609.

Henderson, B. E., Gerkins, V., Rosario, I., Casagrande, J., and Pike, M. C. (1975). *N. Engl. J. Med.* **293**, 790.

Herlant, M. (1975). *In* "The Anterior Pituitary" (A. Tixier-Vidal and M. G. Farquhar, eds.), pp. 1–19. Academic Press, New York.

Hill-Samli, M., and MacLeod, R. M. (1975). *Proc. Soc. Exp. Biol. Med.* **149**, 511.

Hopkins, C. R., and Farquhar, M. G. (1973). *J. Cell Biol.* **59**, 276.

Horrobin, D. F. (1973). "Prolactin: Physiology and Clinical Significance." MTP Medical and Technical Publishing Co., Ltd., Lancaster.

Huggins, C., and Fukunishi, R. (1963). *Radiat. Res.* **20**, 493.

Huggins, C., and Yang, N. C. (1962). *Science* **137**, 257.

Huggins, C., Grand, L. C., and Brillantes, F. P. (1961). *Nature (London)* **189**, 204.

Huggins, C., Moon, R. C., and Morrii, S. (1962). *Proc. Natl. Acad. Sci. U.S.A.* **48**, 379.

Hui, Y. H., DeOme, K. B., and Briggs, G. M. (1971). *J. Natl. Cancer Inst.* **46**, 929.

Hwang, P., Friesen, H., Hardy, J., and Wilansky, D. (1971a). *J. Clin. Endocrinol. Metab.* **33**, 1.

Hwang, P., Guyda, H., and Friesen, H. (1971b). *Proc. Natl. Acad. Sci. U.S.A.* **68**, 1902.

Hwang, P., Guyda, H., and Friesen, H. (1972). *J. Biol. Chem.* **247**, 1955.

Hymer, W. C. (1975). *In* "Ultrastructure in the Pituitary Gland" (A. Tixier-Vidal and M. G. Farquhar, eds.), pp. 137–180. Academic Press, New York.

Hymer, W. C., Snyder, J., Wilfinger, W., Swanson, N., and Davis, J. A. (1974). *Endocrinology* **95**, 107.

Ichinose, R. R., and Nandi, S. (1966). *J. Endocrinol.* **34**, 331.

Ito, A., Moy, P., Kaunitz, H., Kortwright, K., Clarke, S., Furth, J., and Meites, J. (1972). *J. Natl. Cancer Inst.* **49**, 701.

Jacobs, L. A., Snyder, P. J., Wilber, J. F., Utiger, R. D., and Daughaday, W. H. (1971). *Lancet* **3**, 996.

Jensen, E. V. (1974). *N. Engl. J. Med.* **291**, 1252.

Jones, A. E., Fisher, J. N., Lewis, U. J., and Vanderlaan, W. P. (1965). *Endocrinology* **76**, 578.

Jull, J. W. (1958). *In* "Endocrine Aspects of Breast Cancer" (A. R. Currie and C. F. W. Illingworth, eds.), pp. 305–317. Livingstone, Edinburgh.

Kanematsu, S., and Sawyer, C. H. (1963). *Endocrinology* **72**, 243.

Kelly, P. A., Bedirian, K. N., Baker, R. D., and Friesen, H. G. (1973). *Endocrinology* **92**, 1289.

Kelly, P. A., Bradley, C., Shiu, R. P. C., Meites, J., and Friesen, H. G. (1974). *Proc. Soc. Exp. Biol. Med.* **146**, 816.

Kelly, P. A., Shiu, R. P. C., Robertson, M. D., and Friesen, H. G. (1975). *Endocrinology*, **96**, 1187.

Kim, U., and Depowski, M. J. (1975). *Cancer Res.* **34**, 2068.

Kim, U., and Furth, J. (1960a). *Proc. Soc. Exp. Biol. Med.* **103**, 640.

Kim, U., and Furth, J. (1960b). *Proc. Soc. Exp. Biol. Med.* **103**, 643.

Kim, U., and Furth, J. (1960c). *Proc. Soc. Exp. Biol. Med.* **105**, 490.

Kim, U., Clifton, K. H., and Furth, J. (1960). *J. Natl. Cancer Inst.* **24**, 1030.

Kim, U., Furth, J., and Yannopoulos, K. (1963). *J. Natl. Cancer Inst.* **31**, 233.

Klaiber, M. S., Gruenstein, M., Meranze, D. R., and Shimkin, M. B. (1969). *Cancer Res.* **29**, 999.

Kwa, H. G., DeJong-Bakker, M., Engelsman, E., and Cleton, F. J. (1974). *Lancet* **1**, 433.

Kwa, H. G., Cleton, F. J., Touber, J. L., and Robyn, C. (1975). "Workshop on Human Prolactin." Antonie van Leeuwenhoek Ziekenhuis, Amsterdam.

Lacassagne, A. (1961). *Acta Unio Int. Cancrum* **17**, 97.

Lacassagne, A., and Duplan, J. F. (1959). *C. R. Hebd. Seances Acad. Sci.* **249**, 810.

Lagios, M. D. (1974). *Oncology* **29**, 22.

Lawson, D. M., and Gala, R. R. (1975). *Endocrinology* **96**, 313.

Leavitt, W. W., Friend, J. P., and Robinson, J. A. (1969). *Science* **165**, 496.

Lee, A. E. (1971). *J. Endocrinol.* **49**, 353.

Lemon, H. M. (1969). *Cancer* **23**, 781.

Leung, B. S., and Sasaki, G. H. (1973). *Biochem. Biophys. Res. Commun.* **55**, 1180.

Lewis, U. J., Singh, R. N. P., and Seavey, B. K. (1971a). *Biochem. Biophys. Res. Commun.* **44**, 1169.

Lewis, U. J., Singh, R. N., Sinha, Y. N., and Vanderlaan, W. P. (1971b), *J. Clin. Endocrinol. Metab.* **33**, 153.

Li, C. H. (1972). *Proc. Am. Philos. Soc.* **116**, 365.

Li, C. H. (1973). *Calif. Med.* **118**, 55.

Li, C. H., Dixon, J. S., Lo, T. B., Pankov, Y. A., and Schmidt, K. D. (1969). *Nature* (*London*) **224**, 695.

Liebelt, R. A. (1959). *Proc. Am. Assoc. Cancer Res.* **3**, 37.

Lloyd, H. M., Meares, J. D., and Jacobi, J. (1975). *Nature* (*London*) **255**, 497.

Loeb, L., and Kirtz, M. M. (1939). *Am. J. Cancer* **36**, 56.

Lorber, J., Stewart, C. R., and Milford-Ward, A. (1973). *Lancet* **1**, 1187.

Lutterbeck, P. M., Pryor, J. S., Varga, L., and Wenner, R. (1971). *Br. Med. J.* **8**, 228.

Lyons, W. R. (1937). *Proc. Soc. Exp. Biol. Med.* **35**, 645.

Lyons, W. R. (1958). *Proc. R. Soc. London* **149**, 303.

McCann, S. M., Dhariwal, P. S., and Porter, J. C. (1968). *Annu. Rev. Physiol.* **30**, 589.

McCormick, G. M., and Moon, R. C. (1965). *Br. J. Cancer* **19**, 160.

McCormick, W. F., and Halmi, N. (1971). *Arch. Pathol.* **92**, 230.

McGuire, W. L., Chamness, G. C., and Shepherd, R. E. (1974). *Life Sci.* **14**, Part 1, 19.

Machlin, L. J., Jacobs, L. S., Cirulis, N., Kimes, R., and Miller, R. (1974). *Endocrinology* **95**, 1350.

MacLeod, R. M., and Lehmeyer, J. E. (1972). *Lactogenic Horm., Ciba Found. Symp., 1971*, pp. 53–76.

MacLeod, R. M., Bass, M. B., Buxton, E. P., Dent, J. N., and Benson, D. G., Jr. (1966). *Endocrinology* **78**, 267.

MacMahon, B., Cole, P., and Brown, J. B. (1973). *J. Natl. Cancer Inst.* **50**, 21.

MacMahon, B., Cole, P., and Brown, J. B. (1974). *Int. J. Cancer* **14**, 161.

McNatty, K. P., Sawers, R. S., and McNeilly, A. S. (1974). *Nature* (*London*) **250**, 653.

Malarkey, W. B., Jacobs, L. S., and Daughaday, W. H. (1971). *N. Engl. J. Med.* **285**, 1160.

Mason, T. E., Phifer, R. F., Spicer, S. S., Swallow, R. A., and Dreskin, R. B. (1969). *J. Histochem. Cytochem.* **17**, 563.

Meites, J. (1970). "Hypophyseotropic Hormones of the Hypothalamus: Assays and Chemistry." Williams & Wilkins, Baltimore, Maryland.

Meites, J. (1973). *In* "Human Prolactin" (J. L. Pasteel, C. Robyn, and F. J. G. Ebling, eds.), pp. 105–118. Experta Med. Found., Amsterdam.

Meites, J., and Nicoll, C. S. (1966). *Annu. Rev. Physiol.* **28**, 57.

Meldolesi, J., Marini, D., and Marini, M. L. D. (1972). *Endocrinology* **91**, 802.

Meyer, R. K., and Clifton, H. K. (1956). *Endocrinology* **58**, 686.

Mineshita, T., and Yamaguchi, K. (1965). *Cancer Res.* **25**, 1168.

Mittra, I. (1974). *Nature* (*London*) **248**, 525.

Mittra, I., Hayward, J. L., and McNeilly, A. S. (1974). *Lancet* **1**, 889.

Moore, D. H., Sarkar, N. H., Kelly, C. E., Pilsbury, N., and Charney, J. (1969). *Tex. Rep. Biol. Med.* **27**, 1027.

Moore, D. H., Charney, J., and Pullinger, B. D. (1970). *J. Natl. Cancer Inst.* **45**, 561.

Mowles, T. F., Ashkanazy, B., Mix, E., Jr., and Sheppart, H. (1971). *Endocrinology* **89**, 484.

Mühlbock, O. (1956). *Adv. Cancer Res.* **4**, 371.

Mühlbock, O., and Boot, L. M. (1959). *Cancer Res.* **19**, 402.

Nagasawa, H., and Yanai, R. (1971). *Endocrinol. Jpn.* **17**, 536.

Nagataki, S., Shizume, K., and Nakao, K. (1967). *J. Clin. Endocrinol. Metab.* **27**, 638.

Nakane, P. K. (1975). *In* "The Anterior Pituitary" (A. Tixier-Vidal and M. G. Farquhar, eds.), pp. 45–61. Academic Press, New York.

Nakane, P. K., and Pierce, G. B., Jr. (1967). *J. Histochem. Cytochem.* **14**, 929.

Nandi, S., and Bern, H. A. (1960). *J. Natl. Cancer Inst.* **24**, 907.

Niall, H. D., Hogan, M. L., Tregear, G. W., Segré, G. V., Hwang, P., and Friesen, H. (1973). *Recent Prog. Horm. Res.* **29**, 387.

Nicoll, C. S., and Bern, H. A. (1972). *Lactogenic Horm., Ciba Found. Symp., 1971,* pp. 299–317.

Nicoll, C. S., and Meites, J. (1962). *Endocrinology* **70,** 272.

Noble, R. L., and Collip, J. B. (1941). *Can. Med. Assoc. J.* **44,** 1.

Oka, T., and Topper, Y. T. (1972). *Proc. Natl. Acad. Sci. U.S.A.* **69,** 1693.

Olivier, L., Vila-Porcile, E., Racadot, O., Peillon, F., and Racador, J. (1975). *In* "The Anterior Pituitary" (A. Tixier-Vidal and M. G. Farquhar, eds.), pp. 231–276. Academic Press, New York.

Pasteels, J. L. (1962). *C. R. Hebd. Seances Acad. Sci., Ser. D* **254,** 2664.

Pasteels, J. L., Robyn, C., and Ebling, F. J. G., eds. (1973). "Human Prolactin." Excerpta Med. Found., Amsterdam.

Peake, G. T., McKeel, D. W., Jarett, L., and Daughaday, W. H. (1969). *J. Clin. Endocrinol. Metab.* **29,** 1383.

Pelc, S. R. (1968). *Nature (London)* **219,** 162.

Phifer, R. F., Midgley, A. R., and Spicer, S. S. (1972). *In* "Gonadotropins" (B. B. Saxena, C. G. Beling, and H. M. Gandy, eds.), pp. 9–25. Wiley, New York.

Posner, B. I., Kelly, P. A., Shiu, R. P. C., and Friesen, H. G. (1974). *Endocrinology* **95,** 521.

Posner, B. I., Kelly, P. A., and Friesen, H. G. (1975). *Science* **188,** 57.

Racadot, J., Vila-Porcile, E., Peillon, R., and Olivier, L. (1971). *Ann. Endocrinol.* **32,** 298.

Ramirez, V. D., and McCann, S. M. (1964). *Endocrinology* **75,** 206.

Riddle, O., Bates, R. W., and Dykshorn, S. W. (1932a). *Proc. Soc. Exp. Biol. Med.* **29,** 1211.

Riddle, O., Bates, R. W., and Dykshorn, S. W. (1932b). *Anat. Rec.* **54,** 25.

Rivera, E. M. (1966). *Nature (London)* **209,** 1151.

Rivier, C., and Vale, W. (1974). *Endocrinology* **95,** 950.

Robertson, M. C., and Friesen, H. G. (1975). *Endocrinology* **97,** 621.

Rodbard, D., and Bertino, R. E. (1973). *Adv. Exp. Med. Biol.* **36,** 327.

Rogol, A. D., and Rosen, S. W. (1974). *J. Clin. Endocrinol. Metab.* **35,** 714.

Rous, P., and Beard, J. W. (1935). *J. Exp. Med.* **62,** 523.

Rous, P., and Kidd, J. G. (1941). *J. Exp. Med.* **73,** 365.

Salmon, W. D., Jr., and Daughaday, W. H. (1957). *J. Lab. Clin. Med.* **49,** 825.

Sasaki, G. H., and Leung, B. S. (1975). *Cancer* **35,** 645.

Schally, A. V., Arimura, A., and Kastin, A. J. (1973). *Science* **179,** 341.

Shaar, C. J., and Clemens, J. A. (1974). *Endocrinology* **95,** 1202.

Shellabarger, C. J., Aponte, G. E., Cronkite, E. P., and Bond, V. P. (1962). *Radiat. Res.* **17,** 492.

Shiino, M., Sarchol, J. B., and Rennels, E. G. (1974). *Proc. Soc. Exp. Biol. Med.* **147,** 361.

Shiu, R. P. C., Kelly, P. A., and Friesen, H. G. (1973). *Science* **180,** 968.

Simpson, A. A., and Schmidt, G. H. (1971). *J. Endocrinol.* **51,** 265.

Singh, D. V., DeOme, K. B., and Bern, H. A. (1970). *J. Natl. Cancer Inst.* **45,** 657.

Sinha, Y. N., Selby, F. W., and Vanderlaan, W. P. (1973). *J. Clin. Endocrinol. Metab.* **36,** 1039.

Sinha, Y. N., Selby, F. W., and Vanderlaan, W. P. (1974). *Endocrinology* **94,** 757.

Smith, P. E. (1927). *J. Am. Med. Assoc.* **88,** 158.

Smith, V. G., and Convey, E. M. (1975). *Proc. Soc. Exp. Biol. Med.* **149,** 70.

Smithline, F., Sherman, L., and Kolodny, H. D. (1975). *N. Engl. J. Med.* **292,** 784.

Spiegelman, S. (1974a). *J. Am. Med. Assoc.* **230,** 1036.

Spiegelman, S. (1974b). *Cancer Chemother. Rep.* **48,** 595.

Sterental, A., Dominguez, J. M., Weissman, C., and Pearson, O. H. (1964). *Cancer Res.* **23**, 481.

Stockdale, F. E., and Topper, Y. J. (1966). *Proc. Natl. Acad. Sci. U.S.A.* **56**, 1283.

Stockdale, F. E., Jeurgens, W. G., and Topper, Y. J. (1966). *Dev. Biol.* **13**, 266.

Stoll, B. A., ed. (1974a). "Mammary Cancer and Neuroendocrine Therapy." Butterworth, London.

Stoll, B. A. (1974b). *In* "Mammary Cancer and Neuroendocrine Therapy" (B. A. Stoll, ed.), pp. 401–411. Butterworth, London.

Stoudemire, G. A., Stumpf, W. E., and Sar, M. (1975). *Proc. Soc. Exp. Biol. Med.* **149**, 189.

Stricker, P., and Grüter, F. (1928). *C. R. Seances Soc. Biol. Sis Fil.* **99**, 1978.

Stumpf, W. E. (1970). *J. Histochem. Cytochem.* **18**, 21.

Suh, H. K., and Frantz, A. G. (1974). *J. Clin. Invest.* **53**, 79a.

Talwalker, P. K., and Meites, J. (1961). *Proc. Soc. Exp. Biol. Med.* **107**, 880.

Talwalker, P. K., Ratner, A., and Meites, J. (1963). *Am. J. Physiol.* **295**, 213.

Tannenbaum, A. (1959). *In* "The Pathophysiology of Cancer" (F. Homburger, ed.), pp. 517–555. Harper (Hoeber), New York.

Temin, H. M. (1974). *Cancer Res.* **34**, 2835.

Tindal, J. S., Knaggs, G. S., and Turvey, A. (1967). *J. Endocrinol.* **37**, 279.

Tixier-Vidal, A. (1975). *In* "The Anterior Pituitary" (A. Tixier-Vidal and M. G. Farquhar, eds.), pp. 181–229. Academic Press, New York.

Tixier-Vidal, A., and Farquhar, M. G., eds. (1975). "The Anterior Pituitary." Academic Press, New York.

Tixier-Vidal, A., and Picart, R. (1967). *J. Cell Biol.* **35**, 501.

Turkington, R. W. (1972). *J. Clin. Endocrinol. Metab.* **34**, 159.

Turkington, R. W. (1974). *Cancer Res.* **34**, 758.

Upton, A. C., Kimball, A. W., Furth, J., Christenberry, K. W., and Benedict, W. H. (1960). *Cancer Res.* **20**, 1.

Vale, W., Rivier, C., Brazeau, P., and Guillemin, R. (1974). *Endocrinology* **95**, 968.

Vignon, F., and Rochefort, H. (1974). *Hebd. Seances Acad. Sci.* **278**, 103.

Voogt, J. L., and Ganong, W. F. (1974). *Proc. Soc. Exp. Biol. Med.* **147**, 795.

Warchol, J. B., Shiino, M., and Renneis, E. G. (1974). *Experientia* **30**, 1444.

Welsch, C. W., and Meites, J. (1969). *Int. Congr. Physiol. Sci.* p. 466.

Welsch, C. W., and Rivera, E. M. (1972). *Proc. Soc. Exp. Biol. Med.* **139**, 623.

Welsch, C. W., Jenkins, T. W., and Meites, J. (1970a). *Cancer Res.* **30**, 1024.

Welsch, C. W., Nagasawa, H., and Meites, J. (1970b). *Cancer Res.* **30**, 2310.

Wilfinger, W., Snyder, J., Hymer, W. C., Gaffney, E., Bergland, R., and Page, R. (1975). *Proc. Endocrine Soc.* Abstract No. 62, p. 81.

Wolstenholme, G. E. W., and Knight, J., eds. (1972). "Lactogenic Hormones." Churchill-Livingstone, Edinburg and London.

Wynder, E. L., Bross, I. J., and Hirayama, T. (1960). *Cancer* **13**, 559.

Yalow, R. B. (1974). *J. Med. Sci.* **10**, 1185.

Yanai, R., and Nagasawa, H. (1969). *Proc. Soc. Exp. Biol. Med.* **131**, 167.

Yanai, R., and Nagasawa, H. (1971). *Horm. Behav.* **2**, 73.

Yanai, R., and Nagasawa, H. (1971). *Experientia* **27**, 934.

Yang, N. C., Castro, A. J., Lewis, M., and Wong, T. W. (1961). *Science* **134**, 386.

Yokoro, K., and Furth, J. (1961). *Proc. Soc. Exp. Biol. Med.* **107**, 921.

Yokoro, K., and Furth, J. (1962). *J. Natl. Cancer Inst.* **29**, 887.

Evidence for Chemical Communication in Primates

RICHARD P. MICHAEL, ROBERT W. BONSALL, AND
DORIS ZUMPE

*Department of Psychiatry, Emory University School of Medicine,
and Georgia Mental Health Institute, Atlanta, Georgia*

I. INTRODUCTION

During the past 10–15 years an increasing number of field and laboratory studies has documented observations that implicate chemical communication in the behavior of many primate species; in particular, there

are data indicating the role of odors and of olfactory signals. This concept is well established in invertebrates (e.g., moths and butterflies), for which much is known about the glands that emit the chemicals, the identity of the chemical substances involved, and the electrophysiology of the receiving systems in the antennae. Unfortunately, we have only sparse information on these different aspects of the chemical signaling systems in primates and other mammals.

A. PROSIMIANS

Prosimians usually possess one or more areas in which the skin glands are specialized and their secretions, together with saliva, urine, and feces, are variously used to mark objects in the general environment, other animals of the same species (conspecifics), or even parts of the animal's own body. Tree shrews (*Tupaia*) possess specialized throat and chest glands (Sprankel, 1961, 1962) used for marking the environment ("chinning"), probably to determine territory (Vandenbergh, 1963; Conway and Sorenson, 1966; Kaufmann, 1965). Martin (1968) has reported that the female tree shrew is marked by the male during pair bonding, and that newly born young are marked by the mother, probably for litter identification. *Lemur* has scent glands on the forelimbs near the palms and also near the armpits (Sutton, 1887; Pocock, 1918; Montagna, 1962; Montagna and Yun, 1962). In the social *Lemur catta* there is a ritualized form of marking in which the males wipe their brachial and antebrachial glands on their tails, which they then wave over their heads at each other during so-called "stink fights" (Jolly, 1966). These are associated with aggressive, dominance interactions, whose frequency increases at the start of the mating season. This is very short in Madagascar, where there is evidence for estrous synchrony within a given group that perhaps reflects the action of a primer pheromone (Jolly, 1966; Evans and Goy, 1968). Female ring-tailed lemurs (*Lemur catta*) become attractive to males a few days before they become receptive, during which time males follow the females, investigate the genitalia, and attempt to mount. *Avahi* has cutaneous glands at the corner of the jaw (Boulière *et al.*, 1956; Petter, 1962), and sifaka (*Propithecus*) males have a gland at the neck (Petter, 1965). Slow and slender lorises (*Nycticebus* and *Loris*) have brachial glands (Seitz, 1969), and *Tarsius* has epigastric and circumanal glands in addition to glands on the hands and feet (Hill *et al.*, 1952). Marking environmental objects with glandular secretions, urine, and feces is thought to serve territorial demarcation in lemurs (*Lemur*), sifakas (*Propithecus*), mouse lemur (*Microcebus*), and dwarf lemur (*Cheirogaleus*) (Petter, 1962). In the nocturnal, solitary *Loris tardigradus* (Ilse, 1955) and *Nycticebus coucang* (Seitz,

1969) marking probably serves territorial demarcation, sex identification, and individual recognition. Estrous *Loris* emit a characteristic odor (Ramaswami and Anand Kumar, 1962), and the male potto (*Perodicticus potto*) licks the estrous female's vulva and urinates and defecates frequently (Cowgill, 1969). Similar behavior was noted in a male *Tarsius* during sexual excitement (Harrison, 1963). In the family-living *Galago*, chemical communication also appears to be involved in sexual activity. Urine-washing, in which the animal urinates into a cupped hand and rubs its foot in it, is a behavior pattern that *Galago* shares with many prosimians and New World monkeys. The frequency of this behavior in male *Galago*, together with olfactory inspection of females, increases just prior to estrus, when a white vagina overflow commences that further excites the male (*G. senegalensis*: Doyle *et al.*, 1967; *G. crassicaudatus*: Eaton *et al.*, 1973).

B. New World Monkeys

Many New World monkeys also have specialized skin glands. Most Callithricidae and Cebidae studied to date have sternal glands (Epple and Lorenz, 1967); the night monkey (*Aotus*) has, in addition, probable scent glands on the face near the nose and in the anal region (Tachibana, 1936; Hill *et al.*, 1959; Ortmann, 1960; Hanson and Montagna, 1962). Marmosets and tamarins have been studied most intensively with respect to olfactory communication (Muckenhirn, 1967; Epple, 1967, 1971, 1973, 1975; Moynihan, 1970; Snyder, 1972). Many species exhibit marking behavior during aggressive and dominance interactions, and males sniff at the bodies and genital regions of females prior to copulation. In the brown-headed tamarin (*Saguinus fuscicollis*), scent marks appear to carry information about the sex, identity, and social rank of the donor, and, as in the tree shrews, marking of the female by the male appears to accompany pair-bonding. Glandular and urine marking in the night monkey (*Aotus trivirgatus*), howler monkey (*Alouatta villosa*), woolly monkey (*Lagothrix*), spider monkey (*Ateles*), titi monkey (*Callicebus moloch*), capuchins (*Cebus capucinus, C. apella, C. albifrons*), and squirrel monkey (*Saimiri sciureus*) are not well understood, but thought to be related to territoriality (Ullrich, 1954; Nolte, 1958; Bernstein, 1965; Moynihan, 1967; Epple and Lorenz, 1967; Schifter, 1968; Klein and Klein, 1971). In some species, olfactory and gustatory inspection of the female's anogenital region by the male appears to provide some information about her hormonal status. Male *Ateles* frequently sniff at, and ingest, female urine (Klein, 1971; Klein and Klein, 1971). Captive female *Saimiri* urine-wash, and are sniffed at by males, more often when they are sexually receptive (Latta *et al.*, 1967), and, under seminatural conditions, the breeding season in *Saimiri* is characterized by the males frequently sniffing at the anogenital regions or urine marks of females (Baldwin, 1970). Olfactory inspection of the female's anogenital region by the male has also been noted in *Callicebus moloch* (Mason, 1966) and in *Alouatta villosa* (Carpenter, 1934; Altmann, 1959).

C. OLD WORLD MONKEYS AND APES

Among Old World primates, which alone have a true menstrual cycle, specialized skin glands are greatly reduced (*Mandrillus*: Hill, 1944, 1954; the orang-utan, *Pongo*: Schultz, 1921; *Homo*: Schiefferdecker, 1917; Schaffer, 1937; Bunting *et al.*, 1948); however, the fact that olfaction does, nevertheless, play some role, at least in a sexual context, is evidenced by the numerous reports of males sniffing and licking at the female's genitalia: the toque monkey (*Macaca sinica*) produces a vaginal discharge during certain days of the menstrual cycle that is sufficiently odorous to be detected by humans (Jay, 1965). Olfactory, gustatory, and tactile inspection by the male of the female's anogenital region has been reported for several species: macaques and baboons (Hamilton, 1914), bonnet monkey (*M. radiata*: Simonds, 1965; Rahaman and Parthasarathy, 1969), crab-eating monkey (*M. fascicularis*: Ellefson, 1968), pig-tailed macaque (*M. nemestrina*: van Hooff, 1962; Bernstein, 1967), rhesus monkey (*M. mulatta*: Altmann, 1962), stump-tailed macaque (*M. arctoides*: Chevalier-Skolnikoff, 1974), chacma baboon (*Papio ursinus*: Hall, 1962), gelada (*Theropithecus gelada*: Spivak, 1971), vervet monkey (*Cercopithecus aethiops*: Gartlan, 1969), talapoin (*C. talapoin:* Dixson *et al.*, 1973), patas monkey (*Erythrocebus patas:* Hall *et al.*, 1965), chimpanzee (*Pan troglodytes:* van Lawick-Goodall, 1969; Tutin and McGrew, 1973), and *Gorilla gorilla* (Hess, 1973). In comparison with prosimians and platyrrhines, Old World monkeys tend to be larger, more social, more frequently ground-living, and range over wide areas of forest or savannah, and they show very little marking behavior. In anatomical terms, there is a relative reduction in the mass of neural structures related to olfactory processes as one ascends the phylogenetic scale toward man (Fig. 1). Nevertheless, the comparative behavioral data strongly suggest that males of many Old World primate species, regardless of their habitat and social organization, use olfactory cues emitted by the female and thereby obtain an indication of her hormonal status, and the weight of the behavioral evidence clearly indicates that chemical communication, mediated by olfactory pathways, plays a significant part in the reproductive life of these highly complex mammalian forms.

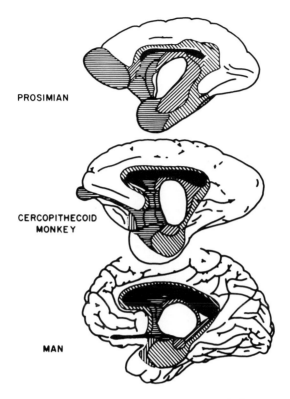

PROSIMIAN

CERCOPITHECOID
MONKEY

MAN

FIG. 1. Note the reduction in the mass of the phylogenetically old brain structures and those associated with olfaction as one ascends the comparative scale from prosimian to man. In this respect, the brain of the rhesus monkey more closely resembles that of man, a microsmatic form, than a prosimian. After Stephan (1963).

II. CHEMICAL COMMUNICATION IN RHESUS MONKEYS

A. THE CONCEPTS OF FEMALE RECEPTIVITY AND ATTRACTIVENESS

The catarrhine monkeys and the apes, alone among mammals, have a clearly defined menstruation with a cycle lasting about 30 days (Michael and Zumpe, 1971). In contrast to the majority of mammals, they do not show well-circumscribed periods of estrus (heat behavior), but will accept the male and copulate throughout the cycle. However, earlier work in both the rhesus monkey (Ball and Hartman, 1935; Carpenter, 1942) and chimpanzee (Yerkes and Elder, 1936; Yerkes, 1939; Young and Orbison, 1944) has indicated that the levels of sexual interaction show some systematic variations with the different phases of the menstrual cycle. It seems that the role of hormonal influences on behavior, although attenuated in these species, is still apparent. Furthermore, studies in the rhesus monkey (Michael and Herbert, 1963; Michael, 1965a, 1971; Michael et al., 1967a; Michael and Welegalla, 1968; Goy and Resko, 1972; Bielert et al., 1976) have shown that well-marked rhythms in mounting behavior by males occur in relation to the menstrual cycles of their female partners, and these rhythms are abolished by bilateral ovariectomy. One of the most notable features of the behavior of anthropoid primates is its variability: not all pairs show the cyclic fluctuations described above, nor does sexual activity invariably decline, immediately and dramatically, to very low levels when the ovaries are ablated. It should be clearly recognized that nonhormonal factors make a significant contribution to the sexual interactions of these species; nevertheless, from the evidence cited above, the importance of the endocrines will be obvious.

We have found it useful to think of female sexuality in primates in terms of two major variables defined as (i) sexual receptivity and (ii) sexual attractiveness (Michael et al., 1967b). Although they are abstractions in themselves, they can be operationally defined in behavioral terms. The state of receptivity in the female depends in large part upon hormonal feedback effects on as yet unidentified brain mechanisms and neural processes (Michael, 1969). In other words, whether the female is receptive or unreceptive to the male depends on how the hormones within her blood stream interact with, and hence activate, brain mechanisms. This is probably true for most birds (Barfield, 1965, 1971; Hutchison, 1967, 1971, 1974; Komisaruk, 1967; Meyer, 1972; Haynes and Glick, 1974) and mammals (Harris et al., 1958; Lisk, 1962, 1967; Harris and Michael, 1964; Michael, 1965b; Davidson, 1966; Palka and Sawyer, 1966; Thiessen and Yahr, 1970; Powers, 1972; Voci and Carlson, 1973; Ciaccio and Lisk, 1973; Morin and Feder, 1974; Owen et al., 1974). What is so different about primates is the extent to which more or less reflex postural responses are modulated by prior experience and by the exigencies of the immediate behavioral context. Sexual activity in the rhesus monkey is not an all-or-nothing phenomenon and the part played by the female's willingness to mate (receptivity) can be distinguished from that due to the male's libido by the frequency and form of her behavioral patterns. Nor can we neglect the overriding influence of individual differences and partner preferences. For example, a moderately receptive female may consistently refuse mating with one male partner while permitting some copulatory activity with another. Female receptivity is, of course, an expression of her internal motivational state, or, in a now outmoded terminology, of her sex "drive." We have to rely on measures of female behavior to make inferences about this, e.g., the frequency with which she makes advances and sexual invitations to the male (Michael and Welegalla, 1968; Michael and Zumpe, 1970a; Zumpe and Michael, 1970) or the rate with which she presses a lever in an operant situation to gain access to a male partner (Michael et al., 1972). These are complex issues that cannot be explored further here.

Much easier to discuss from the behavioral standpoint is the question of female attractiveness. It is easier because we can use changes in the male's behavior to tell us whether or not a given female has a high or low stimulus value in a sexual context. The male rhesus monkeys used to determine female attractiveness should have an intermediate level of sexual potency or libido: for instance, if too immature, their potency may be low and they may be insufficiently responsive to the changing stimulus properties of their female partners. On the other hand, if their sexual potency is very high, for instance, because of sexual deprivation, they may simply ignore changes in the stimulus properties of females with which they are paired, but for obviously different reasons. However, given males whose potencies are in the intermediate range, changes in various indices of male sexual activity (numbers of mounting attempts, mounts, intromissions, ejaculations; ejaculation times; various latency measures, etc.) can be used as reliable indices of changes in the stimulatory properties of their female partners. Obviously, the foregoing is a simplified statement and several additional factors must be held constant, but we have the possibility of experimentally manipulating a female's stimulus properties and then observing the changes this induces in the behavior of her male partners.

Attractiveness and receptivity can vary independently, particularly under experimental conditions. A highly receptive female, if unattractive, will be one that makes many sexual invitations and approaches to the male without their being very effective in eliciting responses. Conversely, a highly attractive but unreceptive female will be one to which males show intense sexual interest although she makes few sexual invitations and frequently refuses their copulatory attempts (e.g., during pregnancy) (Michael and Zumpe, 1970b). When the female is both unreceptive and unattractive there is generally little sexual interaction between the pair and, finally, when attractiveness and receptivity coincide, the interactions are most intense with much grooming and copulatory activity. All these combinations can be observed in nature when the female is intact and having normal menstrual cycles. No doubt many sensory stimuli enter into the determination of a given female's attractiveness for a particular male partner. We cannot as yet characterize the different primate "personalities" (introverted or extroverted, etc.) as we can for the human. Certainly, some females are active and exploratory while others stay with the male quietly. Differences in ages, relative sizes, aggressivity, dominance, and also the frequency and form of sexual displays must enter into the situation. Many of these influences are mediated by visual pathways. But tactile stimulation, both in the form of grooming activity and the nature of the afferent stimulation provided by the vagina during copulation, makes a significant contribution. Finally, there is the afferent stimulation that may be mediated by olfactory pathways. We have emphasized vision and touch in addition to olfaction because it is our view that sexual attraction and arousal in the rhesus monkey depend on several sensory modalities, all of which make a contribution, and none of which, in isolation, is necessarily sufficient. Therefore, to assess the role of olfactory mechanisms and chemical signals, we need to tease apart their contribution from a matrix of other behaviors. An inevitable consequence of this is to give an undue emphasis to the modality under consideration, and it is a highly important task then to restore perspective by determining its importance in the life of the animal under natural conditions.

B. Hormonal Factors and Female Attractiveness

In our neuroendocrine studies of rhesus monkey behavior, pairs of jungle-bred animals of opposite sexes are observed in quiet observation rooms from behind one-way vision mirrors for 60-minute periods. During this time all the behavioral interactions are scored and recorded (Michael et al., 1966). Mating in this species consists of a series of mounts by the male on the female, usually with intromission and pelvic thrusting. The mounting series (about 3–20 mounts) is terminated by a mount in which ejaculation occurs. After ejaculation, there is a pause of some 30 minutes before the start of another mounting series. There may be from zero to as many as seven mounting series, each with an ejaculation, during a 1-hour test period; one or two ejaculations per test would be fairly usual. Between each mount, and also during the postejaculatory pause, animals usually groom each other intensively. To control for individual differences and partner preferences, an experimental animal is provided with more than one partner, and contemporaneous changes in behavior with all partners are looked for. Also, pairs are studied longitudinally and are tested day by day often for many months so that each pair can be used as its own control. Pregnancies are prevented by ligating the fallopian tubes.

1. Ovariectomy, Estrogen, and Progesterone

Sexual interactions between male rhesus monkeys and ovariectomized females decline to very low levels at varying times after ovariectomy.

Injecting females with 5–10 μg of estradiol daily restores male sexual activity in about 3 days, and mounting behavior with ejaculations reappears. Estrogen treatment of the female thus restores the attractiveness (and also the receptivity) that is lacking in long-ovariectomized females (Michael *et al.*, 1967a). When females are treated, in addition, with large doses of progesterone, both the number of mounts and ejaculations made by their male partners decline (Fig. 2) (Michael *et al.*, 1967c); this closely parallels the behavioral situation seen during the early part of the luteal phase when females are intact (Michael, 1968). The effects of progesterone on behavior are extremely interesting because two separate mechanisms are responsible for its depressing effect on sexual activity. The first depends on its action in decreasing female receptivity, which is observed

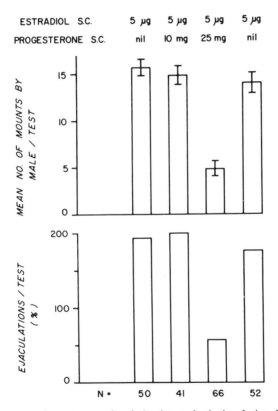

FIG. 2. The suppression of mounting behavior and of ejaculation in male rhesus monkeys when their ovariectomized, estrogen-treated female partners were treated with progesterone. N = number of tests. When values exceed 100%, more than one ejaculation occurred in each test. Vertical bars give standard errors of means (6 pairs). From Michael *et al.* (1968), with permission.

as an increase in the number of female refusals of the male's mounting
attempts. The second depends on its action in decreasing female attractiveness, which is observed as a decline in the number of mounting
attempts made by males: this latter effect is evident only in certain pairs.
Figure 3 shows that a high dose of progesterone results in a dramatic
decline in the number of mounts, and this is due, principally, to a decline
in male mounting attempts, not to a change in female refusals whose
increase is small and nonsignificant (Michael *et al.*, 1968). Since the
male's motivation to approach and mount the female was diminished, this
suggested that some form of distance communication might be operating
in these particular pairs.

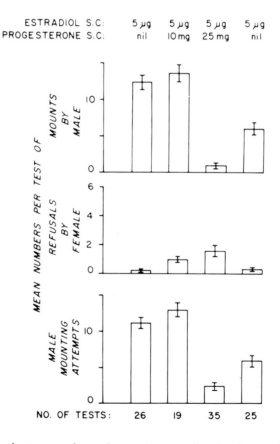

Fɪɢ. 3. High subcutaneous doses of progesterone to females depress the number of
mounts made by males due to decreased numbers of mounting attempts, reflecting
the loss of male interest (3 pairs). Vertical bars give standard errors of means. From
Michael *et al.* (1968), with permission.

2. *Intravaginal Estrogen*

The above experiments certainly do not exclude the role of tactile communication (since animals had contact) nor do they differentiate between visual and olfactory signals. Because the male's olfactory investigation is generally directed at the female's perineum (Fig. 4), it was decided to compare the effects of administering estrogen (1) locally to the vagina, (2) locally to the sexual skin, and (3) systemically by subcutaneous injection. With increasing intravaginal dose rates, graded changes occurred in several behavioral indices, suggesting increasing systemic absorption of estrogen from the vagina. However, this alone could not account for the stimulating effect on male mounting attempts of the 5-μg intravaginal dose, since the effect was significantly greater than the same dose administered subcutaneously (Fig. 5). The sexual invitations of females were not significantly increased by intravaginal estrogen, and therefore the increased sexual interest of males could not easily be attributed to a change in the receptivity of females or in their sexual displays. No changes in the males' behavior were observed when estrogen (2.5 μg per day) was applied directly to the females' sexual skins although they assumed a bright red coloration. From these and other data, it is

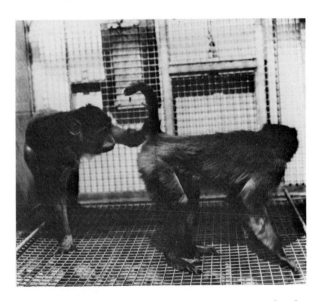

FIG. 4. Olfactory examination of a female rhesus monkey's rear by the male during a test. The male has seized the female by the tail and pulled her toward him. Note the male's facial expression and protruding lips (cf. "Flehmen" face—van Hooff, 1962). From Keverne and Michael (1971), with permission.

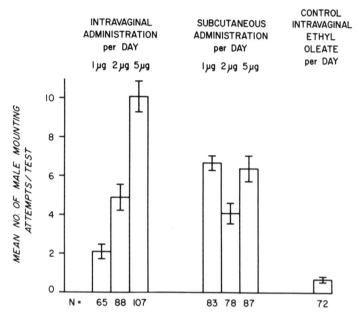

Fig. 5. Comparison of the effects of intravaginal and subcutaneous administration of estrogen to female rhesus monkeys. A graded increase in male mounting attempts occurred with increasing intravaginal dosage, and the 5-μg dose produced a greater effect than the same dose given subcutaneously. N = number of tests. Vertical bars give standard errors. From Michael and Saayman (1968), with permission.

concluded that the sexual skin does not provide a major visual signal in this species (Michael and Saayman, 1968; Dixson *et al.*, 1973; Saayman, 1973; Czaja *et al.*, 1975). Thus, an estrogen-dependent change locally in the vagina appeared to be exerting a stimulating effect on males, and this could have been due either to an olfactory cue or to a tactile one, namely, a change in the quality of the vaginal stimulation of the penis. The demonstration that odors were involved required experiments in which males were both deprived of the tactile information and rendered reversibly anosmic.

C. Olfactory Perception of the Female's Endocrine Status

1. Stimulating Effect of Estrogen

It is necessary, first, to describe briefly our use of operant conditioning procedures. Adult male rhesus monkeys of known sexual potency are first trained to press a lever for food reward on a fixed-ratio schedule in a free-cage situation. When high rates of pressing are consistently achieved, animals are transferred to a large twin-compartment cage equipped with a lifting partition. Operating the lever at least 250 times activates a servomotor that raises the partition giving access to the other side. Initially, the reinforcement is food and, when males are thoroughly familiar with the situation, the reinforcement is a female rhesus monkey. The male is free to press or not, entirely as he feels inclined, and there are no shocks, punishments, or signals of any kind to shape his behavior. The work task is fairly severe, and some males are required to press rapidly up to 600 times to obtain access to the female for a 1-hour period, during which the behavioral interactions are scored. Thirty minutes are allowed for pressing to criterion. If this is not reached, the animals are returned to their home cages, and a few hours later on the same day they are brought together for a 1-hour mating test in a nonoperant situation; in this way, behavioral data are obtained for those days when the operant task is not completed. Each male was paired with three ovariectomized females, and one of these (the control) received estradiol, 10 μg s.c. per day throughout. The other two partners were initially untreated. Males will press regularly for access to estrogen-treated females but do so only intermittently or not at all for long-ovariectomized, untreated ones. This demonstrates that males are prepared to work more consistently for estrogenized than for nonestrogenized partners. Males can be rendered anosmic by plugging the nasal olfactory area with strips of gauze impregnated with bismuth–iodoform–paraffin paste and by cutting the nerve supply to the organ of Jacobson. These gauze plugs can be inserted forcibly above the superior turbinate bones so as to prevent olfaction but leave a clear nasal airway permitting animals to breathe normally (Michael and Keverne, 1968). Earlier experiments with intravaginal estrogen, quoted above, demonstrated that the administration of 5 μg by this route would increase male interest in females after a latency of about 15 days without altering the female's invitational behavior. This treatment was therefore used in these experiments in which males were also made anosmic by the insertion of nasal plugs (Fig. 6, upper and lower left). The two anosmic males illustrated here continued to behave toward the experimental females as though they had not received any estrogen treatment, but continued pressing much as previously for the control females (not illustrated). The sexual behavior observed during the separately conducted mating tests on days when the male failed to press revealed an absence of sexual interest and interaction with experimental females. However, between 5 and 8 days after removal of the nasal plugs, males commenced lever pressing for access to, and started mounting and ejaculating with, experimental females receiving intravaginal estrogen. This time interval is the same

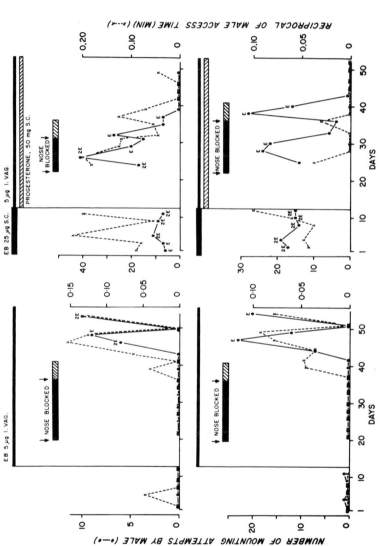

Fig. 6. *Upper and lower left:* Anosmic males fail to respond (increased lever-pressing and mounting attempts) to intravaginal estrogen treatment of their ovariectomized partners until their olfactory acuity returns. *Upper and lower right:* Anosmic males fail to respond (decreased lever-pressing and mounting attempts) to progesterone treatment of their ovariectomized, estrogen-treated partners until their olfactory acuity returns. The recovery period is indicated by the hatched area of the bar after removal of the nasal plugs. Hormone treatments of females in lower graphs are identical to those in upper graphs. E = ejaculation.

as that required for the restoration of olfaction in similarly treated human subjects, and the periods during which olfactory acuity was returning are indicated in Fig. 6 as hatched bars after the nasal plugs were removed. These results indicated that the perception by males of an altered endocrine status of females depended upon an olfactory signal under conditions where there were no changes in visual stimuli. These results have been confirmed in 8 of 10 pairs that have been similarly investigated. We should emphasize that to demonstrate an olfactory signal it was necessary to commence behavioral tests with females in an unattractive, unreceptive condition. The behavior of males with fully estrogenized, control females demonstrated that simply rendering males anosmic would not block their sexual interest in females that they had been successfully mating with immediately previously; the memory of a rewarding past experience was an overriding one.

2. Inhibiting Effect of Progesterone

The results reported in Section II, B, 1 implicated progesterone in the decline in sexual activity occurring during the luteal phase of the menstrual cycle. To demonstrate its adverse effect on the males' behavior in a lever-pressing situation, ovariectomized females were first made attractive by the administration of estrogen intravaginally so that males pressed for access, mounted, and ejaculated regularly. After 14 days of this treatment, females were given in addition large doses of progesterone subcutaneously. In all cases, there were brisk declines in both operant and sexual activity to zero levels (Fig. 7), an effect that could then be reversed by stopping progesterone and starting subcutaneous estrogen treatment. It was obviously of interest to ascertain what role, if any, olfactory communication might play in mediating this effect. Ovariectomized females were therefore first treated with estrogen subcutaneously to make them attractive and receptive, and were then given large doses of progesterone subcutaneously as previously. However, in these experiments, the noses of the males were blocked during the progesterone treatment (Fig. 6, upper and lower right) and, at the time the males' behavior would have been expected to decline to zero levels (Fig. 7), they continued lever-pressing for access to the progesterone-treated females. Furthermore, they mounted and ejaculated despite the females' lack of receptivity, indicated by the high numbers of their refusals. When the nasal plugs were removed, however, lever-pressing and sexual behavior declined to zero levels as olfactory acuity returned. The simplest explanation of these results is that anosmic males fail to detect a negative olfactory signal emanating from progesterone-treated females.

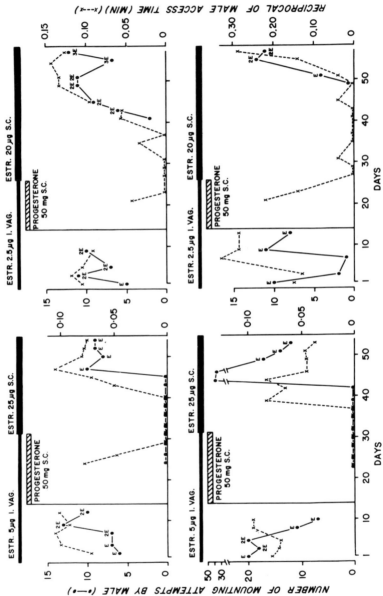

Fig. 7. Inhibitory effect of progesterone (4 pairs). Females first made attractive by estrogen (ESTR.) administration were then treated with progesterone, and there were brisk declines in both the lever-pressing and sexual behavior of their male partners. This effect was reversed by stopping progesterone and increasing the estrogen treatment.

D. Behavioral Effects of Rhesus Monkey Vaginal Secretions

Since olfactory examination of the female's perineum by the male and the behavioral effects of intravaginal estrogen were so striking, we commenced a study of the behavioral effects of vaginal secretions. Secretions were collected by pipette from estrogen-treated donors and then applied to the sexual skin area of long-ovariectomized, recipient females. Males were then given 1-hour mating tests with recipient females in an operant situation (Michael and Keverne, 1969). Males worked consistently for access to, and mated with, control, estrogen-treated females (not illustrated) throughout the 125 days of study. Figure 8 shows that there were very low levels of sexual activity with ovariectomized, untreated female partners (4 ejaculations in 50 tests), and also that the local application of estradiol to the sexual skin was without any consistent effects on the males' behavior (1 ejaculation and one masturbation in 52 tests), although an

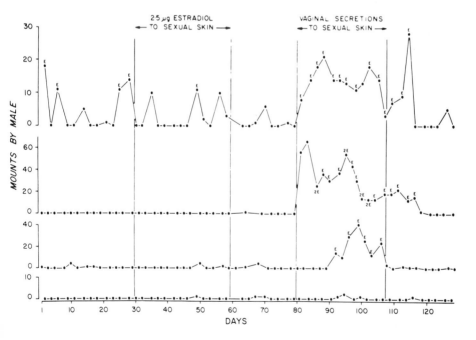

Fig. 8. Effects on the males' mounting and ejaculations of giving their untreated ovariectomized female partners (1) applications of estradiol to the sexual skin, and (2) applications of vaginal secretions collected from estrogen-treated donors. The latter treatment alone increased the males' sexual behavior. E = ejaculation. From Michael and Keverne (1970), with permission.

intense red coloration was produced. Control applications of vaginal secretions from untreated females were regarded as unnecessary, since females provided their own. However, when vaginal secretions collected from an estrogen-treated donor were applied, there was an increase in mounting and ejaculation in three of the four pairs (32 ejaculations in 37 tests), but no effect in the fourth pair. We were careful not to introduce secretions into the recipient's vagina (to avoid changing its stimulatory properties), but rubbed them onto the area of the sexual skin. Since recipient females had been generally unattractive and unreceptive to males for a total of 131 tests conducted over the previous 11 weeks, the immediate onset of lever-pressing and mounting activity in two of the pairs when secretions were applied was a striking effect (Michael and Keverne, 1970), and it certainly encouraged us to pursue the identification of chemical attractants (pheromones) in this material. The stimulation of sexual activity of male rhesus monkeys by the application of estrogen-stimulated secretions to the sexual skin of their partners is shown in Fig. 9 (11 pairs, 449 tests).

Vaginal secretions were next collected from estrogen-treated donor females by lavage with a vaginal pipette containing 1 ml of distilled water. After buffering at pH 4.5 with sodium dihydrogen phosphate, samples were extracted with 2 ml of diethyl ether. Two to three minutes before a behavioral test, a recipient female was trapped in a net and the 2 ml of ether extract were applied to the sexual skin. Thus, the ether-soluble material present in a single vaginal washing from a donor female was transferred to the sexual skin of a recipient. Diethyl ether alone was applied in the same way before tests during the pretreatment period for control purposes.

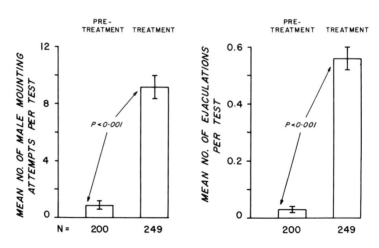

FIG. 9. Illustrating the marked stimulation of male mounting attempts and ejaculations by applying vaginal secretions collected from estrogen-treated donors to the sexual skin of their ovariectomized female partners (11 pairs, 449 tests).

The results for all 5 pairs studied are shown in Fig. 10. There were highly significant ($P < 0.001$) increases in mounting attempts, in ejaculations, and in male grooming times during treatments of recipient females with ether extracts (Keverne and Michael, 1971). It was noticeable that the "on" effects were generally abrupt while the "off" effects of withdrawing the treatment were much less so. As primates have a good memory, we attributed this difference to the influence of past experience and to the reinforcing effect on subsequent behavior of a previously rewarding consummatory event. However, it should be emphasized that there could scarcely have been more rigorous test conditions for assessing the behavioral effects of these ether extracts because females, which had been ovariectomized more than 6 months previously, were totally unreceptive and made large numbers of refusals throughout. We concluded from these results that a major portion of the behavioral activity in estrogen-stimulated vaginal secretions was ether-soluble.

III. Identification of Behaviorally Active Chemicals in Vaginal Secretions

A. Behavioral Effects of Separated Fractions of Vaginal Secretions

The behavioral assay described above was used to test for sex-attractant activity in fractions of vaginal secretions separated by conventional liquid- and gas-phase techniques. The acidic nature of the behaviorally

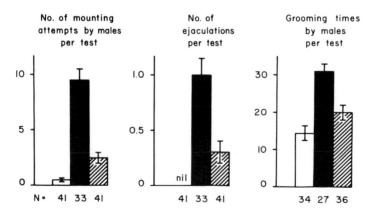

Fig. 10. Behavioral effects of ether extracts of estrogen-stimulated vaginal secretions. When these were applied to ovariectomized recipient females, there were highly significant increases in mounting attempts, ejaculations, and grooming activity by their male partners. White columns = pretreatment; black columns = during treatment; hatched columns = after withdrawal of treatment; N = number of tests. Vertical bars give standard errors. From Keverne and Michael (1971).

active constituents of the ether extracts was demonstrated by treating them with 2 ml of aqueous 0.01 N sodium hydroxide, acidifying the aqueous layer and reextracting it with ether. This second extract retained behavioral activity; a result that suggested the active constituents were acidic because ether-soluble neutral and basic components, for example, all but phenolic steroids, were removed by this procedure. Further fractionation of the acidic components was obtained by ion-exchange chromatography. The ether extracts of 40 vaginal secretions were combined and washed with 5 ml of 0.01 N sodium hydroxide. The alkaline layer was titrated to pH 7.4 and eluted through a 10 × 150 mm column of DEAE-cellulose (Whatman DE-52) with 50 mM pH 7.4 sodium phosphate buffer. The eluate was continuously monitored for ultraviolet absorbance at 280 nm and was collected in 2-ml fractions. Fractions were combined according to their elution volume relative to that of a strongly absorbing phenolic component, acidified with hydrochloric acid, and extracted into ether for behavioral testing (Fig. 11). The fractions containing the phenolic com-

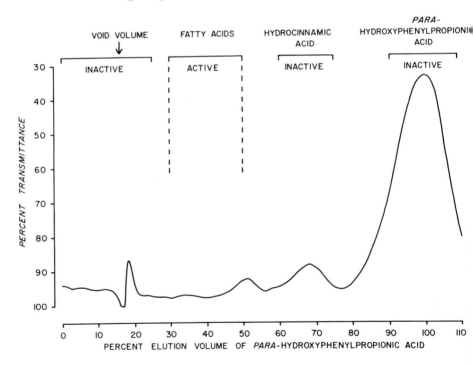

FIG. 11. Elution profile at 280 nm on DEAE-cellulose of alkaline reextracts of vaginal secretions from ovariectomized, estrogen-treated rhesus monkeys. The fractions were tested for behavioral activity; that containing fatty acids was found to be active and was subjected to further analysis by gas chromatography and mass spectrometry. From Curtis et al. (1971), with permission.

ponent had no effect on the male when applied to the recipient female, nor did either the void volume fraction or fractions containing a sweet-smelling component eluted at 60–75% of the elution volume of the phenolic component. The phenolic component and the sweet-smelling substance were methylated and identified by mass spectrometry as p-hydroxyphenylpropionic acid (HPPA) and phenylpropionic acid (hydrocinnamic acid, HCA). The only components that were sufficient in themselves to stimulate the sexual activity of the male in the behavioral assay were eluted at 30–50% of the elution volume of HPPA. In 12 pretreatment tests when ether alone was applied, there were 6 mounting attempts and no ejaculations compared with 52 mounting attempts and 12 ejaculations in the 12 tests when the fraction was applied (Curtis *et al.*, 1971). Their elution properties corresponded with those of unsubstituted monocarboxylic acids. Thus, for further fractionation by gas chromatography, column packings suitable for the analysis of free fatty acids were chosen. A Perkin-Elmer Model F11 with dual-column flame ionization detection and linear temperature programming was fitted with 3-foot × ¼-inch columns packed with 5% Carbowax 20 M-terephthalic acid on AWDMCS Chromosorb W. Gas chromatograms of ether extracts of vaginal secretions from ovariectomized donors are shown in Fig. 12. The peaks were much larger in secretions from donors who were receiving 10 μg of estradiol benzoate subcutaneously per day than in those from ovariectomized untreated donors. Peaks 1–5 were trapped from a pool of 48 secretions from estrogen-treated donors into ether cooled in Dry Ice (average recovery 62.5%) and were tested for sex-attractant activity in the behavioral assay. Figure 13 shows the effect of the trapped fraction on the sexual behavior of male rhesus monkeys when it was applied to the sexual skin of their ovariectomized, unreceptive partners. There were 10 mounting attempts but no ejaculation in 22 tests before treatment compared with 213 mounting attempts ($P < 0.001$) and 14 ejaculations ($P < 0.001$) in the 26 treatment tests (Michael *et al.*, 1971).

B. Identification of Active Components

The gas chromatographic retention times (86, 131, 152, 203, and 251 units) of the five peaks in the trapped fraction were compared with the following aliphatic acids: acetic (87 U), propanoic (131 U), methylpropanoic (152 U), butanoic (203 U), and methylbutanoic (251 U), and a synthetic mixture of these acids coinjected with some of the natural extract showed no difference between the two. Preparative gas chromatography and mass spectrometry were used to confirm these identifications. The chromatographic effluent corresponding to each of the five peaks was trapped in a U tube at −70°C and transferred to the direct insertion probe

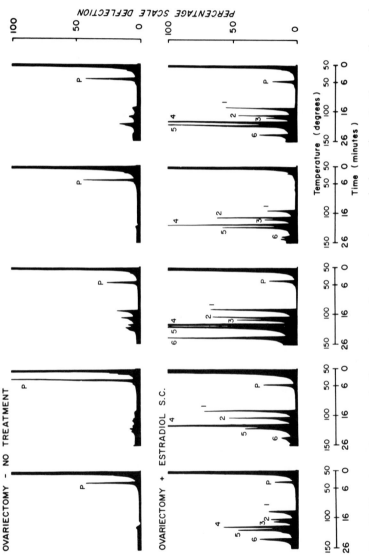

FIG. 12. Gas chromatograms of ether extracts of rhesus monkey vaginal secretions. In the secretions collected from five ovariectomized, untreated females, the volatile acid content was low (top set). In the secretion collected from five ovariectomized females during treatment with estradiol (bottom set), the volatile acid content showed an 8-fold increase. The right-hand chromatograms (top and bottom) are from the same animal before and during treatment with estradiol. Peak P, after the solvent front, is authentic n-pentanol added to the extracting ether as a concentration marker. Peaks 1–6 are aliphatic acids. From Michael et al. (1971), with permission. Copyright 1971 by the American Association for the Advancement of Science.

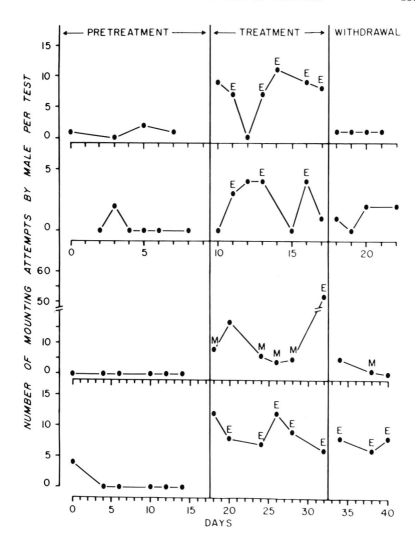

Fɪɢ. 13. Shows the effect of fractions trapped from the gas chromatograph on the sexual behavior of male rhesus monkeys when they were applied to the sexual skin of their ovariectomized, unreceptive partners. E = ejaculation. M = masturbation to ejaculation. From Michael *et al.* (1971), with permission. Copyright 1971 by the American Association for the Advancement of Science.

of an AEI-MS9 mass spectrometer. The spectra so obtained were identical
to those of authentic acids trapped by the same method. A mixture of
these acids was then made up to match the concentrations present in a pool
of 24 ether extracts of vaginal secretions collected from three ovariectomized donors treated with estrogen. The mixture contained 9.2 μg of acetic,
8.8 μg of propanoic, 4.2 μg of methylpropanoic, 12.2 μg of butanoic, and
8.3 μg of methylbutanoic acids per 1 ml of ether. Two milliliters of this
mixture, the approximate equivalent of 1.5 secretions, were applied to the
sexual skin of an ovariectomized female and tested with three males for
sex-attractant activity (Fig. 14). Mounting attempts increased from 15
during 19 tests when ether alone was applied to 170 in 16 tests when the

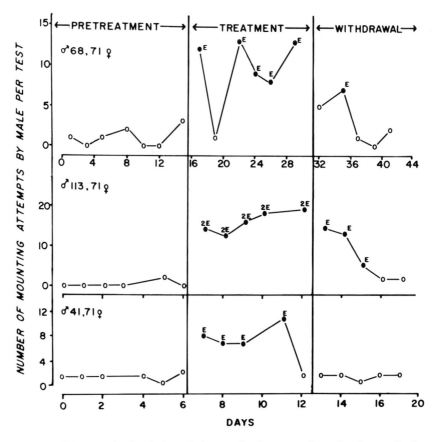

Fig. 14. The sexual stimulation of three male rhesus monkeys by the application
of a synthetic mixture of authentic fatty acids to the sexual skin of an ovariectomized,
recipient female: a significant increase in mounting activity and in ejaculations occurred. E = ejaculation. From Michael *et al.* (1972), with permission.

mixture was used ($P < 0.001$): there were no ejaculations during the control period compared with 19 during tests with the mixture of authentic acids ($P < 0.001$). This confirmed our working hypothesis that the volatile fatty acids were responsible, at least in part, for the sex-attractant activity of vaginal secretions. A sixth acid, methylpentanoic acid, has now been identified in vaginal secretions: its gas chromatographic retention time was identical to that of peak 6 (Fig. 12).

A new synthetic mixture of acetic (157 μg), propanoic (43.6 μg), methylpropanoic (14.3 μg), butanoic (88.8 μg), and methylbutanoic (25.2 μg) acids in 2 ml of ether was prepared to match the concentration in a pool of secretions from three ovariectomized, estrogen-treated donors, and this has been tested in 13 pairs of rhesus monkeys made up from 7 males and 5 females. Six of the seven males showed positive responses in at least one series of applications. The mixture stimulated the males' sexual behavior with all but one of the females. None of the three males tested with this female showed any response to the synthetic mixture although they did when it was applied to other recipients. This suggested that the response of males is determined both by the sex-attractant activity of the material applied and by individual differences between females that are independent of olfactory signals: these latter, largely unknown, factors clearly influence the "sensitivity" of the assay. The multiplicity of factors determining primate sexual behavior virtually preclude a linear dose-response relationship, a problem shared with many bioassays, and valid comparisons of the activity in different samples and fractions can be attempted only on a within-pair basis. The data clearly demonstrate that the volatile fatty acids in vaginal secretions have sex-attractant properties, but the possibility certainly remains that other components are either independently active or augment the activity of the acids.

IV. Volatile Fatty Acids in Different Mammalian Species

A. Nonhuman Primates

The above findings stimulated us to search for similar substances in the vaginal secretions of other primate species. The animals were all intact and were not treated with hormone preparations. Vaginal secretions were obtained by lavage with 1 ml of water and were then either frozen until analysis or diluted with methanol to stop bacterial action. Samples in methanol were made alkaline with 0.01 N NaOH to reduce the volatility of the fatty acids and the methanol was distilled off. The remaining aqueous layer was treated in the same way as samples that had been stored frozen. Each was made acid with HCl or NaH_2PO_4 (pH < 4.5) and extracted with 2 ml of ether containing n-pentanol as a concentration marker. The ether extract was concentrated to about 50 μl by distillation and 2–4 μl of this solution was analyzed by gas chromatography (Perkin-Elmer F-11) on FFAP or Carbowax-terephthalic acid columns. Peak areas were calculated manually or by an automatic peak area integrator (Perkin-Elmer Model I), and the mass of each acid in the original extract was computed from these areas by relating them to the area of the concentration marker peak and to calibration constants determined with authentic acids processed in parallel with the samples. The minimum detection limits per secretion were about 1μg for acetic and 0.1 μg for the other acids, and the coefficient of variation was less than 20% for all acids. Figure 15 shows the amounts of the acids found in two New World (*Saimiri* and *Cebus*) and six Old World species including four macaques. The patterns of acid content seem to differ somewhat for different species, but their occurrence in primates is quite general. Although the behavioral activity of these acids has been demonstrated only in the rhesus monkey, their detection in several other primate species, together with the prevalence of genital sniffing, suggests that an investigation of chemical communication in other primates would be worthwhile.

B. HUMAN

The relationship between olfaction and human sexual behavior has long been subject to comment and speculation (Comfort, 1971), but scientific data on its significance are lacking. To develop our research in this direction we collected secretions from 28 women attending an infertility clinic at the Samaritan Hospital for Women, London. However, only two of the 28 contained acids in similar quantities to those found in a preliminary study on secretions provided by the cooperative wives of colleagues. It was possible that this difference arose because women presenting themselves at a clinic often take excessive measures to clean themselves by washing and douching. We therefore felt it necessary to study a nonclinic population of healthy women more systematically. Subjects were recruited by a female psychologist from a population of university students. Any who reported a history of gynecological disorders were excluded. The rest signed a consent form which protected their human rights and were allotted a code number to preserve their anonymity. Data on menstruation dates and use of contraceptives or vaginal deodorants were collected by the psychologist, but the design was a double-blind one, and data were not revealed to the chemists analyzing the samples until after the study had been completed.

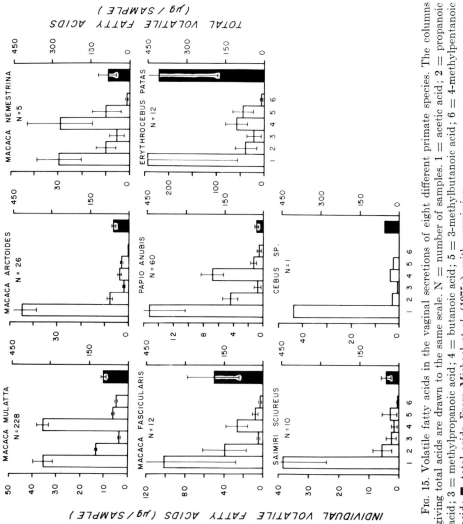

Fig. 15. Volatile fatty acids in the vaginal secretions of eight different primate species. The columns giving total acids are drawn to the same scale. N = number of samples. 1 = acetic acid; 2 = propanoic acid; 3 = methylpropanoic acid; 4 = butanoic acid; 5 = 3-methylbutanoic acid; 6 = 4-methylpentanoic acid; ■, total acids. From Michael et al. (1975a), with permission.

So that the subjects could reliably and comfortably obtain samples of their own vaginal secretions, a new collection procedure was devised. Commercial tampons were reduced to 1 cm in length, washed in hot methanol in a Soxhlet extractor for 2 hours, dried at 110°C, and hermetically sealed in polyethylene bags. This procedure removed waxes and other extractable matter that would have interfered with the chemical analysis and also protected the tampons from contamination. Each subject was given a kit containing 16 tampons and 15 numbered snap-cap bottles each containing 20 ml of methanol, and was instructed to wear a tampon for 6–8 hours on alternate days and, on removal, to drop it immediately into the bottle. The methanol both prevented bacterial action and started the extraction process. The extra tampon served as a control blank and, on receipt in the laboratory, it was processed in parallel with the samples (Fig. 16). Tampons were packed individually into glass columns and washed with methanol in chromatographic fashion. Eluates were combined with the methanol from the sample bottle, mixed with 100 μl of 0.1 N sodium hydroxide to reduce the volatility of the fatty acids, and evaporated to dryness. Residues were taken up in 1 ml of water, washed with 4 ml of ether to remove neutral and basic components, acidified (below pH 2.0), and reextracted with 4 ml of ether containing n-pentanol as a concentration marker. This solution was concentrated and analyzed in the same manner as the ether extracts of vaginal secretions obtained by lavage. The method has been extensively validated (Michael *et al.*, 1975b). Some control tampons were found to contain low levels of acetic acid only (mean $12.8 \pm 1.7 \mu$g, $N = 31$). The use of these tampons under the specified conditions had no discernible effect on the chemistry of the secretions.

All of the 47 women produced acetic acid in at least some of their samples, and only 16 of the 635 samples contained no detectable volatile fatty acids. Sixty-eight percent of the samples contained only acetic acid, and all the samples from 16 women contained only this acid. Fifty-six samples contained more than 10 μg of acids (propanoic, methylpropanoic, butanoic, methylbutanoic, and methylpentanoic) in addition to acetic, and the 14 women who produced these samples were arbitrarily designated "producers." Figure 17 shows a comparison of the mean acid profile of these samples with that of similarly selected samples from intact rhesus monkeys. The proportions of the acids were similar, but there was a higher level of acetic in the human material. However, whereas 90% of secretions from monkeys contained 10 μg or more of acids in addition to acetic, only 8.8% of samples from humans did so. Results obtained by lavage and by tampon are not strictly comparable, but our early results with lavage in the human suggest that this difference may have been due to differences

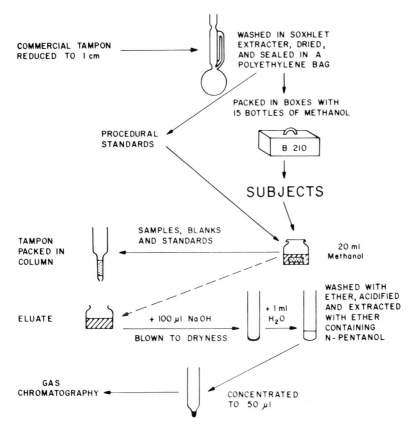

FIG. 16. New method by which human subjects can reliably and comfortably collect samples of their own vaginal secretions. The initial steps of the extraction procedure are shown (R. W. Bonsall, unpublished).

in hygiene. Using a tampon technique, comparable results on the concentrations and incidence of these acids have been obtained in women, and their identification has been confirmed by mass spectrometry (Preti and Huggins, 1975).

C. INFRAPRIMATE MAMMALS

The occurrence of these volatile fatty acids is not confined to primates or to the vagina, and they are widely distributed in nature. Thus, they have been found in the rumen of the sheep (El-Shazly, 1952a,b), in the human colon (*Homo sapiens*: Gompertz *et al.*, 1973), in the preputial gland of the pig (Patterson, 1968), and in the anal glands of the red fox

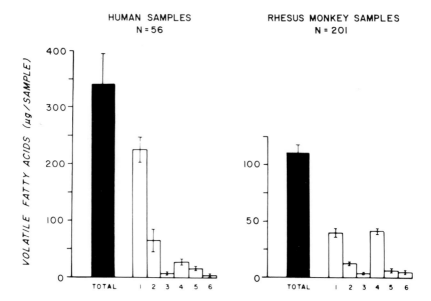

Fɪɢ. 17. Comparison of the volatile fatty acid content of vaginal secretions from women and rhesus monkeys. The overall pattern of the different acids was not dissimilar, but there were clear species differences. 1, acetic; 2, propanoic; 3, methylpropanoic; 4, butanoic; 5, methylbutanoic; 6, methylpentanoic. Vertical bars = standard errors of the means. From Michael et al. (1975b), with permission.

(*Vulpes vulpes*: Albone and Fox, 1971), mongoose (*Herpestes auropunctatus*: Gorman et al., 1974), guinea pig (Berüter et al., 1974), and cat (R. P. Michael, unpublished). Not all these reports are quantitative, but all demonstrated the presence of acetic, propanoic, methylpropanoic, butanoic, and methylbutanoic acids. Observations on the mongoose and cat have implicated the anal glands in chemical communication, but further work is required to establish whether the acids are responsible for the behavioral activity of the secretions.

V. Factors Influencing the Volatile Fatty Acid Content and
Behavioral Activity of Vaginal Secretions

A. Effect of Estradiol

Vaginal lavages obtained from ovariectomized monkeys that are not receiving hormone treatments contain very little solid matter and have barely detectable levels of volatile fatty acids (Figs. 12 and 18A). On the other hand, lavages from ovariectomized monkeys on long-term daily

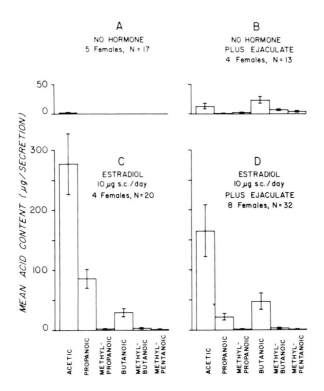

FIG. 18. The effects of estradiol and of ejaculate on volatile fatty acids in the vaginal secretions of ovariectomized rhesus monkeys. Estrogen caused a marked elevation of the acid content. Ejaculate increased the levels in untreated, but not in estrogenized, females. N = number of samples.

treatment with 10 μg of estradiol benzoate subcutaneously (Figs. 12 and 18C) contain mucus and solid debris and have elevated levels of acids. Since estrogen treatment increases the attractiveness of ovariectomized females (see above), these observations lend weight to the hypothesis that the volatile fatty acids are responsible for the sex attractant activity of the vaginal secretions. The time-course of the effect of estrogen treatment (10 μg/day) on volatile fatty acid content showed a significant increase on day 6 of treatment (Fig. 20); this coincided with an increase in the mucus content and solid debris of the secretions. However, it was not until day 17 of treatment that maximal levels were found.

B. EFFECT OF PROGESTERONE

Large doses of progesterone (25–50 mg per day) administered to ovariectomized, estrogen-treated females markedly reduced their sexual attractiveness, an effect mediated via olfactory pathways (Fig. 6, upper and lower right). Progesterone administration had a graded dose-response effect on the acid content of vaginal secretions of ovariectomized, estrogen-treated female rhesus monkeys (Fig. 19). At 2 mg per day, the progesterone was without any discernible effect; at 5 mg per day, the content of the different fatty acids was reduced more or less uniformly by 50%; and at 25 mg per day, the levels were reduced almost to those of ovariectomized, untreated females. The time-course of the progesterone effect on vaginal acids is shown in Fig. 20. A characteristic of this effect was the rapidity with which the acid content was reduced: thus, at the 25-mg dosage, levels dropped almost to zero after 28 hours of treatment. Somewhat paradoxically, the initial effect of progesterone on acid content, within 4 hours of the first treatment, was a stimulatory one: this was consistent for the four females studied, and its significance is discussed below.

Having shown that the secretions of an ovariectomized donor treated with estrogen possessed sex-attractant properties, we wished to determine whether the additional administration of progesterone would reduce them. In experiments conducted in collaboration with D. E. B. Keverne, four pairs of rhesus monkeys were studied during mating tests in an operant conditioning situation as previously described. In 32 pretreatment tests, males never lever-pressed for access to the ovariectomized, recipient females, and there were only 40 mounting attempts and one ejaculation;

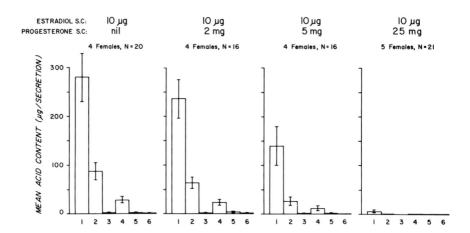

Fig. 19. The graded inhibitory effects of progesterone on the volatile fatty acids in estrogen-stimulated secretions. Secretions were collected after 17 days of estrogen and 1 day of progesterone treatment. N = number of samples. Vertical bars give standard errors. Abscissas: 1, acetic acid; 2, propranoic acid; 3, methylpropanoic acid; 4, butanoic acid; 5, methylbutanoic acid; 6, methylpentanoic acid.

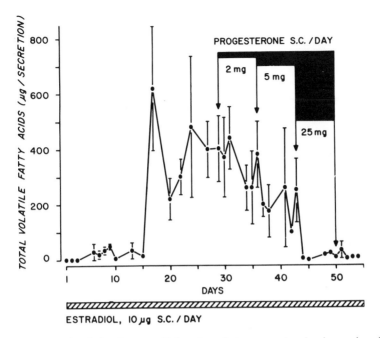

FIG. 20. The stimulation by estradiol and graded suppression by increasing doses of progesterone of the volatile fatty acid content of vaginal secretions collected from ovariectomized rhesus monkeys. Each point is the mean of 4 samples from 4 females. Vertical bars give standard errors.

these occurred in one test with one pair. In 76 treatment tests, when secretions from an estrogenized donor were applied, males lever-pressed for access on 29 occasions, made a total of 597 mounting attempts, and had 21 ejaculations (Fig. 21). When progesterone (25 mg per day) was administered to the donor female in addition to the estradiol, males stopped lever-pressing, and made only 114 mounting attempts, and one ejaculation in 40 tests. Thus, progesterone treatment completely suppressed the sex-attractant activity of the donor secretions.

C. Effect of Testosterone

While both estrogens and androgens increase female receptivity, androgens have little effect on female attractiveness (Michael, 1972). Five ovariectomized females received subcutaneous injections of 0.5 mg of testosterone propionate per day, and vaginal secretions were collected after 10 days of treatment; this dosage had previously been shown to stimulate increased female invitations. The mean ($\pm$ SE) values ($N = 10$)

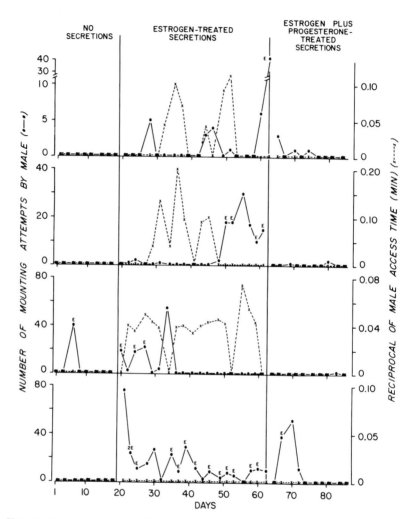

FIG. 21. The effects of estradiol (10 μg s.c. per day) and of progesterone (25 mg s.c. per day) treatments of ovariectomized donor rhesus monkeys on the sexual and operant behavior of males. Estrogen-treated secretions stimulated males, and estrogen plus progesterone-treated secretions were without effect, when applied to their ovariectomized partners (4 pairs).

of the different volatile fatty acids were as follows: acetic, 2.5 ± 1.3 μg; propanoic, 0.3 ± 0.1 μg; methylpropanoic, 0.5 ± 0.4 μg; butanoic, 3.4 ± 2.7 μg; methylbutanoic, 2.7 ± 2.1 μg; and methylpentanoic 0.4 ± 0.3 μg: this represents a minimal increase over pretreatment levels (Fig. 18). These findings are in keeping with our observations that androgen-stimulated increases in the female's sexual behavior are relatively unsuccessful in eliciting responses from males.

D. Effect of Ejaculate

Lavages from ovariectomized females receiving no hormone treatment ordinarily contain very low levels of volatile fatty acids, but lavages from recipient females used in the behavioral bioassay tests, taken after tests in which the male ejaculated, contained considerable amounts of solid matter, and some had acid levels in the range of estrogenized females. However, the mean values were considerably lower than, and the relative concentrations of the individual acids were somewhat different from, those of estrogenized females (Fig. 18B). Secretions taken from females treated with estradiol but kept in isolation from males were compared with those from similarly treated females receiving daily ejaculations (Fig. 18C and D). The total acid contents of the two groups were similar, but there were differences in the proportions of individual acids. In particular, butanoic acid was increased when ejaculate was present in both the untreated and estrogen-treated groups. The significance of these differences in composition is at present unknown, but it is possible that ejaculate could alter the female's attractiveness under a variety of conditions.

VI. Source of Sex-Attractant Acids

A. Microbiology

The volatile fatty acid content of vaginal secretions from estrogenized donors was found to increase after incubation at 37°C *in vitro*. This effect was prevented by autoclaving and by adding penicillin, but not by adding streptomycin. The acid content of autoclaved secretions could be increased by inoculation with fresh secretions, and serial inoculations of autoclaved secretions were equally effective (Bonsall and Michael, 1971; Michael *et al.*, 1972). These observations together with the characteristic shape of the incubation curve strongly suggested acid synthesis by the vaginal microflora, and that the secretions were acting as a substrate. Tryptone soya broth and other media were found to serve equally well as substrates. In an attempt to identify the organisms responsible, the following microbes were isolated from the vaginal secretions of estrogenized rhesus monkeys: *Lactobacillus delbruckii, L. bulgaricus, Staphylococcus albus, Strepto-*

coccus faecalis, Proteus mirabilis, and diphtheroid organisms (identifications were made in the Department of Bacteriology, St. Mary's Hospital, London). None of these microorganisms in pure culture was able to produce acids in tryptone soya broth in the same proportions as inocula with fresh secretions. It seemed, therefore, that either a natural mixture of the identified organisms was involved or we had failed to isolate those actually responsible. This problem needs further study.

The finding that microorganisms were necessary for the production of volatile fatty acids in vaginal secretions suggested that a similar mechanism might account for their widespread occurrence in other mammals. Some bacteriology has been conducted on the anal gland secretions of the mongoose (Gorman *et al.,* 1974), where these acids are found. All the microorganisms, *Peptococcus, Peptostreptococcus plagarumbelli, Bacillus cereus,* and unidentified Eubacteria or Catenabacteria, were capable of producing some of the acids from litmus milk medium, but only *Peptococcus* synthesized all of them. It seems likely, therefore, that many bacteria may be involved in acid synthesis, and that the prevailing flora of the vagina or gland may determine to some extent the proportions of acids produced. In view of these findings, the very high levels (about 20 mg) of acids reported in human vaginal secretions (Waltman *et al.,* 1973) may well be accounted for by bacterial activity occurring *in vitro* after collection.

B. Biochemistry

A biosynthetic route in bacteria for the production of volatile fatty acids from amino acids has been known for over 40 years (Stickland, 1934, 1935a,b; Nisman, 1954). The reaction, commonly called the Stickland reaction after its discoverer, involves the coupling of reductive deamination to oxidative deamination and decarboxylation of an amino acid as an anaerobic source of energy. A consequence of this is that 2 moles of the reduction product are produced for every 1 mole of the oxidation product. The classic example of this was the catabolic action of *Clostridium sporogenes* on valine to produce methylbutanoic acid (2 parts) and methylpropanoic acid (1 part). While *Clostridium* is an unlikely candidate for the production of acids in the healthy vagina, the close 1:2 relationship between the concentration of these two isoacids in different secretions and, in particular, during the primate menstrual cycle (see below) is highly suggestive of the Stickland reaction. Figure 22 shows a hypothetical scheme for the biosynthesis of acids from protein, lipid, and carbohydrate by the Stickland reaction and other anaerobic, catabolic pathways. The finding that the presence of ejaculate can change the pattern of acid production suggests that the substrate also may influence the proportions of acids present.

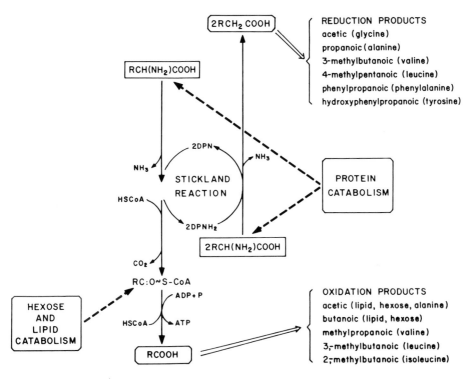

Fig. 22. Hypothetical scheme for the biosynthesis of volatile fatty acids by the Stickland reaction. Products of reductive deamination (top) preserve the carbon skeleton of the substrate (glycine, alanine, etc.) whereas the products of oxidative deamination and decarboxylation lose one carbon atom as carbon dioxide. Carbohydrate and lipid catabolites contribute to the acyl-CoA pool. All the acids listed are found in natural secretions (see text). DPN = diphosphopyridine nucleotide; other hydrogen acceptors could substitute. HSCoA, coenzyme A. From Michael *et al.* (1975b), with permission.

VII. Variations in Volatile Acid Content and in Sex-Attractant Properties of Vaginal Secretions During the Menstrual Cycle

A. Rhesus Monkey

The average volatile acid content of vaginal secretions from intact rhesus monkeys during normal menstrual cycles was within the range found in secretions from ovariectomized, estrogen-treated females. To determine whether the behavioral activity of secretions varied during the menstrual cycle, lavages from three intact monkeys were applied in sequence to ovariectomized recipient females for behavioral testing. Samples were collected daily by lavage with 1 ml of distilled water. In 42 pretreatment tests with control applications of distilled water, a total of 50 mounting attempts (MA) occurred with no ejaculations (E), whereas in 71 treatment tests with donor secretions there were 674 mounting attempts ($P < 0.001$) and 29 ejaculations. Thus, secretions from intact females had sex-attractant activity. However, the relationship between the day of the menstrual cycle when the secretions were collected and the males' response differed for each donor (Table I). Secretions from the first donor (28-day cycle) caused a marked mid-cycle increase in the males' behavior; those from the second donor (32-day cycle) caused an increase throughout all but the first part of the cycle; and those from the third donor (27-day cycle) caused both mid-cycle and late luteal stimulation.

One quarter of each of the secretions from two of the females was used for chemical analysis, and there was a clear relationship between behavioral activity and volatile fatty acid content. Because a linear dose-response effect is lacking, the data were treated by searching for a significant interaction between tests with a positive behavioral change and a set minimum volatile acid content in the secretion applied. A positive behavioral effect consisted of four or more mounting attempts per test (exceeding the pretreatment mean by one standard deviation). When the secretions applied contained less than 45 μg of acids, there were only four positive responses in 15 tests (26.7%) compared with thirty positive responses in 34 tests (88.2%) in which secretions with more than 45 μg of acids were applied. This interaction was highly significant by chi square

TABLE I

SEXUAL ACTIVITY OF VAGINAL SECRETIONS COLLECTED DURING THE MENSTRUAL CYCLES OF RHESUS MONKEYS[a]

Cycle of donor (days)		Days before menstruation of donor							
		32–29	28–25	24–21	20–17	16–13	12–9	8–5	4–1
28	MA	—	2.0	29.7	36.7	24.0	0	0.8	11.7
	E	—	0	0.33	0.67	1.0	0	0	0.33
32	MA	0	0.5	3.5	5.3	4.7	5.3	7.0	2.0
	E	0	0	0.5	1.0	0.67	0.5	1.0	0.25
27	MA	—	3.3	17.0	9.0	4.8	5.7	22.0	11.0
	E	—	0	0	0	0	0	0.5	0.25

[a] The numbers in the body of the table give mounting attempts (MA) and ejaculations (E) of males paired with recipient female rhesus monkeys to which donor secretions were applied. Each value is a mean for 2–4 tests.

testing ($P < 0.001$). Thus, the males were detecting and responding consistently when secretions contained more than 45 μg of acids, and these preliminary results provide further evidence for their physiological significance.

To obtain more definitive data on the relationship between the acid content of vaginal secretions and the phase of the menstrual cycle, five female rhesus monkeys were studied during 31 menstrual cycles. Vaginal secretions ($N = 390$) and plasma samples ($N = 492$) were collected on alternate days, except near mid-cycle when daily blood samples were drawn. Females were behaviorally tested with males throughout the period of study (results reported elsewhere). Plasma steroids (estradiol, progesterone, testosterone, and dihydrotesterone) were assayed simultaneously in duplicate on 0.5 ml of plasma samples by a method involving chromatography on Sephadex LH-20 (Bonsall and Michael, in preparation). Three-day means for estradiol and progesterone are shown with the cycles lined up on the day of the estradiol peak (day 0) (Fig. 23). The acid content of the vaginal secretions varied considerably both between females and from day to day in each female. The mean totals were high throughout the cycle and well within the range for ovariectomized estrogen-treated females. There were two acid peaks, one in the mid-follicular phase and a second, larger one, in the mid-luteal phase. Straight-chain acids, in general, followed the same pattern, but the branched-chain acids were relatively higher at the beginning of the cycle (Fig. 23). These more extensive data confirmed our original findings (Bonsall and Michael, 1971).

These findings immediately present one with a paradox, for high levels of estrogen appear to be associated with a reduction in the acid content of secretions. This contrasts with what we know about the stimulatory effect of estrogens both on the behavior of males and on the acid content of secretions when administered to ovariectomized females. One possible hypothesis to account for this emerges from a consideration of the dynamics of the system. We postulate that the concentration of acids in a secretion is determined by (1) the availability of substrate and (2) the time for which the substrate is exposed to the anaerobic activity of bacteria in the vagina. Thus, in the ovariectomized, untreated female the availability of suitable substrate will be the limiting factor in the amounts of acids produced. In intact females, however, secretions contain cell debris and other solid matter throughout the menstrual cycle, especially when ejaculate is present. With excess substrate, the acid content of the lavage will be determined solely by the time the secretion has been exposed to bacterial degradation. Fluid secretions such as occur at midcycle, passing more rapidly through the vagina, will prevent an accumulation of acids within the vagina, but present a much larger amount externally for the male's detection. Thus, a

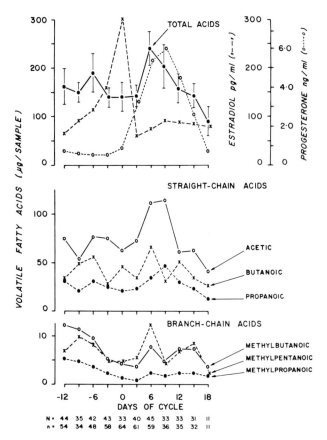

Fig. 23. Simultaneous determinations of volatile fatty acids in vaginal secretions, and estradiol and progesterone in plasma samples, from 5 female rhesus monkeys during 31 menstrual cycles. The data are lined up on the day of the estradiol peak (day 0) and calculated as 3-day means. N = number of vaginal secretions, n = number of plasma samples, and vertical bars (total acids) give standard errors.

negative relationship between the content of acids in the vagina (and in the lavage) and the vapor concentration available for detection may hold: the analogy would be between a single plasma determination and a production rate. This hypothesis can offer an explanation for an effect of progesterone in sometimes initially stimulating the acid content of lavages (Fig. 20). When substrate production is abruptly halted and the flow properties of the secretion are suddenly reduced, bacterial action will increase the acid content of the next lavage. The hypothesis predicts that, at mid-cycle, the vapor concentration of acids available to the male will be increased despite reduced vaginal content, and this possibility needs to be tested experimentally.

The specialized area of sexual skin, which is a morphological feature of several macaque and baboon species that also show the quadrupedal presentation posture, becomes reddened and hotter under the influence of estrogen. These primate species therefore possess an excellent radiating surface for maximizing the volatilization of airborne chemical signals; the relation between posture and olfaction has been considered by Andrew (1964).

B. Anubis Baboon

Two mature female baboons were used as donors of vaginal secretions during six menstrual cycles. Lavages were collected with 1 ml of distilled water, as with the rhesus monkey, using a longer pipette to allow full insertion into the vagina during sexual swelling. One of the baboons would present sexually at the front of her cage when the sex skin was swollen to facilitate collection of secretions but needed restraint after detumescence. Secretions collected during three of the cycles were analyzed for volatile acids, and these are shown in Fig. 24. As with the rhesus monkey, the acid content showed considerable day-to-day variability, but the relationship to the phase of the cycle was much clearer than in the rhesus. Most of the

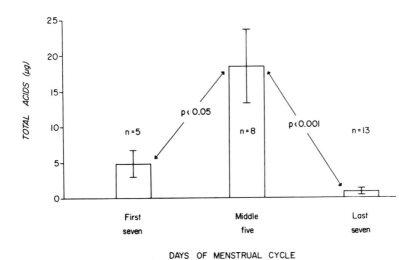

Fig. 24. Changes in the volatile fatty acid content of vaginal secretions throughout the course of three menstrual cycles of anubis baboons (*Papio anubis*). There was a significant increase in total acids in the 5 days immediately before deflation of the sexual skin as compared with the periods immediately after and immediately before the first day of menstruation. n = number of samples. Vertical bars give standard errors. From Michael *et al.* (1972), with permission.

secretions with low acid levels were confined to the early and late stages of the cycle.

Secretions collected during the other three baboon cycles were tested for their sex-attractant properties using 4 pairs of rhesus monkeys. Application of the baboon secretions to recipient rhesus females, in the same sequence they were collected, markedly stimulated the sexual activity of the male rhesus partners. Mounting attempts by males were few in tests before treatment (14 in 35 tests), and no ejaculations occurred. During tests when baboon secretions were applied, mounting attempts by the males increased (363 in 68 tests) ($P < 0.001$), and there were 19 ejaculations ($P < 0.001$). Furthermore, most of the sexual activity of the male rhesus monkeys occurred during the mid-cycle period of the donors when their sexual skin swelling was maximal. Thus, transfer of vaginal secretions from the intact baboon to the ovariectomized rhesus monkey stimulated the male rhesus monkey's sexual behavior in a cyclic manner that reflected the pattern of fatty acid content of baboon secretions during the menstrual cycle. Field studies have suggested that olfactory cues are important in the reproductive behavior of baboons (Saayman, 1971), and the presence of fatty acids in vaginal secretions may be relevant in this regard. Cross-species sexual behavior has long been observed in the laboratory (Hamilton, 1914) and occurs in the wild. There are hybrids among macaques (Chiarelli, 1968) and baboons (Maples and McKern, 1967; Kummer, 1968), and between *Hylobates moloch* and *Symphalangus syndactylus* (D. Shafer, personal communication). A pheromone system common to several primates could even explain the sexual interest between species as widely divergent as the baboon and the chimpanzee (van Lawick-Goodall, 1968).

C. HUMAN

Figure 25 (top graph) shows the volatile fatty acid content of the samples collected from 47 human subjects by the tampon method described above (Section IV, B). Data are arranged according to successive 3-day periods of the menstrual cycle (day 1 being the first day of menstruation). Samples showed high levels of volatile fatty acids in the second quarter, and a progressive decline during the second half of the cycle. This variation was statistically significant ($P < 0.02$) (Michael et al., 1975b; Michael, 1975), but most of it could be attributed to the subgroup of women who produced samples containing more than 10 μg of acids other than acetic. These women were termed "producers." Acetic acid was present in relatively large amounts throughout the menstrual cycle, but showed the smallest proportional variation of the individual acids. The contribution made by the C_3–C_6 acids to the mid-cycle increase in total content is shown by the hatched area (Fig. 25). Acetic acid has a relatively high olfactory detection threshold in humans compared with the less volatile, branched-chain fatty acids (Amoore, 1970). Thus, the greatest variation in content during the menstrual cycle was shown by the more odoriferous C_3–C_6 acids and in women who produced them in relatively large amounts (Fig. 25).

Fifteen of the subjects in this study were using oral contraceptives, mostly of the combined estrogen–progestagen type, when samples were being provided. This fact was unknown at the time of analysis. Samples

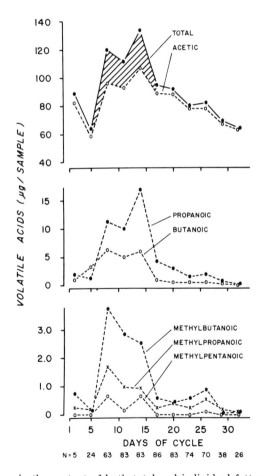

FIG. 25. Changes in the content of both total and individual fatty acids in vaginal secretions in successive 3-day periods of the cycles of 47 women. Hatched area (top graph) shows the contribution of acids other than acetic to the increase near mid-cycle. N = number of samples. From Michael *et al.* (1975b), with permission.

from these subjects had a lower mean volatile fatty acid content than the others (Michael *et al.*, 1974) and showed no significant rhythmic variation in content during the menstrual cycle (Fig. 26).

A clear distinction should be made between the quantitative results obtained by lavage and those obtained by tampon: a single vaginal washing reflects only the acids contained in the vagina at the moment of collection, but exposure of a tampon to vaginal fluids for 6 hours provides a measure of the total production during that period. Secretions collected by lavage from rhesus monkeys during the menstrual cycle showed two peaks, but secretions collected by tampon from women had only one peak at mid-cycle. If our hypothesis on the dynamics of acid production is correct, and rhesus monkeys and humans have similar patterns of acid production during the menstrual cycle, then the single mid-cycle peak would be predicted with this tampon method.

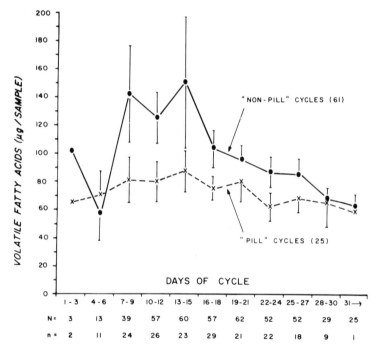

FIG. 26. Changes in the content of volatile fatty acids in secretions from women using oral contraceptives and from women with normal cycles arranged according to successive 3-day periods of the menstrual cycle. The rise before mid-cycle was abolished in women taking oral contraceptives. N = number of "nonpill" samples. n = number of "pill" samples. Vertical bars give standard errors. From Michael *et al.* (1974), with permission. Copyright 1974 by the American Association for the Advancement of Science.

Volatile fatty acids are generally regarded as unpleasant when present in a test tube, and certainly do not possess the qualities normally associated with perfumes. However, in recent studies (Doty *et al.*, 1975) in which an assessment was made by a panel of testers of the "pleasantness" and intensity of the odors of human vaginal secretions collected on tampons, those collected near the time of ovulation were generally regarded as least unpleasant or intense. The relationship between these data and ours on volatile fatty acid content is unclear, but without doubt many other compounds, both identified and unidentified (Preti and Huggins, 1975), contribute to the odor of human vaginal secretions. Women producers have a mechanism regulating the amount of volatile acids in their vaginal secretions, and the levels of these increased at a time when mating would be most likely to have a fertile outcome. In contrast, the nonfertile cycles of women taking oral contraceptives did not show these changes. In a clinical trial of 62 couples (N. Morris and R. Udry, personal communication), the twelve couples who exhibited a cyclic pattern of sexual behavior during the menstrual cycle also showed an increased frequency of sexual intercourse ($P < 0.01$) when a mixture of volatile fatty acids, instead of control substances (perfume or alcohol), was applied to the woman. They concluded that their data did not reject the hypothesis that an olfactory signal influenced the desire of some men for coitus. Thus, if chemical communication is a factor in human sexuality, its role clearly varies from couple to couple. The question should be asked whether or not, in the human, an olfactory mechanism is a vestigial one that has been so diluted by social factors, learning and experience, as to become of minor importance. In the present state of knowledge, we still lack unequivocal evidence for olfactory communication of sexual status in the human.

VIII. Summary

We have reviewed some of the extensive literature documenting the importance of olfaction in the life of numerous primate species under natural conditions. The emission and reception of olfactory signals is clearly apparent from the observation of their behavior patterns. Our own research in the rhesus monkey under laboratory conditions has led us to the view that the male receives information about the hormonal status of his female partner via olfactory pathways. Males made temporarily anosmic failed to detect increases in the attractive properties of their partners, but did so when their olfactory acuity returned. Similarly, males were unaware of the decline in the attractive properties of their female partners, due to the administration of progesterone, when anosmic, but immediately became aware of their changed hormonal condition when their olfactory acuity returned. To demonstrate the role of olfactory mechanisms in the behavioral interactions of the pair, it was necessary to conduct experiments to exclude the role of visual signals (sexual displays, and changes in sexual skin coloration), and also to exclude the role of afferent (tactile) stimulation. Nevertheless, mating activity can proceed normally in anosmic males with prior experience of receptive females. All sensory modalities no doubt contribute importantly to sexual arousal in primates.

The olfactory signal appeared to be present in the vaginal secretions of estrogen-treated females. The behaviorally active components were extractable into ether and had acidic properties: they were identified by gas chromatography and mass spectrometry as a series of volatile, short-chain aliphatic acids. For convenience, we have called them copulins. The same compounds have been found in the vaginal secretions of seven other species of New and Old World primates, and in the human female. In ovariectomized rhesus monkeys, levels of acids were very low, but they increased 8-fold with estrogen treatment. Progesterone, on the other hand, rapidly suppressed the acid content of secretions, and this was associated with a loss of their attractant properties when they were tested for behavioral activity. Vaginal secretions contaminated with ejaculate sometimes showed an increased acid content and a changed proportion of the individual acids, probably because it acted as a substrate for the microflora known to synthesize these acids. A biosynthetic pathway, involving the Stickland reaction and other anaerobic, catabolic processes, has been proposed for their production. The acid content of vaginal lavages from rhesus monkeys showed two peaks during the menstrual cycle, one in the follicular phase and the other in the luteal phase. However, at the time of the plasma estradiol peak, when sexual activity is normally high, there was a dip in the acid content of secretions. We hypothesize that the increased fluidity and volume of secretions at mid-cycle prevents accumulation of acids in the vagina and maximizes the amounts carried externally for the male's detection. In anubis baboons, however, which possess a large sexual skin swelling at mid-cycle, the acid content of secretions showed a maximum at this time. When baboon secretions were collected sequentially during the cycle and then applied to ovariectomized rhesus females, the rhesus males paired with them also showed maximal sexual activity during the mid-cycle phase of the baboon females. Vaginal secretions collected from healthy women by a tampon methed, which gave an indication of production rates rather than a measure of acid content, also showed a mid-cycle peak of volatile acids. A small subgroup of these women, termed "producers," were mainly responsible for the cyclic changes of the group. Another subgroup of women taking oral contraceptives showed no significant variations during the menstrual cycle. There is no direct evidence that copulins serve as sex-attractants in the human, but some women possess a mechanism for increasing the content of odoriferous compounds in their secretions at the time of maximum fertility, and other, as yet unidentified, compounds may well be involved.

ACKNOWLEDGMENTS

The work described here was supported by grants from the Medical Research Council (U.K.), the Foundations' Fund for Research in Psychiatry, the Population Council, the Grant Foundation and Grant MH 19506, U.S. Public Health Service. We also wish to acknowledge the support of the Georgia Department of Human Resources.

REFERENCES

Albone, E. S., and Fox, M. W. (1971). *Nature (London)* **233**, 569.

Altmann, S. A. (1959). *J. Mammal.* **40**, 317.

Altmann, S. A. (1962). *Ann. N.Y. Acad. Sci.* **102**, 338.

Amoore, J. E. (1970). "Molecular Basis of Odor." Thomas, Springfield, Illinois.

Andrew, R. J. (1964). *In* "Evolutionary and Genetic Biology of Primates" (J. Buettner-Janusch, ed.), Vol. 2, p. 227. Academic Press, New York.

Baldwin, J. D. (1970). *Primates* **11**, 317.

Ball, J., and Hartman, C. G. (1935). *Am. J. Obstet. Gynecol.* **29**, 117.

Barfield, R. J. (1965). *Am. Zool.* **5**, 203.

Barfield, R. J. (1971). *Endocrinology* **89**, 1470.

Bernstein, I. S. (1965). *Folia Primatol.* **3**, 211.

Bernstein, I. S. (1967). *Primates* **8**, 217.

Berüter, J., Beauchamp, G. K., and Muetterties, E. L. (1974). *Physiol. Zool.* **47**, 130.

Bielert, C., Czaja, J. A., Eisele, S., Scheffler, G., Robinson, J. A., and Goy, R. W. (1976). *J. Reprod. Fertil.* **46**, 179.

Bonsall, R. W., and Michael, R. P. (1971). *J. Reprod. Fertil.* **27**, 478.

Boulière, F., Petter, J. J., and Petter-Rousseaux, A. (1956). *Mem. Inst. Sci. Madagascar, Ser. A* **10**, 299.

Bunting, H., Wislocki, G. B., and Dempsey, E. W. (1948). *Anat. Rec.* **100**, 61.

Carpenter, C. R. (1934). *Comp. Psychol. Monogr.* **10**, 1.

Carpenter, C. R. (1942). *J. Comp. Psychol.* **33**, 113.

Chevalier-Skolnikoff, S. (1974). *Arch. Sex. Behav.* **3**, 95.

Chiarelli, B. (1968). *Cytologia* **33**, 1.

Ciaccio, L. A., and Lisk, R. D. (1973). *Neuroendocrinology* **13**, 21.

Comfort, A. (1971). *Nature (London)* **230**, 432.

Conaway, C. H., and Sorenson, M. W. (1966). *Symp. Zool. Soc. London* **15**, 471.

Cowgill, U. M. (1969). *Folia Primatol.* **11**, 144.

Curtis, R. F., Ballantine, J. A., Keverne, E. B., Bonsall, R. W., and Michael, R. P. (1971). *Nature (London)* **232**, 396.

Czaja, J. A., Eisele, S. G., and Goy, R. W. (1975). *Fed. Proc., Fed. Am. Soc. Exp. Biol.* **34**, 1680.

Davidson, J. M. (1966). *Endocrinology* **79**, 783.

Dixson, A. F., Everitt, B. J., Herbert, J., Rugman, S. M., and Scruton, D. M. (1973). *Symp. Int. Congr. Primatol., 4th, 1972,* Vol. 2, p. 36.

184   RICHARD P. MICHAEL ET AL.

Doty, R. L., Ford, M., Preti, G., and Huggins, G. R. (1975). *Science* **190**, 1316.
Doyle, G. A., Pelletier, A., and Bekker, T. (1967). *Folia Primatol.* **7**, 169.
Eaton, G. G., Slob, A., and Resko, J. A. (1973). *Anim. Behav.* **21**, 309.
Ellefson, J. (1968). Ph.D. Thesis, University of California, Berkeley.
El-Shazly, K. (1952a). *Biochem. J.* **51**, 640.
El-Shazly, K. (1952b). *Biochem. J.* **51**, 647.
Epple, G. (1967). *Folia Primatol.* **7**, 37.
Epple, G. (1971). *Proc. Int. Congr. Primatol., 3rd, 1970,* Vol. 3, p. 166.
Epple, G. (1973). *J. Reprod. Fertil., Suppl.* **19**, 447.
Epple, G. (1975). *In* "Primate Behavior, Developments in Field and Laboratory Research" (L. A. Rosenblum, ed.), Vol. 4, p. 195. Academic Press, New York.
Epple, G., and Lorenz, R. (1967). *Folia Primatol.* **7**, 98.
Evans, C. S., and Goy, R. W. (1968). *J. Zool.* **156**, 181.
Gartlan, J. S. (1969). *J. Reprod. Fertil., Suppl.* **6**, 137.
Gompertz, D., Brooks, A. P., Gaya, H., and Spiers, A. S. D. (1973). *Gut* **14**, 183.
Gorman, M. L., Nedwell, D. B., and Smith, R. M. (1974). *J. Zool.* **172**, 389.
Goy, R. W., and Resko, J. A. (1972). *Recent. Prog. Horm. Res.* **28**, 707.
Hall, K. R. L. (1962). *Proc. Zool. Soc. London* **139**, 283.
Hall, K. R. L., Boelkins, R. C., and Goswell, M. J. (1965). *Folia Primatol.* **3**, 22.
Hamilton, G. V. (1914). *J. Anim. Behav.* **4**, 295.
Hanson, G., and Montagna, W. (1962). *Am. J. Phys. Anthropol.* **20**, 421.
Harris, G. W., and Michael, R. P. (1964). *J. Physiol. (London)* **171**, 275.
Harris, G. W., Michael, R. P., and Scott, P. P. (1958). *In* "The Neurological Basis of Behavior" (G. E. W. Wolstenholme and M. O'Connor, eds.), p. 236. Churchill, London.
Harrison, B. (1963). *Malay. Nat. J.* **17**, 218.
Haynes, R. L., and Glick, B. (1974). *Poult. Sci.* **53**, 27.
Hess, J. P. (1973). *In* "Comparative Ecology and Behavior of Primates" (R. P. Michael and J. H. Crook, eds.), p. 507. Academic Press, New York.
Hill, W. C. O. (1944). *Nature (London)* **153**, 199.
Hill, W. C. O. (1954). *J. Anat.* **88**, 582.
Hill, W. C. O., Porter, A., and Southwick, M. D. (1952). *Proc. Zool. Soc. London* **122**, 79.
Hill, W. C. O., Appleyard, H. M., and Auber, L. (1959). *Trans. R. Soc. Edinburgh* **63**, 535.
Hutchison, J. B. (1967). *Nature (London)* **216**, 591.
Hutchison, J. B. (1971). *J. Endocrinol.* **50**, 97.
Hutchison, J. B. (1974). *In* "The Neurosciences: Third Study Program" (F. O. Schmidt and F. G. Worden, eds.), p. 593. MIT Press, Cambridge, Massachusetts.
Ilse, D. R. (1955). *Anim. Behav.* **3**, 118.
Jay, P. (1965). *In* "Behavior of Nonhuman Primates" (A. M. Schrier, H. F. Harlow, and F. Stollnitz, eds.), Vol. 2, p. 525. Academic Press, New York.
Jolly, A. (1966). "Lemur Behavior." Univ. of Chicago Press, Chicago, Illinois.
Kaufmann, J. H. (1965). *Folia Primatol.* **3**, 50.
Keverne, E. B., and Michael, R. P. (1971). *J. Endocrinol.* **51**, 313.
Klein, L. L. (1971). *Folia Primatol.* **15**, 233.
Klein, L. L., and Klein, D. (1971). *Int. Zoo Yearb.* **11**, 175.
Komisaruk, B. R. (1967). *J. Comp. Physiol. Psychol.* **64**, 219.
Kummer, H. (1968). "Social Organization of Hamadryas Baboons." Univ. of Chicago Press, Chicago, Illinois.

Latta, J., Hopf, S., and Ploog, D. (1967). *Primates* **8**, 229.

Lisk, R. D. (1962). *Am. J. Physiol.* **203**, 493.

Lisk, R. D. (1967). *Endocrinology* **80**, 754.

Maples, W. R., and McKern, T. W. (1967). *Baboon Med. Res., Proc. Int. Symp., 2nd, 1965*, p. 13.

Martin, R. D. (1968). *Z. Tierpsychol.* **25**, 409.

Mason, W. A. (1966). *Tulane Stud. Zool.* **13**, 23.

Meyer, C. C. (1972). *J. Comp. Physiol. Psychol.* **79**, 8.

Michael, R. P. (1965a). *Proc. R. Soc. Med.* **58**, 595.

Michael, R. P. (1965b). *Br. Med. Bull.* **21**, 87.

Michael, R. P. (1968). *In* "Endocrinology and Human Behaviour" (R. P. Michael, ed.), p. 69. Oxford Univ. Press, London and New York.

Michael, R. P. (1969). *Prog. Endocrinol., Proc. Int. Congr. Endocrinol., 3rd, 1968* Excerpta Med. Found. Int. Congr. Ser. No. 184, p. 302.

Michael, R. P. (1971). *In* "Frontiers in Neuroendocrinology" (L. Martini and W. F. Ganong, eds.), p. 359. Oxford Univ. Press, London and New York.

Michael, R. P. (1972). *Acta Endocrinol. (Copenhagen) Suppl.* **166**, 322.

Michael, R. P. (1975). *J. Steroid Biochem.* **6**, 161.

Michael, R. P., and Herbert, J. (1963). *Science* **140**, 500.

Michael, R. P., and Keverne, E. B. (1968). *Nature (London)* **218**, 746.

Michael, R. P., and Keverne, E. B. (1969). *J. Endocrinol.* **46**, xx.

Michael, R. P., and Keverne, E. B. (1970). *Nature (London)* **225**, 84.

Michael, R. P., and Saayman, G. S. (1968). *J. Endocrinol.* **41**, 231.

Michael, R. P., and Welegalla, J. (1968). *J. Endocrinol.* **41**, 402.

Michael, R. P., and Zumpe, D. (1970a). *Behaviour* **26**, 168.

Michael, R. P., and Zumpe, D. (1970b). *Anim. Behav.* **18**, 1.

Michael, R. P., and Zumpe, D. (1971). *In* "Comparative Reproduction of Nonhuman Primates" (E. S. E. Hafez, ed.), p. 205. Thomas, Springfield, Illinois.

Michael, R. P., Herbert, J., and Welegalla, J. (1966). *J. Endocrinol.* **36**, 263.

Michael, R. P., Herbert, J., and Welegalla, J. (1967a). *J. Endocrinol.* **39**, 81.

Michael, R. P., Saayman, G. S., and Zumpe, D. (1967b). *Nature (London)* **215**, 554.

Michael, R. P., Saayman, G. S., and Zumpe, D. (1967c). *J. Endocrinol.* **39**, 309.

Michael, R. P., Saayman, G. S., and Zumpe, D. (1968). *J. Endocrinol.* **41**, 421.

Michael, R. P., Keverne, E. B., and Bonsall, R. W. (1971). *Science* **172**, 964.

Michael, R. P., Zumpe, D., Keverne, E. B., and Bonsall, R. W. (1972). *Recent Prog. Horm. Res.* **28**, 665.

Michael, R. P., Bonsall, R. W., and Warner, P. (1974). *Science* **186**, 1217.

Michael, R. P., Bonsall, R. W., and Warner, P. (1975a). *In* "Olfaction and Taste" (D. A. Denton and J. P. Coghlan, eds.), p. 417. Academic Press, New York.

Michael, R. P., Bonsall, R. W., and Kutner, M. (1975b). *Psychoneuroendocrinology* **1**, 153.

Montagna, W. (1962). *Ann. N.Y. Acad. Sci.* **102**, 190.

Montagna, W., and Yun, S. J. (1962). *Am. J. Phys. Anthropol.* **20**, 95.

Morin, L. P., and Feder, H. H. (1974). *Brain Res.* **70**, 71.

Moynihan, M. (1967). *In* "Primate Ethology" (D. Morris, ed.), p. 236. Weidenfeld and Nicolson, London.

Moynihan, M. (1970). *Smithsonian Contrib. Zool.* **28**, 1.

Muckenhirn, N. A. (1967). Ph.D. Thesis, University of Maryland, College Park.

Nisman, B. (1954). *Bacteriol. Rev.* **18**, 16.

Nolte, A. (1958). *Behaviour* **12**, 183.

Ortmann, R. (1960). *Handb. Zool.* **8** (3), No. 7, 1.
Owen, K., Wallace, P., and Thiessen, D. (1974). *Physiol. Behav.* **12,** 755.
Palka, Y. S., and Sawyer, C. H. (1966). *J. Physiol. (London)* **185,** 251.
Patterson, R. L. S. (1968). *J. Sci. Food Agric.* **19,** 434.
Petter, J. J. (1962). *Ann. N.Y. Acad. Sci.* **102,** 267.
Petter, J. J. (1965). *In* "Primate Behaviour" (I. DeVore, ed.), p. 292. Holt, New York.
Pocock, R. I. (1918). *Proc. Zool. Soc. London* **1,** 19.
Powers, J. B. (1972). *Brain Res.* **48,** 311.
Preti, G., and Huggins, G. R. (1975). *J. Chem. Ecol.* **1,** 361.
Rahaman, H., and Parthasarathy, M. D. (1969). *Primates* **10,** 149.
Ramaswami, L. S., and Anand Kumar, T. C. (1962). *Naturwissenschaften* **49,** 115.
Saayman, G. S. (1971). *Folia Primatol.* **15,** 36.
Saayman, G. S. (1973). *Symp. Int. Congr. Primatol., 4th, 1972,* Vol. 2, p. 64.
Schaffer, J. (1937). *Wien. Klin. Wochenschr.* **50,** 790.
Schiefferdecker, P. (1917). *Biol. Zentralbl.* **37,** 534.
Schifter, H. (1968). *Zool. Garten (Leipzig)* **36,** 107.
Schultz, A. H. (1921). *J. Mammal.* **2,** 194.
Seitz, E. (1969). *Z. Tierpsychol.* **26,** 73.
Simonds, P. E. (1965). *In* "Primate Behavior" (I. DeVore, ed.), p. 175. Holt, New York.
Snyder, P. A. (1972). *In* "Saving the Lion Marmoset: Proceedings of the Wild Animal Propagation Trust Golden Lion Marmoset Conference" (D. D. Bridgwater, ed.), p. 23. Wild Animal Propagation Trust, Wheeling, West Virginia.
Spivak, H. (1971). *Z. Tierpsychol.* **28,** 279.
Sprankel, H. (1961). *Z. Wiss. Zool.* **165,** 186.
Sprankel, H. (1962). *Zool. Anz., Suppl.* **25,** 198.
Stephan, H. (1963). *Prog. Brain Res.* **3,** 111.
Stickland, L. H. (1934). *Biochem. J.* **28,** 1746.
Stickland, L. H. (1935a). *Biochem. J.* **29,** 889.
Stickland, L. H. (1935b). *Biochem. J.* **29,** 896.
Sutton, J. B. (1887). *Proc. Zool. Soc. London* p. 369.
Tachibana, O. (1936). *Kaibogaku Zasshi* **7,** 98.
Thiessen, D. D., and Yahr, P. (1970). *Physiol. Behav.* **5,** 275.
Tutin, C. E. G., and McGrew, W. C. (1973). *Am. J. Phys. Anthropol.* **38,** 195.
Ulrich, W. (1954). *Z. Tierpsychol.* **11,** 150.
Vandenbergh, J. G. (1963). *Folia Primatol.* **1,** 99.
van Hooff, J. A. R. A. M. (1962). *Symp. Zool. Soc. London* **8,** 97.
van Lawick-Goodall, J. (1968). *Anim. Behav. Monogr.* **1,** 161.
van Lawick-Goodall, J. (1969). *J. Reprod. Fertil., Suppl.* **6,** 353.
Voci, V. E., and Carlson, N. R. (1973). *J. Comp. Physiol. Psychol.* **83,** 388.
Waltman, R., Tricomi, V., Wilson, G. E., Lewin, A. H., Goldberg, N. L., and Chang, M. M. Y. (1973). *Lancet* **2,** 496.
Yerkes, R. M. (1939). *Q. Rev. Biol.* **14,** 115.
Yerkes, R. M., and Elder, J. H. (1936). *Comp. Psychol. Monogr.* **13,** No. 5.
Young, W. C., and Orbison, W. D. (1944). *J. Comp. Physiol. Psychol.* **37,** 107.
Zumpe, D., and Michael, R. P. (1970). *Anim. Behav.* **18,** 293.

Hormonal Regulation of Spermatogenesis*

VIDAR HANSSON,† RICARDO CALANDRA,† KENNETH PURVIS,†
MARTIN RITZEN,‡ AND FRANK S. FRENCH§

I. Introduction

The hormonal regulation of spermatogenesis involves an interplay of sex steroids and pituitary gonadotropic hormones acting on specific cells of the testis. Several reviews have brought together earlier work on spermatogenesis (Bishop and Walton, 1960; Clermont and Harvey, 1967; Courot et al., 1970; Steinberger, 1971; Steinberger and Steinberger, 1973). Recent research has led to the identification of target cells for pituitary hormones and steroid hormones within the testis and to the elucidation of molecular mechanisms for hormone action. In his review of the hormonal control of mammalian spermatogenesis, Steinberger (1971) concluded that "knowledge of the biochemical parameters of the hormonal action on spermatogenesis is too meager even for a limited attempt to formulate

* Financial support has been obtained from the WHO, NIH, Norwegian Research Council for Science and the Humanities (NAVF), Norwegian Society for Fighting Cancer, and Swedish Medical Research Council.

† Institute of Pathology, Rikshospitalet, Oslo, Norway

‡ Pediatric Endocrinology Unit, Karolinska Sjukhuset, Stockholm, Sweden

§ Department of Pediatrics, Laboratory of Reproductive Biology, University of North Carolina, Chapel Hill, North Carolina

a working hypothesis." However, during the last 3 or 4 years much has been learned about how hormones regulate the functions of cells within the testis and about the interactions between extratubular and intratubular cells. Also important mechanisms involved in the hormonal control of Sertoli cells and the interaction between Sertoli cells and germ cells have been revealed (Dufau and Means, 1974; French et al., 1975).

Smith demonstrated in 1927 that hypophysectomy prevents testicular development and spermatogenesis (Smith, 1927). This early work (Smith, 1927, 1930) led to the concept that the testis is stimulated by pituitary hormones. As a result of the important work of Greep and co-workers (1936; Greep and Fevold, 1937), it became evident that gonadotropic activity from the pituitary was due to two different substances: luteinizing hormone (LH), which stimulated interstitial cells, and follicle-stimulating hormone (FSH), which acted on the seminiferous tubules to promote spermatogenesis. The precise role of FSH became less clear when it was shown that testosterone in the absence of the pituitary was capable of maintaining spermatogenesis (Walsh et al., 1937; Nelson and Merckel, 1938; Ahmad et al., 1973). The function of FSH in regulating spermatogenesis remains an area of controversy.

Until recently, much of the work on the hormonal regulation of spermatogenesis had been limited to morphological studies. These types of studies failed to establish whether hormonal stimulation of spermatogenesis was mediated through stimulation of Sertoli cells or by a direct effect on germ cells. Identification of target cells for the various hormones within the seminiferous tubules has been complicated by the intimate relationship between Sertoli cells and germ cells. In 1971 it was proposed that the various stages of spermatogenesis may require different hormones, and that testosterone was important mainly for the completion of meiosis (Steinberger, 1971). The primary spermatocytes were therefore possible target cells for androgen. FSH, on the other hand, was reported to act on the maturation of the spermatids (Steinberger, 1971). When a specific marker of Sertoli cell secretory function was identified, i.e., testicular androgen-binding protein (ABP) (French and Ritzen, 1973a,b), it became possible to determine which hormonal effects on spermatogenesis might be mediated by Sertoli cells (Hansson et al., 1973, 1974b, 1975a,b; French et al., 1974; Hagenas et al., 1974, 1975). In addition, new techniques have been developed to separate testicular cells so that studies can be carried out to determine the direct effects of hormones on isolated cells (Meistrich et al., 1973; Fritz et al., 1974, 1975; Sanborn et al., 1975; Steinberger et al., 1975). Finally, the dry-mount autoradiographic technique developed by Stumpf (Stumpf and Sar, 1975) has recently been applied to the testis (Sar et al., 1975).

These developments have expanded our knowledge of the actions of FSH, LH, and androgens on the various cells in the testis. In the present paper we review some of the recent literature on the hormonal regulation of spermatogenesis with a focus primarily on the interactions of peptide and steroid hormones and their cellular localization. Most of the studies reported have been carried out in the rat or mouse.

II. HORMONES AND HORMONAL TARGET CELLS IN THE TESTIS

The extratubular compartment of the testis consists of Leydig cells dispersed in a loose connective tissue among blood and lymph vessels (Fawcett, 1973). In addition, the tubules are surrounded by peritubular cells, which are similar to smooth muscle cells and are probably important for the contractions of the seminiferous tubules (Clermont, 1958; Ross, 1967; Bressler and Ross, 1972). Within the tubule, adjacent Sertoli cells embrace the developing germ cells and interconnect to form the blood–testis barrier (Fawcett, 1975). Spermatogonia are localized outside the blood–testis barrier whereas the spermatocytes and various stages of the spermatids are localized in the adluminal compartment (Dym and Fawcett, 1970; Tindall et al., 1975). The localization of hormone action in the testis is outlined in Table I, which shows the major cell types of the testis and the hormones stimulating these cells. It should be remembered that Table I may be incomplete in that the responsiveness of different cell types to hormones may vary at different ages as well as under different hormonal conditions. The information discussed in this chapter was derived mainly from experiments on rats.

TABLE I

HORMONES AND HORMONAL TARGET CELLS IN THE TESTIS

Cell type	Hormone[a]
Leydig cells	LH
	Estradiol-17β
	Testosterone/DHT
	Prolactin
	FSH ?
Peritubular cells	Testosterone/DHT
Sertoli cells	FSH
	Testosterone/DHT
Germinal cells	Testosterone/DHT ?

[a] DHT, dihydrotestosterone; FSH, follicle-stimulating hormone; LH, luteinizing hormone.

II. LEYDIG CELLS

A. LUTEINIZING HORMONE (LH)

The classical studies which indicated that LH [or interstitial cell-stimulating hormone (ICSH)] is the main stimulatory hormone of Leydig cell development and androgen biosynthesis have been carefully reviewed by Hooker (1970). Further evidence that LH is acting directly on the Leydig cells comes from the identification of specific receptors for LH and human chorionic gonadotropin (hCG) on Leydig cell membranes (Catt et al., 1974) and from the observation that LH or hCG stimulates testosterone biosynthesis in isolated Leydig cells (Catt et al., 1974; Bahl et al., 1974; Moyle and Ramachandran, 1973). The LH/hCG receptor has been studied using membrane preparations (Catt et al., 1971, 1972a,b; Bahl et al., 1974) and solubilized membrane components (Dufau et al., 1974; Charreau et al., 1974). LH and hCG bind to membrane receptors on isolated Leydig cells in vitro and stimulate an immediate increase in adenyl cyclase activity and testosterone production (Moyle and Ramachandran, 1973; Catt et al., 1974).

A common receptor site for LH and hCG is present on Leydig cells. Binding of labeled hCG or LH is confined to interstitial cells, since no specific binding to tubular elements has been demonstrated. The equilibrium constant of associations is K_a 2 to 6×10^{10} M^{-1} at 0°C. Binding of LH and hCG to Leydig cell receptors has been shown to be temperature dependent. Binding occurs rapidly at 37°C and is dependent upon the relative concentrations of hormone and receptor sites (Catt et al., 1974). After sucrose gradient centrifugation of fragmented interstitial cells, LH and hCG receptors are associated with vesicular membranes (Tsuruhara et al., 1972). Localization of LH receptors on the plasma membrane is supported by the ability of Sepharose-coupled LH to activate testicular steroidogenesis in vitro (Dufau et al., 1971; Catt et al., 1974).

hCG binding to receptors in Leydig cells is accompanied by stimulation of testosterone synthesis; however, the levels of testosterone plateau when only a small proportion (less than 1%) of the total binding sites are occupied (Moyle and Ramachandran, 1973; Catt et al., 1974; Mendelson et al., 1975; Moyle et al., 1976). Stimulation of cyclic AMP (cAMP, adenosine 3',5'-monophosphate) is not detectable until testosterone production is almost maximal (Catt et al., 1974; Mendelson et al., 1975; Moyle et al., 1976). This observation has caused some to question the role of receptor binding and cAMP in the steroidogenic action of LH or hCG on the Leydig cells.

Bahl *et al.* (1974) and Moyle *et al.* (1976) have shown that glycosidase-treated hCG derivatives inhibit the binding of ^{125}I-labeled hCG to Leydig cell receptors and are potent inhibitors of the hCG-stimulated adenyl cyclase. In the presence of an excess of glycosidase-treated analogs, stimulation of cAMP was completely suppressed, while the steroidogenic response was still at a maximum. Thus, there may be two types of receptor sites on the plasma membrane for hCG—one that promotes steroidogenesis and another for cAMP production. Somewhat similar data have been provided by Catt *et al.* (1974) and Mendelson *et al.* (1975). It appears that the majority of the hCG receptors in the Leydig cells are coupled to adenylate cyclase in the cell membrane. However, the absence of increased adenylate cyclase activity during stimulation of testosterone synthesis by low levels of LH or hCG has raised the possibility that other membrane-associated responses may operate during the initial phase of gonadotropin-induced steroidogenesis in Leydig cells. Furthermore, the lag period between LH or hCG binding to receptor and stimulation of testosterone synthesis (Rommerts *et al.*, 1972; Catt *et al.*, 1974) suggests that several metabolic events may occur before enhancement of steroidogenesis becomes apparent. LH-induced testosterone synthesis appears to depend on both RNA and protein synthesis (Catt *et al.*, 1974). This action of LH thus differs from that of ACTH on the adrenals. In the adrenals, steroid production is postulated to be mediated by cytoplasmic events, the requirements for protein synthesis being met by translation of already existing messenger RNA molecules (Garren *et al.*, 1971).

B. ESTROGENS

It is well established that estrogens inhibit the secretion of FSH and LH from the pituitary. Moreover, evidence indicates there may be direct effects of estradiol on Leydig cells as well. Stumpf (1969) and Sar *et al.* (1975) have reported autoradiographic evidence for specific localization of radioactivity in nuclei of Leydig cells in immature rat testis after administration of radioactive estradiol-17β *in vivo* (Fig. 1). Similar accumulation of radioactivity was not seen in the peritubular cells, Sertoli cells, or germ cells. More recently, biochemical studies have demonstrated that interstitial tissue of rat testis contains high concentrations of estrogen receptors both in cytoplasm and in nuclei (Mulder *et al.*, 1973, 1974). These estradiol-17β receptors have physiochemical and binding properties similar to those of estrogen receptors in other estrogen target tissue, such as uterus (Jensen and DeSombre, 1973). Estrogen receptors were not found in seminiferous tubules. Leydig cell receptors for estradiol-17β have a sedimentation coefficient of 8 S and an equilibrium association constant

(K_a) of 10^{10} M^{-1}. Higher concentrations of estrogen receptors have been found in testicular interstitial tissue than in other tissues of the male rat. Mulder *et al.* (1974) calculated approximately 140 femtomoles per milligram of protein. This is 10–20 times higher than the estrogen receptor content of prostate or epididymis, and approximately twice as high as that of the anterior pituitary.

Like other steroid receptor complexes, estradiol-receptor complexes were shown to be translocated into Leydig cell nuclei, from which they could be extracted with 0.4 *M* KCl (Mulder *et al.*, 1973, 1974). The salt-extractable complex migrated with a sedimentation coefficient of 5 S when analyzed by sucrose gradient centrifugation. Estrogen receptors in Leydig cells are specific for estradiol and diethylstilbestrol, and have lower affinities for estrone, dihydrotestosterone (DHT), and testosterone (Mulder *et al.*, 1974). The physiological meaning of the nuclear uptake of estradiol by testicular interstitial cells is not yet clear. Testicular estradiol receptors are not limited to the rat, since Mulder *et al.*, (1974) have demonstrated their presence in mouse and monkey testicular tissue as well. Preliminary experiments in our laboratories indicate estradiol receptors in the human testis. However, no attempt has been made to localize these receptors in specific cell types (R. Calandra, K. Purvis, and V. Hansson, unpublished).

Several investigators (Steinberger, 1973; Danutra *et al.*, 1973; Jones *et al.*, 1975) have observed that estradiol inhibits testosterone secretion in the rat prior to a detectable decrease in the blood levels of LH. Following the injection of estradiol-17β, reduction in blood testosterone is observed within hours, whereas an effect on LH levels occurs much later. Pretreatment with estradiol also reduces the hCG-stimulated testosterone response (Jones *et al.*, 1975). Estradiol appears to inhibit the action of LH on the Leydig cells, and this may represent one mechanism whereby Leydig cell responsiveness to LH is regulated.

The major site of estrogen production in the testis has not yet been established. Studies by de Jong *et al.* (1973, 1974) have shown that estradiol concentrations in rat testis interstitial tissue are much higher than those of the seminiferous tubules. Although the main production of testosterone is in the interstitial compartment, estradiol has been reported to be produced primarily in the seminiferous tubules (de Jong *et al.*,

---

FIG. 1. Autoradiogram of testis of immature hypophysectomized rat 1 hour after injection of ^{3}H-labeled 17β-estradiol, showing nuclear concentration of silver grain in the Leydig cells. From Sar *et al.* (1975).

FIG. 2. Autoradiogram of testis of hypophysectomized rat 3 hours after injection of ^{3}H-labeled testosterone, showing nuclear concentration of silver grains in tubular, peritubular, and interstitial cells. From Sar *et al.* (1975).

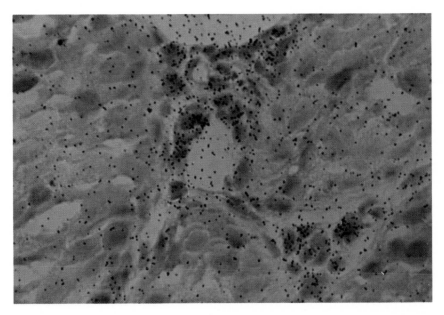

FIG. 1.

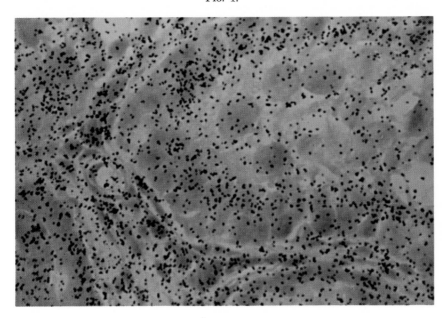

FIG. 2.

1974). On the other hand, the data of Payne and Kelch (1975) indicate that the major site of estradiol synthesis in both the rat and human testis is in the interstitial tissue. In contrast, Armstrong *et al.* (1975) have shown that Sertoli cells in culture can aromatize testosterone to estradiol. This process is stimulated by FSH. It is also well known that Sertoli cell tumors occasionally cause feminization of their "hosts" (Huggins and Moulder, 1945). Therefore, it must be concluded that the site of estradiol production in the testis remains uncertain. It is clear, however, that estrogens act on Leydig cells and that they may serve as local regulators of Leydig cell sensitivity to LH. Further studies will be necessary in order to understand the precise mechanism whereby estrogens regulate Leydig cell metabolism.

C. Androgens

The possibility that the Leydig cell, the primary source of testosterone, might be a target cell for its own product, is intriguing. Studies performed with rats and mice with the syndrome of testicular feminization (Tfm) (Chan *et al.*, 1969; Vanha-Perttula *et al.*, 1970) have demonstrated that a large fraction of the testicular volume of the Tfm rat is composed of Leydig cells. Increased activities of several Leydig cell enzymes have been observed histochemically. At the same time, however, Tfm rats have increased peripheral plasma LH levels in the presence of low testosterone concentrations in the spermatic vein (Bardin *et al.*, 1973). The paradox of decreased testosterone secretion combined with elevated plasma LH suggests a defect in androgen biosynthesis in Leydig cells of the Tfm rat. The reason for this is a dramatic reduction of LH receptors on the Leydig cells from the Tfm testis (K. Purvis and V. Hansson, unpublished). It is possible that androgen stimulation of Leydig cells is important for normal induction of LH receptors on the Leydig cell membranes.

When pregnenolone was incubated with testis from adult Tfm rats in comparison with normal rats of the same strain, normal rats converted this substrate primarily to testosterone. In contrast, testis from Tfm rats formed little testosterone but produced a large quantity of androstenedione. These observations on mature Tfm rats indicated that the Leydig cells of androgen-insensitive rats have a reduced ability to convert androstenedione to testosterone and suggested that the 17β-hydroxysteroid dehydrogenase is defective. Incubations of testis from immature Tfm rats (1 month old) confirmed the presence of low 17β-hydroxysteroid dehydrogenase activity indicating that the defect is not altogether postnatally acquired (Aronin *et al.*, 1974). Studies by Coffey *et al.* (1972) demonstrated further that the testis of adult Tfm rats retains the high 5α-reductase activity (converts testosterone to 5α-dihydrotestosterone) characteristic of immature animals, whereas in normal rats this enzyme activity decreases after puberty (Coffey et al., 1972; Van der Molen et al., 1975). Therefore, the low blood levels of testosterone in the Tfm rat might result from rapid metabolism of testosterone within the testis as well as a diminished rate of testosterone synthesis.

The question remains whether the defective testicular steroidogenesis and the end-organ insensitivity in the Tfm rat constitutes a linked genetic defect or whether the enzyme deficiency may be a phenotypic expression of the androgen insensitivity. The fact that the decrease in 17β-hydroxysteroid dehydrogenase activity was limited to the testis suggested the latter of these possibilities (Schneider and Bardin, 1970; Bardin et al., 1971). The androgen-insensitive Tfm/y mouse also has a defect in 17β-hydroxysteroid dehydrogenase (Bardin et al., 1973). Although absence of 17β-hydroxysteroid dehydrogenase activity occurs as a genetic abnormality in man (Saez et al., 1971), it seems likely that defective activity of this enzyme may also result from a lack of androgen stimulation. These data suggest that androgen action on the Leydig cell may be required for the maintenance of normal testosterone synthesis (Bardin et al., 1973).

Blackburn et al. (1973) have performed extensive morphological studies on Leydig cell differentiation in Tfm/y mice and found evidence for maturational arrest. Lack of development occurred in the presence of high LH levels. Both light microscopical and histochemical evidence indicated adequate LH stimulation. Mitochondrial proliferation reflected the hyperstimulation with LH. On the other hand, many structural features expected in a fully differentiated or hyperstimulated Leydig cell were absent. The Leydig cell cytoplasm in the Tfm animals contained numerous lipid globules. Although increased in number, mitochondria were uniformly round rather than pleomorphic and contained numerous tubulovesicular rather than lamellar cristae. Leydig cells from Tfm/y mice contained relatively little endoplasmatic reticulum and the tubulovesicular, lamellar and whorllike configurations typical of the normal mouse Leydig cell were not present (Bardin et al., 1973; Blackburn et al., 1973). Microvilli and intracellular canaliculi, which are characteristic of the well-differentiated cell in normal animals, were also absent. In general, the cytodifferentiation of Leydig cells of Tfm/y mice was similar to that of normal Leydig cells shortly after birth.

Although the defect in steroid biosynthesis as well as the apparent arrest in Leydig cell differentiation in Tfm/y mice might result from cryptorchidism (Schneider and Bardin, 1970), a more attractive explanation is that androgen action is required for the postnatal maturation of Leydig cells. If so, the androgen biosynthesis initiated by gonadotropin stimulation at the time of puberty would contribute to normal Leydig cell differentiation (Bardin et al., 1973).

Recent studies have demonstrated the presence of androgen receptors in interstitial cells in the hypophysectomized rat testis. Stumpf, Sar, and collaborators (Sar *et al.*, 1975) have reported autoradiographic data showing distinct nuclear accumulation of testosterone and DHT in extratubular cells, including Leydig cells (Fig. 2). Localization of labeled androgens in interstitial cell nuclei is prevented by previous injections of unlabeled testosterone or an antiandrogen, cyproterone acetate (Sar *et al.*, 1975). The specific localization of silver grains in Leydig cell nuclei is absent in androgen-insensitive Tfm/y rats (Sar *et al.*, 1975). Also, biochemical techniques have been used to demonstrate specific intracellular receptors for testosterone and DHT, in extratubular cells. Wilson and Smith (1975) compared receptor binding of androgen in isolated seminiferous tubules to that of the remaining interstitial tissue (containing also considerable amounts of tubular elements). Careful teasing out of the tubules from the 50-day-old testes did not cause an increase in specific activity of androgen receptors in the purified tubules compared to that of the remaining tissue (interstitial tissue + tubules). If androgen receptors were localized exclusively within the seminiferous tubules, the highly purified tubular preparation should contain more receptors per milligram of cytosol protein than the remaining tissue. However, it was found that the remaining interstitial tissue contained at least the same or higher content of androgen receptors (Wilson and Smith, 1975). Thus, studies on LH receptors and androgen biosynthesis, Leydig cell morphology, as well as androgen receptors (which are clearly different from the estrogen receptors) in the Leydig cell strongly suggest that androgens directly affect Leydig cell function.

D. PROLACTIN

Administration of prolactin to hypophysectomized rats and mice potentiates the effect of LH on the restoration of spermatogenesis (Woods and Simpson, 1961; Bartke, 1971). Since the same dose of prolactin did not augment the effect of testosterone propionate on spermatogenesis, it was concluded that prolactin did not act directly on the germinal epithelium, but potentiated the effect of LH on testosterone production in Leydig cells (Bartke, 1971). This conclusion has been supported by other studies in hypophysectomized rats. It has been shown that the plasma levels of testosterone, the incorporation of ^{14}C-labeled acetate into testosterone by testicular minces *in vitro*, and the endogenous mass of testosterone in these incubations, were all significantly greater in rats treated with both prolactin and LH than in those treated with LH alone (Hafiez *et al.*, 1972a,b). Administration of prolactin alone had no detectable effect on testicular steroidogenesis. Similar synergistic effects of LH and prolactin in stimulating Leydig cells have been reported by Balin and Schwartz (1972) and by Johnson (1974). Recent autoradiographic data also suggest that radioiodinated prolactin can become localized in the Leydig cells of the mouse testis (Rajaniemi et al., 1974).

It should be stressed that stimulation of testicular steroidogenesis by prolactin has been demonstrated only in laboratory mice and rats, and there is no evidence that prolactin has similar effects in other species. Reports that injection of prolactin in the bull and rabbit did not affect plasma testosterone levels or the response to LH (Smith and Hafs, 1973; Smith et al., 1973) do not rule out a role for prolactin in the regulation of testicular function in these species, since the animals studied were not hypophysectomized. As shown by Hafiez et al. (1972a), prolactin potentiates the effect of LH in hypophysectomized rats, but has no detectable effect on plasma testosterone levels in intact males (Bartke, 1976). Similarly, prolactin did not potentiate the effects of LH on testosterone production in decapsulated testis from intact rats in vitro or in Leydig cell preparations from intact mice (Van Damme et al., 1973, 1974). Another indication pointing to the Leydig cells as target cells for prolactin is the fact that prolactin-deficient, hereditary dwarf mice are sterile and can be made fertile by prolactin administration (Bartke, 1976). Furthermore, inhibitors of prolactin secretion (ergocornine and 2-bromo-α-ergokryptine) cause a reduction of seminal vesicle weight as well as plasma testosterone (Bartke, 1976).

Aragona and Friesen (1975) have recently shown the presence of specific prolactin receptors in rat testis. Similar results have been obtained in our laboratory (Charreau et al., 1976). The concentration of prolactin receptors in the testis is considerably lower than in prostate and exhibits significant age changes. Very low numbers of prolactin receptors are present at 21 days of age, increasing to a maximum at approximately 70 days of age (Aragona and Friesen, 1975). We have recently shown that prolactin receptors are localized to the interstitial cells (Charreau et al., 1976). Thus, in light of the studies cited above, demonstrating significant effects of prolactin on LH-induced steroidogenesis, and the presence of prolactin receptors in interstitial tissue, prolactin may be considered as an important pituitary hormone regulating Leydig cell function.

The mechanism by which prolactin activates Leydig cells is not known. In the prostate, binding of prolactin to membrane receptors is associated with an increase in the retention of testosterone in the prostate (Farnsworth, 1972) as well as the metabolism of testosterone to DHT (Oseko et al., 1973). It is currently believed that these changes are induced via stimulation of membrane-bound adenylate cyclase and the formation of cAMP (Golder *et al.*, 1972). Treatment with prolactin-producing ectopic pituitary grafts or with purified prolactin increases the concentration of esterified cholesterol in the testes of mice. Moreover, treatment of normal intact male mice with prolactin inhibitors reduces the testicular concentration of esterified cholesterol as well as plasma testosterone and the weights of the accessory sex glands (Bartke, 1976). Still much has to be learned about the action of prolactin in the testis, but the studies performed so far point to the Leydig cell as the target cell for prolactin as well as for other hormones.

E. FOLLICLE-STIMULATING HORMONE (FSH)

Several investigators have reported an effect of FSH on testosterone secretion in the testis (Lostroh, 1969; Connell and Eik-Nes, 1968). Since Leydig cells are responsible for the secretion of testosterone, Leydig cell function may also be affected by FSH. Studies by Johnson and Ewing (1971) demonstrated that FSH augments testosterone secretion in the perfused rabbit testis following stimulation with LH. The fact that FSH stimulates testosterone secretion in the presence of saturating concentrations of LH suggests that these gonadotropic hormones act at different sites or by different mechanisms (Johnson and Ewing, 1971). FSH augmentation of LH has also been suggested with respect to stimulation of cytochrome P-450 (Purvis and Menard, 1975) and 5α-reductase (Nayfeh *et al.*, 1975) in interstitial cells of rat testis. Whereas Bhalla and Reichert (1974) found specific binding of FSH to Leydig cell membranes, this was not found by Means and Huckins (1974). Moreover, by incubating decapsulated testes *in vitro* Dufau *et al.* (1972) and Van Damme *et al.* (1975). failed to show any synergistic action of LH and FSH on testosterone production. Thus, it remains controversial whether FSH has any direct effect on Leydig cells. It is quite possible that the conflict in the data may be due to different methodology, species differences, or Leydig cell responsiveness to FSH during only a limited period of development.

Although LH is the principal stimulus of Leydig cells, androgens, estrogens, FSH, and prolactin may have important complementary roles in regulating the differentiation and function of these cells. Much still has to be learned about the hormone regulation of androgen biosynthesis in Leydig cells, and, since testosterone must be considered a principal stimulus for the spermatogenic process, the regulation of androgen biosynthesis in Leydig cells is a very important aspect of the hormonal control of spermatogenesis.

IV. Peritubular Cells

Androgens

It is generally accepted that the myoid cells or peritubular cells are responsible for the contractile activity of the seminiferous tubules (Clermont, 1958; Lacy and Rotblat, 1960; Leeson and Leeson, 1963; Ross and Long, 1966). There are marked variations in the organization of the peritubular tissue between different species (Fawcett et al., 1973). The pattern of development of the myoid cells has been investigated by several authors, who suggest that an intact pituitary testicular axis is required for normal differentiation of these cells (Bressler and Ross, 1972; Hovatta, 1972a,b; de Krester et al., 1975). Peritubular cells have also been identified in the normal human testis (Ross and Long, 1966; Bustos-Obregon and Holstein, 1973). From studies of the immature testes of patients with hypogonadotropic hypogonadism, it was demonstrated that the peritubular tissue was poorly organized, but during treatment with FSH and LH this tissue attained a normal adult appearance (de Kretser and Burger, 1972). The relative lack of organization of the peritubular tissue found in immature testicular biopsies obtained from patients with hypogonadotropic hypogonadism (de Kretser and Burger, 1972) suggests that the development of this region is directly or indirectly dependent on the secretion of FSH and LH. The development of the peritubular tissue appears to be dependent on androgen. Bressler and Ross (1972) noted that myoid cell differentiation occurs in testicular tissue implanted into hypophysectomized, testosterone-treated hosts. These studies are supported by the results of Hovatta (1972a,b), who used the antiandrogen cyproterone acetate in tissue culture studies and demonstrated an effect on the peritubular tissue of the rat testis. De Kretser et al. (1975) speculated that the development of the myoid cells and extracellular microfibrillar system appears to depend on gonadotropin secretion by the pituitary gland. They therefore suggested that a hyalinization process may result from the stimulation of components of the peritubular tissue by the elevated levels of gonadotropic hormone evident in the majority of patients with severe germinal cell depletion (de Kretser et al., 1974). However, no evidence indicating direct effects on gonadotropins on the peritubular tissue has been demonstrated. On the contrary, neither FSH nor LH binds to isolated peritubular cells (Steinberger et al., 1975; Fritz et al., 1975). Another very likely explanation is that the reduced levels of intratesticular androgens may be responsible for the disorganization of the peritubular tissue. It is known that a large percentage of patients with oligospermia or azospermia have low testosterone levels in spite of elevated LH. Thus, reduced androgen levels may cause disorganization of the peritubular tissues with decreased uptake of androgens into the seminiferous tubules (de Kretser et al., 1975).

The most direct evidence for androgen action on peritubular cells comes from autoradiographic studies (Sar et al., 1975). As illustrated in Fig. 2, there is a distinct localization of androgens (both testosterone and DHT) in peritubular cells in the hypophysectomized rat testis. Nuclear accumulation of androgens can be inhibited by previous injection of unlabeled androgens as well as the antiandrogen cyproterone acetate. Similar concentrations of radioactivity in peritubular cell nuclei cannot be seen in rats with the syndrome of testicular feminization (Sar et al., 1975), in which the testicular content of intracellular androgen receptors is greatly reduced (Smith et al., 1975). Certain indications that testosterone or active metabolites of testosterone are regulating the tubular contractions have also recently been presented (Urry, 1975). Low doses of testosterone propionate that reduce the intratesticular levels of androgen were shown to inhibit tubular contractions, whereas high doses stimulated tubular contraction, probably as a result of direct androgen effects on peritubular cells in the presence of suppressed gonadotropins. Similar biphasic effects of testosterone on androgen-dependent intratesticular processes have been demonstrated (Weddington et al., 1976; Berndtson et al., 1974; Ludvig, 1950). Thus, morphological studies after hormone withdrawal and stimulation both in vivo and in vitro, as well as autoradiographic studies, now clearly suggest that the development and function of myoid cells are dependent on androgen.

V. SERTOLI CELLS

A. FOLLICLE-STIMULATING HORMONE

FSH, like other protein hormones, is believed to produce its effect through interaction with specific binding sites located on the plasma membrane of its target cell (Means, 1975). Much of the current evidence seems to indicate that protein hormones do not enter the target cells, and that binding of the hormone to surface receptors is sufficient to activate intracellular mechanisms leading eventually to specific biological responses. Specific receptors for FSH have been identified in the testis (Means and Vaitukaitis, 1972; Schwartz et al., 1973; Bhalla and Reichert, 1974; Rabin, 1974). Radioreceptor assays for FSH have been used to quantify FSH binding sites during development, after hypophysectomy and during different hormonal treatments (Steinberger et al., 1974; Desjardins et al.,

1974). An adenylate cyclase system, functioning supposedly as the catalytic subunit of the FSH receptor (Rodbell *et al.*, 1971), has been described in testicular tissue (Murad *et al.*, 1969; Kuehl *et al.*, 1970) and appears to be located within the seminiferous tubules. Moreover, FSH has been shown to stimulate RNA and protein synthesis in the testis (Means, 1971, 1974, 1975; Reddy and Villee, 1975).

Although biochemical effects of FSH on the testis were established early, there have until recently been few attempts to localize the FSH-sensitive target cells. In 1965 Murphy proposed that an injection of FSH increased the secretory activity of Sertoli cells and, in fact, suggested that this effect might be used as a bioassay for the hormone in the testis (Murphy, 1965a,b). Subsequently, studies from Mancini and colleagues yielded evidence that FSH conjugated to electron-dense substances, such as ferritin or isothiocyanate, interacted with the supporting Sertoli cells and/or spermatogonia (Mancini *et al.*, 1967; Castro *et al.*, 1970). All these observations are compatible with current views that the Sertoli cell is an FSH target cell in the testis. However, the importance of these early studies was diminished by disadvantages inherent in the techniques used. For example, the hormones injected were only partially purified preparations, and their contaminants may have caused nonspecific localization. Hormones were labeled directly with fluorescent dyes or with ferritin (molecular weight of about 6,000,000) using a conjugation process that caused more than 50% loss of the biological activity of the FSH preparation. In addition, steric hindrance may have interfered with normal binding and transport to the target cells within the testis. Finally, extremely high doses were injected in order to obtain clear localization of FSH in the testis, a fact that casts further doubt on the specificity of the results.

The availability of better labeling techniques for glycoproteins using tritium or radioiodine (Vaitukaitis *et al.*, 1971; Leidenberger and Reichert, 1972) encouraged further studies on the identification of FSH target cells in the testis. Midgley (1972) and co-workers carried out light microscopic autoradiography studies after the topical application of ^{125}I-labeled FSH to unfixed frozen sections. They confirmed that FSH localizes within the seminiferous tubules, although cellular or subcellular localization was not established (Desjardins *et al.*, 1974).

Several lines of research during the last 3 years have established that Sertoli cells are target cells for FSH in the testis. One important discovery was the demonstration and characterization of testicular androgen-binding protein (ABP), which is produced by the Sertoli cell and secreted into the testicular fluid (for review, see Hansson *et al.*, 1975a). ABP disappears both from the testis and epididymis after hypophysectomy and reappears after treatment with pituitary gonadotropins. (Hansson *et al.*, 1973,

1974a,b, 1975b,c; Fritz *et al.*, 1974). In the immature rat, ABP in the caput epididymis decreases to undetectable levels within 5 days after hypophysectomy, but in the mature rat a somewhat slower decline has been found (Hansson *et al.*, 1975c). Within 24 hours after injection of FSH into immature hypophysectomized rats, ABP accumulation can be measured both in the testis and caput epididymis. The levels in the epididymis reach a plateau within 2–4 days, and further treatment does not produce a proportional increase in ABP content (Hansson *et al.*, 1975b). When hypophysectomized rats are injected with different doses of FSH, ABP concentration in the caput epididymis is dose dependent. The sensitivity of this ABP response is comparable to that of the ovarian weight augmentation assay (Steelman–Pohley assay) (Hansson *et al.*, 1975b). Sertoli cell response to FSH administration was found to be specific when measured by the amount of ABP in the epididymis. Other pituitary hormones, androgen (2 mg/3 days), or estrogen (500 μg/3 days) had no effect when administered for the same length of time (Hansson *et al.*, 1974b; Hansson *et al.*, 1975 a,b). The ability of the different FSH preparations to induce ABP secretion from Sertoli cells or to increase ovarian weight are depicted in Fig. 3. The preparation with the highest potency in the Steelman–Pohley assay (HHG-B1) is also the most potent preparation in inducing ABP. Furthermore, the different FSH preparations showed the same relative potencies in the two systems. These findings provided evidence that FSH was the hormone stimulating Sertoli cell production of ABP.

Recent studies by Means and Tindall (1975) have convincingly shown an ABP response to FSH at a short time (1 hour) after hormone administration to prenatally X-irradiated rats (Sertoli cell-enriched testis). The turnover of ABP in the testis is very rapid; 4 hours after the injection of FSH, ABP concentrations in the testis return to control levels. Such rapid effects of FSH on ABP levels in the immature rat testis have been confirmed in our laboratories (Kotite *et al.*, 1976) using ovine FSH (NIH-FSH-S10) as well as highly purified human FSH (LER 1577 and LER 1563).

In our early studies, ABP was measured in epididymis 1–3 days after hormone administration and always at least 12 hours after the last hormone injection (Hansson *et al.*, 1975b). The rapid effects of FSH on ABP in the testis (Means and Tindall, 1975) probably reflect FSH-induced synthesis and breakdown of ABP within the Sertoli cells, while the amount measured in epididymis after a longer period of stimulation results both from synthesis and secretion.

All the studies on FSH effects on ABP suggest that the Sertoli cell is a target cell for FSH. Recent experiments using Sertoli cell cultures confirm this conclusion. Several effects of FSH have been demonstrated in cultured

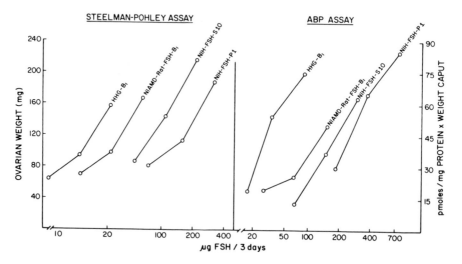

Fig. 3. Comparison of ovarian weight and androgen-binding protein (ABP) response in caput epididymis after administration of different follicle-stimulating hormone (FSH) preparations for 3 days. Steelman–Pohley assays were performed on immature, intact rats weighing 50–60 gm. In the ABP "assays," animals were hypophysectomized at 28 days of age, and treatment was started 2 days later. Each point of the curves represents mean values of 4 animals. From Hansson et al. (1975b).

Sertoli cells including incorporation of ³H-labeled thymidine into nuclear DNA (Griswold et al., 1975), characteristic morphological changes (Tung and Fritz, 1975), and stimulation of the conversion of testosterone to estradiol-17β (Armstrong et al., 1975). Several laboratories have shown that FSH stimulates the formation of cAMP in isolated Sertoli cells in culture (Steinberger et al., 1975; Fritz et al., 1975; Steinberger, 1975). Moreover, Means and Huckins (1974) demonstrated specific binding of ³H-labeled FSH to membrane receptors of seminiferous tubules devoid of germ cells with a subsequent stimulation of cAMP formation, protein kinase and mRNA formation. Finally, FSH stimulation of ABP production *in vitro*, both in organ culture (Ritzen et al., 1975) and in cell cultures (Fritz et al., 1975; Steinberger, 1975) have been reported. Thus, independent studies in several laboratories now strongly suggest that the Sertoli cell is a main target for FSH in the testis. It is less clear, however, whether or not additional target sites exist in other cells of the testis and if all the testicular effects of FSH can be accounted for by the responses induced in the Sertoli cell.

For a more detailed description of FSH action on the Sertoli cell, two recent books should be consulted (Dufau and Means, 1974; French et al., 1975).

B. Androgens

The Sertoli cell appears to be a target cell not only for FSH, but also for androgens (Hansson et al., 1974a,b; Weddington et al., 1975; Hansson et al., 1975a,b; Ritzen et al., 1975). The sensitivity of the Sertoli cell to FSH, as measured by ABP response, decreases dramatically after hypophysectomy, but can be maintained by pretreatment with high doses of testosterone propionate (Hansson et al., 1974a). When hypophysectomized immature rats are treated with 2 mg of testosterone daily beginning at day after hypophysectomy, Sertoli cell sensitivity to FSH is increased compared to that seen in the 2-day hypophysectomized controls (Hansson et al., 1974a). Thus, in prepubertal animals, androgens dramatically influence the sensitivity of the Sertoli cell to FSH. The secretory function of the Sertoli cell during this time period is therefore dependent on FSH and androgens.

Another series of studies also points to the Sertoli cell as a target cell for androgens. When various doses of testosterone propionate (TP 10–10,000 μg/day) were given daily to 21-day-old rats for 10 days, a biphasic effect was observed both on testis weight and on ABP levels in the testis and epididymis (Weddington et al., 1976). At low doses (10–100 μg of TP per day), there was a reduction in testis weight as well as in ABP levels. This was accompanied by a decrease in serum FSH and LH. At higher doses of TP (200–10,000 μg), there was a stimulation both of testis weight and ABP levels in spite of suppressed serum gonadotropins. These effects of TP on Sertoli cell secretion of ABP further support the idea that the Sertoli cell, in addition to being a target cell for FSH, also is a target cell for androgens (Weddington et al., 1976).

We also have noted that androgen alone, in the absence of the pituitary, can maintain Sertoli cell function in hypophysectomized rats when it is given immediately after hypophysectomy (Hansson et al., 1974a, 1975a,c; Weddington et al., 1975). That androgen alone is capable of maintaining ABP production is reminiscent of the early observation that androgen is capable of maintaining spermatogenesis. It suggests that when androgen treatment maintains spermatogenesis it also maintains Sertoli cell function.

We looked to see whether androgen alone was capable of initiating Sertoli cell secretory function when treatment following hypophysectomy was delayed until the seminiferous tubular epithelium was regressed. Rats were hypophysectomized at 28 days of age and 10 days later 4 mg of TP was given daily for 8 days. No increase in ABP was detected in the caput epididymis, and only slightly increased levels of ABP were found in the testis. Under the same conditions, the Sertoli cell remained responsive to FSH (Weddington et al., 1975). The finding that TP alone is less effective in initiating than in maintaining Sertoli cell function may explain why it is less capable of initiating spermatogenesis under similar conditions. A similar discrepancy between the ability of androgens to maintain Sertoli cell secretion and its inability to reinitiate Sertoli cell secretion of ABP after posthypophysectomy regression has been demonstrated in adult hypophysectomized rats (Hansson et al., 1975c, 1976). These findings reemphasize the importance of the Sertoli cell in spermatogenesis and indicate that spermatogenesis requires a functional Sertoli cell as well as androgen. Thus it seems that after a long period of hypophysectomy, the Sertoli cell is transformed into a state of relative androgen insensitivity at least with respect to ABP production (Hansson et al., 1975c, 1976). It is not known which factor or factors are needed to restore normal androgen sensitivity of the Sertoli cell.

In one set of experiments, we treated adult animals after 60 days of posthypophysectomy regression with FSH for 5 days, in order to obtain maximum ABP secretion before continuing the treatment with TP alone (Hansson et al., 1975a,b). The question asked was: At the time when the secretory function of the Sertoli cell is already established by FSH, will testosterone then be capable of taking over and maintaining the secretory function of the Sertoli cell? Our studies seem to indicate that this is not the case (Hansson et al., 1975c). After stopping FSH treatment, there was a gradual decrease in ABP content both in the testis and in the epididymis, in spite of continuing testosterone treatment, indicating that testosterone propionate alone was not capable of maintaining the secretory function of Sertoli cells at the level established by FSH under these experimental conditions. This could be due to the fact that 5 days of FSH treatment is too short a time for restoring the components that are necessary for optimal androgen sensitivity. However, the possibility that factors other than FSH might be needed to normalize Sertoli cell response to androgens cannot be excluded.

Since androgens have such marked effects on the Sertoli cell, as measured by ABP production, it was of great interest to examine whether ABP was present in the androgen-insensitive (Stanley Gumbreck) rat (Tfm rat) (Hansson et al., 1975a,c). As illustrated in Table II, the Tfm rat testis contained almost 10 times as much ABP as that of the normal littermates when calculated per milligram of protein. Also, when calculated as ABP per testis, the Tfm rats contained more ABP than the normal rat. This clearly showed that ABP is formed even in the absence of androgen stimulation. Whether or not ABP production in the Tfm testis is higher or lower than that of the normal littermates was studied in vitro by incu-

TABLE II

Content and Concentration of Testicular Androgen-Binding Protein (ABP) in Testis of Rats with Testicular Feminization (Tfm) and in Normal Littermates[a]

Animal	ABP pmoles/mg protein, mean ± SD	ABP (pmoles/testis, mean ± SD)	n
Control	0.41 ± 0.07	34.3 ± 6.7	(6)
Tfm	2.89 ± 0.51	63.7 ± 14.8	(6)

[a] Testes were homogenized in 4 volumes of 50 mM Tris-HCl buffer, pH 7.4, containing 1 mM EDTA (TE buffer) and 105,000 g supernatants were prepared. The cytosols were diluted with equal volumes of TE-buffer containing 20 % (v/v) glycerol and 10 mM ^{3}H-labeled dihydrotestosterone (DHT) (44 Ci/mmole). Binding was measured by steady-state electrophoresis with 2 nM ^{3}H-labeled DHT in the gels. n, Number of individual animals per group.

bating the testes from Tfm rats and their normal littermates in short-time organ cultures as described previously (Ritzen et al., 1975). Following the initial release of preformed ABP, the production rate in the Tfm testis between 4 and 20 hours of incubation was only one-third of that in the normal littermates (calculated as ABP production per testis). These studies indicate that ABP production in the Sertoli cell of the Tfm testis is lower than in those of normal littermates. The most likely explanation for this is that androgen stimulation of the Tfm testis is insufficient to maintain the normal secretory function of the Sertoli cells (E. M. Ritzen, L. Hagenas, and V. Hansson, unpublished results). The high content of ABP in the testes from Tfm rats as compared to normal rats must result from the absence of an epididymis. A block in the outflow of testicular fluid would allow a large amount of ABP to accumulate in the testis even at a low production rate.

Acute responsiveness of Sertoli cell to testosterone has been recently demonstrated by Means et al. (1976) and Kotite et al. (1976). These authors showed that after injection of 1 mg of testosterone, there was a rapid increase in the testicular content of ABP reaching a maximum concentration after approximately 1–2 hours. This effect of testosterone was inhibited by cycloheximide, and preliminary evidence also suggests that actinomycin D also results in a reduced stimulatory effect of testosterone (Means et al., 1976). Thus, it appears that testosterone stimulation of ABP in the Sertoli cell requires transcriptional events as well as protein synthesis (Means et al., 1976). Although these in vitro studies pointed to the Sertoli cell as a target cell for androgens, the possibility remained that the hormone injected in vivo might exert its effect indirectly through other organs. Ritzen *et al.* (1975) have now demonstrated that ABP synthesis in testis organ culture can be stimulated by testosterone. Thus, testosterone acts directly on the testis to stimulate Sertoli cell production of ABP.

Another indication that androgens are acting directly on the Sertoli cell has come from the demonstration that androgen receptors appear to be localized to these cells (Fig. 2) (Sar *et al.*, 1975; Wilson and Smith, 1975). Androgen receptors in rat testis have physicochemical properties similar to receptors in rat ventral prostate and epididymis and different from ABP (Table III). Moreover, Wilson *et al.* (1976) have shown these androgen receptors to have nearly identical binding properties *in vitro*. In each organ the receptors are specific for testosterone and DHT with slightly higher affinity for DHT than for testosterone. Androgen receptors in the testis are absent in the rat with the syndrome of testicular feminization as demonstrated both by biochemical and autoradiographic techniques (Sar *et al.*, 1975; Smith *et al.*, 1975).

To what extent other hormones have direct actions on the Sertoli cell is still controversial. Recent studies in our laboratories (Ritzen *et al.*, 1975), have shown that fetal calf serum is capable of stimulating ABP production in short-term organ cultures *in vitro* as well as, if not better, than testosterone and/or FSH. The stimulatory effect of fetal calf serum on ABP production *in vitro* cannot be explained by its content of androgens and gonadotropins. In addition, we have found recently that ABP production both *in vivo* (V. Hansson, unpublished data) and *in vitro* (E. M. Ritzen, unpublished data) can be stimulated by a small peptide with a molecular weight of approximately 1000 daltons. This peptide is isolated from human urine (O. Trygstad, unpublished data) and has been shown to have biological effects both on Leydig cells and on Sertoli cells. Although this peptide has not been fully characterized, this result indicates that new hormones involved in the regulation of Sertoli cell function are yet to be discovered. Current concepts in the hormonal regulation of Sertoli cell function are depicted in Fig. 4.

VI. Germ Cells

Androgens

The androgen dependence of spermatogenesis reflects the androgen dependence of germ cells. However, the intimate relationship between Sertoli cells and germ cells makes it difficult to determine whether hormonal effects on germ cells are mediated through the Sertoli cell or by direct actions on germ cells. So far, only indirect evidence indicates that germ cells also contain androgen receptors. Autoradiographic studies (Sar *et al.*,

TABLE III

PHYSICOCHEMICAL PROPERTIES OF RECEPTORS IN RAT TESTIS, EPIDIDYMIS, AND PROSTATE AND IN ANDROGEN-BINDING PROTEIN[a]

Property	Cytoplasmic receptors			ABP
	Testis	Epididymis	Prostate	
Sedimentation coefficient	4 S and 7–10 S			4.6 S
Stokes radius	>80 Å			47 Å
Molecular weight	>200,000			~87,000
PAGE (3½ % gels)	R_f 0.4–0.5			R_f 0.75
Dissociation rate of bound DHT	$t_{1/2}$ 0° > 1 day			$t_{1/2}$ 0°, 6 min
Steroid specificity	DHT > T	DHT > T	DHT > T	DHT > T
Heating at 50°, 30 min	−	−	−	+
Sulfhydryl agent PCMPS (1 mM)	−	−	−	+
Charcoal	−	−	−	+
Protease	−	−	−	−

[a] Minus sign indicates binding destroyed; plus sign indicates binding intact; DHT, dihydrotestosterone; T, testosterone; PAGE, polyacrylamide gel electrophoresis; PCMPS, p-chloromercuric phenylsulfonate.

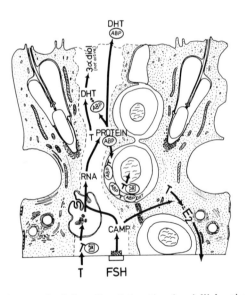

FIG. 4. Hormonal control of Sertoli cell function by follicle-stimulating hormone (FSH) and androgens. Both hormones are important for the production and secretion of androgen-binding protein (ABP). FSH is in addition important for aromatization of testosterone (T) to estradiol (E₂) in the Sertoli cells. DHT, dihydrotestosterone.

1975) suggested labeling of several cell types within the germinal epithelium. However, these studies were carried out in hypophysectomized rats, so that only Sertoli cells, spermatogonia and spermatocytes were present in the germinal epithelium. Although considerable problems exist in evaluating the different cell types in freeze-dried sections, more labeling appears to be present in the seminiferous tubules than can be explained simply by association with Sertoli cells (Fig 2) (Sar et al., 1975). The content of androgen receptors in normal hypophysectomized rat testis was compared with that in hypophysectomized rats of the same age whose germinal cells had been selectively destroyed by prenatal X-irradiation (Wilson and Smith, 1975). The concentration of receptors in germ cell-free testes (calculated per milligram of protein) was similar to that of the nonirradiated controls, which contained germ cells. Calculated on a total testis basis, there was a considerable loss of receptors concomitant with the loss of germ cells (spermatogonia and spermatocytes). However, the possibility that prenatal X-irradiation may reduce the number of androgen receptors in the Sertoli cells has not been excluded. Additional evidence for androgen receptors in germ cells has recently been presented by Sanborn et al. (1975). After separation of the different cell types in the testis, a nuclear exchange assay was used to demonstrate specific nuclear exchange of testosterone and DHT. However, an increase in specific nuclear binding sites following incubation with unlabeled testosterone (indicating nuclear translocation) was not demonstrated, and the characteristics of the nuclear androgen-binding component have yet to be determined.

A recent publication by Lyon et al. (1975) may be interpreted as evidence that androgen does not act directly on germ cells. These workers made male mice chimeric for androgen-resistant (Tfm/y) and normal (+/y) genotypes by the technique of embryo aggregation. They determined whether spermatozoa were formed from the Tfm/y component and the extent to which these spermatozoa were fertile (Lyon et al., 1975). Out of the 57 chimeric animals produced, two fertile males were of the Tfm/y⟷+/y genotype and both produced numerous offspring from their Tfm/y component. This indicated that the requirement for testosterone in spermatogenesis does not involve the cell-autonomous action of the Tfm locus in the germ cells. If the Tfm locus is not involved in androgen action on the germ cells, the androgen message to the germ cells may be mediated through the Sertoli cell. These data support, but do not conclusively prove, that the response to androgen of the seminiferous epithelium is entirely mediated by testicular somatic cells (Lyon et al., 1975).

From the current concept of androgen action in mammalian cells, it is difficult to find a role for steroid hormones in stimulating more mature types of germinal cells like the late spermatids and spermatozoa. Steroid hormone complexes are believed to act primarily through transcription and secondarily on protein synthesis. In haploid cells without transcriptional capability, new concepts of steroid hormone action need to be established before androgen action on mature germ cells can become an attractive theory.

VII. Summary

Androgenic hormones provide a major stimulus for spermatogenesis. Production of testosterone by Leydig cells is regulated by ICSH. Leydig cell development and steroidogenic function may require a direct action of testosterone or dihydrotestosterone. Prolactin and FSH enhances Leydig cell responsiveness whereas estrogen appears to inhibit Leydig cell response to ICSH with respect to steroidogenesis.

Androgens stimulate peritubular cell differentiation and the development of tubular contractions.

Androgens and FSH regulate Sertoli cell function. It seems reasonable to conclude that most hormonal effects on spermatogenesis are mediated through the Sertoli cell.

REFERENCES

Ahmad, N., Haltmeyer, G. C., and Eik-Nes, K. B. (1973). *Biol. Reprod.* **8**, 411.

Aragona, C., and Friesen, H. G. (1975). *Endocrinology* **97**, 677.

Armstrong, D. T., Moon, Y. S., Fritz, I. B., and Dorrington, J. H. (1975). *In* "Hormonal Regulation of Spermatogenesis" (F. S. French *et al.*, eds.), pp. 85–96. Plenum, New York.

Aronin, P. A., Coffey, J. C., French, F. S., and Nayfeh, S. N. (1974). *Steroids* **24**, 139.

Bahl, P., Marz, L., and Moyle, W. R. (1974). *In* "Hormone Binding and Target Cell Activation in the Testis" (M. L. Dufau and A. R. Means, eds.), pp. 125–144. Plenum, New York.

Balin, M., and Schwartz, N. B. (1972). *Am. Zool.* **12**, 19.

Bardin, C. W., Bullock, L., Blackburn, W. R., Sherins, R. J., and Vanha-Perttula, T. (1971). *In* "The Clinical Delineation of Birth Defects" (D. Bergsma, ed.), Vol. III, p. 185. Williams & Wilkins, Baltimore, Maryland.

Bardin, C. W., Bullock, L. P., Sherins, R. J., Mowszowics, I., and Blackburn, W. R. (1973). *Recent Prog. Horm. Res.* **29**, 65.

Bartke, A. (1971). *J. Endocrinol.* **49**, 311.

Bartke, A. (1976). *In* "Sperm Action" (P. O. Hubinot and M. L'Hermite, eds.), pp. 136–152. S. Karger, Basel.

Berndtson, W. E., Desjardins, C., and Ewing, L. L. (1974). *J. Endocrinol.* **62**, 125.

Bhalla, V. K., and Reichert, L. E., Jr. (1974). *J. Biol. Chem.* **249**, 43.

Bishop, M. W. H., and Walton, A. (1960). *In* "Marshall's Physiology of Reproduction" (A. S. Parkes, ed.), 3rd ed., Vol. 1, Part B, p. 1. Longman's Green, New York.

Blackburn, W. R., Chung, K. W., Bullock, L., and Bardin, C. W. (1973). *Biol. Reprod.* **9**, 9.

Bressler, R. S., and Ross, M. H. (1972). *Biol. Reprod.* **6**, 148.

Bustos-Obregon, E., and Holstein, A. F. (1973). *Z. Zellforsch. Mikrosk. Anat.* **141**, 413.

Castro, A. E., Seiguer, A. C., and Mancini, R. E. (1970). *Proc. Soc. Exp. Biol. Med.* **133**, 582.

Catt, K. J., Dufau, M. L., and Tsuruhara, T. (1971). *J. Clin. Endocrinol. Metab.* **32**, 860.

Catt, K. J., Dufau, M. J., and Tsuruhara, T. (1972a). *J. Clin. Endocrinol. Metab.* **34**, 123.

Catt, K. J., Tsuruhara, T., and Dufau, M. L. (1972b). *Biochim. Biophys. Acta* **279**, 194.

Catt, K. J., Tsuruhara, T., Mendelson, C., Ketelslegers, J. M., and Dufau, M. L. (1974). *In* "Hormone Binding and Target Cell Activation in the Testis" (M. L. Dufau and A. R. Means, eds.), pp. 1–30. Plenum, New York.

Chan, F., Allison, J. E., Stanley, A. J., and Gumbreck, L. G. (1969). *Fertil. Steril.* **20**, 482.

Charreau, E. H., Dufau, M. L., and Catt, K. J. (1974). *J. Biol. Chem.* **249**, 4189.

Charreau, E. H., Attramadal, A., Purvis, K., Calandra, R., and Hansson, V. (1976). *In* "The Testis in Normal and Infertile Men: Morphology, Physiology, and Pathology" (P. Troen and H. Nankin, eds.). Raven, New York (in press).

Clermont, Y. (1958). *Exp. Cell Res.* **15**, 435.

Clermont, Y., and Harvey, S. C. (1967). *Ciba Found. Colloq. Endocrinol.* [*Proc.*] **16**, 173.

Coffey, J. C., Aronin, P., French, F. S., and Nayfeh, S. N. (1972). *Steroids* **19**, 433.

Connell, G. M., and Eik-Nes, K. B. (1968). *Steroids* **12**, 507.

Courot, M., Hochereau-de-Reviers, M. T., and Ortavant, R. (1970). *In* "The Testis" (A. D. Johnson, W. R. Gomes, and N. L. Van Demark, eds.), Vol. 1, pp. 339–432. Academic Press, New York.

Danutra, V., Harper, M. C., Boyns, A. R., Cole, E. N., Brownsey, B. G., and Griffiths, K. (1973). *J. Endocrinol.* **57**, 207.

de Jong, F. H., Hey, A. H., and Van der Molen, H. J. (1973). *J. Endocrinol.* **57**, 277.

de Jong, F. H., Hey, A. H., and Van der Molen, H. J. (1974). *J. Endocrinol.* **60**, 409.

de Kretser, D. M., and Burger, H. G. (1972). *In* "Gonadotropins" (B. B. Saxena, C. G. Beling, and H. M. Gandy, eds.), pp. 640–656. Wiley (Interscience), New York.

de Kretser, D. M., Burger, H. G., and Hudson, B. (1974). *J. Clin. Endocrinol. Metab.* **38**, 787.

de Kretser, D. M., Kerr, J. B., and Paulsen, C. A. (1975). *Biol. Reprod.* **12**, 317.

Desjardins, C., Zeleznik, A. J., Midgley, R., and Reichert, L. E. (1974). *In* "Hormone Binding and Target Cell Activation in the Testis" (M. L. Dufau and A. R. Means, eds.), pp. 221–235. Plenum, New York.

Dufau, M. L., and Means, A. R., eds. (1974). "Hormone Binding and Target Cell Activation in the Testis." Plenum, New York.

Dufau, M. L., Catt, K. J., and Tsuruhara, T. (1971). *Biochim. Biophys. Acta* **252**, 574.

Dufau, M. L., Catt, K. J., and Tsuruhara, T. (1972). *Endocrinology* **90**, 1032.

Dufau, M. L., Charreau, E., Ryan, D., and Catt, K. J. (1974). *In* "Hormone Binding and Target Cell Activation in the Testis" (M. L. Dufau and A. R. Means, eds.), pp. 47–77. Plenum, New York.

Dym, M., and Fawcett, D. W. (1970). *Biol. Reprod.* **3**, 308.

Farnsworth, W. E. (1972). *In* "Prolactin and Carcinogenesis" (A. R. Boyns and K. Griffiths, eds.), pp. 217–228. Alpha Omega Alpha Publ., Cardiff, Wales.

Fawcett, D. W. (1973). *Adv. Biosci.* **10**, 83.

Fawcett, D. W. (1975). *Handb. Physiol. Sect. 7: Endocrinol.* **5**, 21–55.

Fawcett, D. W., Neaves, W. B., and Flores, M. N. (1973). *Biol. Reprod.* **9**, 500.

French, F. S., and Ritzen, E. M. (1973a). *J. Reprod. Fertil.* **32**, 479–483.

French, F. S., and Ritzen, E. M. (1973b). *Endocrinology* **93**, 88–95.

French, F. S., McLean, W. S., Smith, A. H., Tindall, D. J., Weddington, S. C., Petrusz, P., Sar, M., Stumpf, W. E., Nayfeh, S. N., Hansson, V., Trygstad, O., and Ritzen, E. M. (1974). *In* "Hormone Binding and Target Cell Activation in the Testis" (M. L. Dufau and A. R. Means, eds.), pp. 265–285. Plenum, New York.

French, F. S., Hansson, V., Ritzen, E. M., and Nayfeh, S. N., eds. (1975). "Hormonal Regulation of Spermatogenesis." Plenum, New York.

Fritz, I. B., Kopec, B., Lam, K., and Vernon, R. G. (1974). *In* "Hormone Binding and Target Cell Activation in the Testis" (M. L. Dufau and A. R. Means, eds.), pp. 311–327. Plenum, New York.

Fritz, I. B., Louis, B. G., Tung, P. S., Griswold, M., Rommerts, F. G., and Dorrington, J. H. (1975). *In* "Hormonal Regulation of Spermatogenesis" (F. S. French *et al.*, eds.), pp. 367–382. Plenum, New York.

Garren, L. D., Gill, G. N., Masui, H., and Walton, G. M. (1971). *Recent Prog. Horm. Res.* **27**, 433.

Golder, M. P., Boyns, A. R., Harper, M. E., and Griffiths, K. (1972). *Biochem. J.* **128**, 725.

Greep, R. O., and Fevold, H. L. (1937). *Endocrinology* **21**, 611.

Greep, R. O., Fevold, H. L., and Hisaw, F. L. (1936). *Anat. Rec.* **65**, 261.

Griswold, M., Mably, E., and Fritz, I. B. (1975). *In* "Hormonal Regulation of Spermatogenesis" (F. S. French *et al.*, eds.), pp. 413–420. Plenum, New York.

Hafiez, A. A., Lloyd, C. W., and Bartke, A. (1972a). *J. Endocrinol.* **52**, 327.

Hafiez, A. A., Bartke, A., and Lloyd, C. W. (1972b). *J. Endocrinol.* **53**, 223.

Hagenas, L., Ritzen, E. M., French, F. S., and Hansson, V. (1974). *J. Steroid Biochem.* **5**, 382.

Hagenas, L., Ritzen, E. M., Ploen, L., Hansson, V., French, F. S., and Nayfeh, S. N. (1975). *Mol. Cell. Endocrinol.* **2**, 339.

Hansson, V., Reusch, E., Trygstad, O., Torgersen, O., French, F. S., and Ritzen, E. M. (1973). *Nature (London)*, New Biol. **246**, 56.

Hansson, V., French, F. S., Weddington, S. C., Nayfeh, S. N., and Ritzen, E. M. (1974a). *In* "Hormone Binding and Target Cell Activation of the Testis" (M. L. Dufau and A. R. Means, eds.), pp. 287–290. Plenum, New York.

Hansson, V., Trygstad, O., French, F. S., McLean, W. S., Smith, A. A., Tindall, D. J., Weddington, S. C., Petrusz, P., Nayfeh S. N., and Ritzen, E. M. (1974b). *Nature (London)* **250**, 387.

Hansson, V., Ritzen, E. M., French, F. S., and Nayfeh, S. N. (1975a). *Handb. Physiol. Sect. 7: Endocrinol.* **5**, 173.

Hansson, V., Weddington, S. C., Petrusz, P., Ritzen, E. M., Nayfeh, S. N., and French, F. S. (1975b). *Endocrinology* **97**, 469.

Hansson, V., Weddington, S. C., Naess, O., Attramadal, A., French, F. S., Kotite, N., Nayfeh, S. N., Ritzen, M., and Hagenas L. (1975c). *In* "Hormonal Regulation of Spermatogenesis" (F. S. French *et al.*, eds.), pp. 323–336. Plenum, New York.

Hansson, V., Ritzen, E. M., and French, F. S. (1976). *In* "The Human Semen and Fertility Regulation in the Male" (E. S. E. Hafez, ed.). Mosby, St. Louis Missouri (in press).

Hooker, C. W. (1970). *In* "The Testis" (A. D. Johnson, W. R. Gomes, and N. L. Van Demark, eds.), Vol. 1, pp. 483–550. Academic Press, New York.

Hovatta, O. (1972a). *Z. Zellforsch. Mikrosk. Anat.* **130**, 171.

Hovatta, O. (1972b). *Z. Zellforsch. Mikrosk. Anat.* **131**, 299.

Huggins, C., and Moulder, P. V. (1945). *Cancer Res.* **5**, 510.

Jensen, E. V., and DeSombre, E. R. (1973). *Science* **182**, 126.

Johnson, B. H., and Ewing, L. L. (1971). *Science* **173**, 635.

Johnson, D. C. (1974). *Proc. Soc. Exp. Biol. Med.* **145**, 610.

Jones, T. M., Fang, V. S., Landau, R. L., and Rosenfield, R. (1975). *Program 57th Meet. Endocrine Soc.* Abstract No. 196, p. 148.

Kotite, N., Morris, M. A., Petrusz, P., Hansson, V., Nayfeh, S. N., and French, F. S. (1976). *Program 58th Meet. Endocrine Soc.* Abstract No. 362, p. 237.

Kuehl, F. A., Jr., Pantanelli, D. J., Tarnoff, J., and Humes, J. L. (1970). *Biol. Reprod.* **2**, 154.

Lacy, D., and Rotblat, J. (1960). *Exp. Cell Res.* **21**, 49.

Leeson, C. R., and Leeson, T. S. (1963). *Anat. Rec.* **147**, 243.

Leidenberger, F., and Reichert, L. E., Jr. (1972). *Endocrinology* **91**, 135.

Lostroh, A. J. (1969). *Endocrinology* **76**, 438.

Ludvig, D. J. (1950). *Endocrinology* **46**, 453.

Lyon, M. F., Glenister, P. H., and Lamoreux, M. L. (1975). *Nature (London)* **258**, 620.

Mancini, R. E., Castro, A., and Seiguer, A. C. (1967). *J. Histochem.* **15**, 516.

Means, A. R. (1971). *Endocrinology* **89**, 981.

Means, A. R. (1974). *Life Sci.* **15**, 371.

Means, A. R. (1975). *Handb. Physiol. Sect. 7: Endocrinol.* **5**, 203–218.

Means, A. R., and Huckins, C. (1974). *In* "Hormone Binding and Target Cell Activation in the Testis" (M. L. Dufau and A. R. Means, eds.), pp. 145–165. Plenum, New York.

Means, A. R., and Tindall, D. J. (1975). *In* "Hormonal Regulation of Spermatogenesis" (F. S. French *et al.*, eds.), pp. 383–398. Plenum, New York.

Means, A. R., and Vaitukaitis, J. (1972). *Endocrinology* **90**, 39.

Means, A. R., Fakunding, J. L., Huckins, C., Tindall, D. J., and Vitale, R. (1976). *Recent Prog. Horm. Res.* **32** (in press).

Meistrich, M. L., Bruce, W. R., and Clermont, Y. (1973). *Exp. Cell Res.* **79**, 213.

Mendelson, C., Dufau, M., and Catt, K. (1975). *J. Biol. Chem.* **250**, 8818.

Midgley, A. R., Jr. (1972). In "Gonadotropins" (B. B. Saxena, C. G. Beling, and H. M. Gandy, eds.), p. 248. Wiley (Interscience), New York.

Moyle, W. R., and Ramachandran, J. (1973). *Endocrinology* **93**, 127.

Moyle, W. R., Bahl, O. P., and Marz, L. (1975). *J. Biol. Chem.* **250**, 9163.

Mulder, E., Brinkman, A. O., Lamers-Stahlhofen, G., and Van der Molen, H. J. (1973). *FEBS Lett.* **31**, 131.

Mulder, E., Van Beurden-Lamers, W. M. O., de Boer, W., Brinkmann, A. O., and Van der Molen, H. J. (1974). *In* "Hormone Binding and Target Cell Activation in the Testis" (M. L. Dufau and A. R. Means, eds.), pp. 343–355. Plenum, New York.

Murad, F., Strauch, B. S., and Vaughan, M. (1969). *Biochim. Biophys. Acta* **177**, 591.

Murphy, H. D. (1965a). *Proc. Soc. Exp. Biol. Med.* **118**, 1202.

Murphy, H. D. (1965b). *Proc. Soc. Exp. Biol. Med.* **120**, 671.

Nayfeh, S. N., Coffey, J. C., Hansson, V., and French, F. S. (1975). *J. Steroid Biochem.* **6**, 329.

Nelson, W. O., and Merckel, C. E. (1938). *Proc. Soc. Exp. Biol. Med.* **38**, 737.

Oseko, F., Slaunwhite, W. R., Jr., Farnsworth, W. E., Gonder, M. J., and Seal, V. S. (1973). *Program 55th Meet. Endocrine Soc.* Abstract No. 51.

Payne, A. H., and Kelch, R. P. (1975). *In* "Hormonal Regulation of Spermatogenesis" (F. S. French *et al.*, eds.), pp. 97–108. Plenum, New York.

Purvis, J. L., and Menard, R. H. (1975). *In* "Hormonal Regulation of Spermatogenesis" (F. S. French *et al.*, eds.), pp. 65–84. Plenum, New York.

Rabin, D. (1974). *In* "Hormone Binding and Target Cell Activation in the Testis" (M. L. Dufau and A. R. Means, eds.), pp. 193–200. Plenum, New York.

Rajaniemi, H., Oksanen, A., and Vanha-Perttula, T. (1974). *Horm. Res.* **5, 6.**

Reddy, P. R. K., and Villee, C. A. (1975). *Biochem. Biophys. Res. Commun.* **63,** 1063.

Ritzen, E. M., Hagenas, L., Hansson, V., and French, F. S. (1975). *In* "Hormonal Regulation of Spermatogenesis" (F. S. French *et al.*, eds.), pp. 353–366. Plenum, New York.

Rodbell, M., Birnbaumer, L., Pohl, S. L., and Krans, H. M. J. *In* "Proteins and Peptides" (M. Margoulies and F. C. Greenwood, eds.), Int. Congr. Ser. No. 241, p. 199. Excerpta Med. Found., Amsterdam.

Rommerts, F. F. G., Cooke, B. A., Van der Kemp, J. W. C. M., and Van der Molen, H. J. (1972). *FEBS Lett.* **24,** 251.

Ross, M. H. (1967). *Am. J. Anat.* **121,** 523.

Ross, M. H., and Long, I. R. (1966). *Science* **153,** 1271.

Saez, J. M., Frederich, A., De Peretti, E., and Bertrand, J. (1971). *In* "The Clinical Delineation of Birth Defects" (D. Bergsma and V. A. McKusick, eds.), Part 7, p. 185. Williams and Wilkins, Baltimore.

Sanborn, B. M., Elkington, J. S. H., Steinberger, A., Steinberger, E., and Meistrich, L. (1975). *In* "Hormonal Regulation of Spermatogenesis" (F. S. French *et al.*, eds.), pp. 293–309. Plenum, New York.

Sar, M., Stumpf, W. E., McLean, W. S., Smith, A. A., Hansson, V., Nayfeh, S. N., and French, F. S. (1975). *In* "Hormonal Regulation of Spermatogenesis" (F. S. French *et al.*, eds.), pp. 311–319. Plenum, New York.

Schneider, G., and Bardin, C. W. (1970). *Endocrinology* **87,** 864.

Schwartz, S., Bell, J., Rechnitz, S., and Rabinowitz, D. (1973). *Eur. J. Clin. Invest.* **3,** 475.

Smith, A. A., McLean, W. S., Nayfeh, S. N., French, F. S., Hansson, V., and Ritzen, E. M. (1975). *In* "Hormonal Regulation in Spermatogenesis" (F. S. French *et al.*, eds.), pp. 257–280. Plenum, New York.

Smith, O. W., and Hafs, H. D. (1973). *Proc. Soc. Exp. Biol. Med.* **142,** 804.

Smith, O. W., Mongkonpunya, K., Hafs, H. D., Convey, E. M., and Oxender, W. D. (1973). *J. Anim. Sci.* **37,** 979.

Smith, P. E. (1927). *J. Am. Med. Assoc.* **88,** 158.

Smith, P. E. (1930). *Am. J. Anat.* **45,** 205.

Steinberger, A., and Steinberger, E. (1973). *In* "The Regulation of Mammalian Reproduction" (S. J. Segal *et al.*, eds.), pp. 139–150. Thomas, Springfield, Illinois.

Steinberger, A., Thanki, K. H., and Siegal, B. (1974). *In* "Hormone Binding and Target Cell Activation in the Testis" (M. L. Dufau and A. R. Means, eds.), pp. 177–191. Plenum, New York.

Steinberger, A., Elkington, J. S. H., Sanborn, B. M., Steinberger, E., Heindel, J. J., and Lindsey, J. N. (1975). *In* "Hormonal Regulation of Spermatogenesis" (F. S. French *et al.*, eds.), p. 399. Plenum, New York.

Steinberger, E. (1971). *Phys. Rev.* **51,** 1.

Steinberger, E. (1973). *Acta Endocrinol. (Copenhagen), Suppl.* **177,** 388.

Steinberger, E. (1975). *In* "Hormonal Regulation of Spermatogenesis" (F. S. French *et al.*, eds.), pp. 337–366. Plenum, New York.

Stumpf, W. E. (1969). *Endocrinology* **85,** 31.

Stumpf, W. E., and Sar, M. (1975). *In* "Methods in Enzymology" (B. W. O'Malley and J. G. Hardman, eds.), Vol. 36, pp. 135–136. Academic Press, New York.

Tindall, D. J., Vitale, R., and Means, A. R. (1975). *Endocrinology* **97**, 636.

Tsuruhara, T., van Hall, E. V., Dufau, M. L., and Catt, K. J. (1972). *Endocrinology* **91**, 463.

Tung, P. S., and Fritz, I. B. (1975). *In* "Hormonal Regulation of Spermatogenesis" (F. S. French *et al.*, eds.), pp. 495–508. Plenum, New York.

Urry, L. (1975). *In* "International Conference of Andrology" Wayne State University, Detroit, Michigan.

Vaitukaitis, J., Hammond, J., Ross, G. T., Hickman, J., and Ashwell, G. (1971). *J. Clin. Endocrinol. Metab.* **32**, 290.

Van Damme, M.-P., Robertson, D. M., Romani, P., and Diczfalusy, E. (1973). *Acta Endocrinol. (Copenhagen)* **74**, 642.

Van Damme, M.-P., Robertson, D. M., and Diczfalusy, E. (1974). *Acta Endocrinol. (Copenhagen)* **77**, 655.

Van der Molen, H. J., Grootegoed, J. A., de Greed Bijleveld, M. J., Rommerts, F. F. G., and van der Vusse, G. J. (1975). *In* "Hormonal Regulation of Spermatogenesis" (F. S. French *et al.*, eds.), pp. 3–23. Plenum, New York.

Walsh, E. L., Cuyler, W. K., and McCullagh, P. (1934). *Am. J. Physiol.* **107**, 508.

Weddington, S. C., Hansson, V., Ritzen, E. M., Hagenas, L., French, F. S., and Nayfeh, S. N. (1975). *Nature (London)* **254**, 145.

Weddington, S. C., Hansson, V., Varaas, T., Verjans, H. L., Eik-Nes, K. B., Ryan, W. H., French, F. S., and Ritzen, E. M. (1976). *Mol. Cell. Endocrinol.* (in press).

Wilson, E. M., and Smith, A. (1975). *In* "Hormonal Regulation of Spermatogenesis" (F. S. French *et al.*, eds.), pp. 281–286. Plenum, New York.

Wilson, E. M., Moussali, C., and French, F. S. (1976). *Program 58th Meet. Endocrine Soc.* Abstract No. 297, p. 205.

Woods, M. C., and Simpson, M. E. (1961). *Endocrinology* **69**, 91.

A New Concept: Control of Early Pregnancy by Steroid Hormones Originating in the Preimplantation Embryo

ZEEV DICKMANN, SUDHANSU K. DEY,
AND JAYASREE SEN GUPTA

Department of Gynecology and Obstetrics and Ralph L. Smith
Human Development Research Center, University of Kansas
Medical Center, Kansas City, Kansas

I. INTRODUCTION

This review is concerned with the part of pregnancy that extends from fertilization through implantation of the blastocyst. The embryo during this period is referred to as the preimplantation embryo, here abbreviated PIE. Since there is no placenta during this period, we will not discuss the placenta as a source of steroid hormones.

As far back as the beginning of the twentieth century, it was already known that pregnancy (with emphasis on early pregnancy) is maintained by substances that the ovaries secrete into the blood stream. The evidence for this was that ovariectomy during early pregnancy led to abortion or resorption of the embryos (Frankel, 1903; Marshall and Jolly, 1905). The fact that the ovarian secretions were the steroid hormones progesterone and estrogen was established about a quarter of a century later. Since the adrenals have the capacity to synthesize steroids, the question arose whether adrenal steroids play a part in the maintenance of pregnancy. The answer to this question was no. Adrenalectomy during early pregnancy caused no adverse effects if the animal was given a proper salt diet (see Deanesly, 1966). Accordingly, for dozens of years, it had been axiomatic that the ovary is the only source of progesterone and estrogen required for the maintenance of early pregnancy. This axiom was challenged by us in a 1973 paper (Dickmann and Dey, 1973) in which we proposed that there is a second source of steroid hormones—the preimplantation embryo. On the basis of additional experimental results, this idea was then further developed and led us to formulate a new concept, which states: *The preimplantation embryo (PIE) has the capacity to synthesize steroid hormones which are prime regulators of the following phenomena: (1) Morula to blastocyst transformation, (2) shedding and dissolution of the zona pellucida, (3) implantation of the blastocyst, and (4) a variety of as yet undefined metabolic activities in morulae and blastocysts* (Dickmann, 1975; Dickmann *et al.*, 1975).

We have been examining the validity of this concept by addressing ourselves to three general questions: (a) Does the PIE contain steroid hormones? (b) If it does, are these steroids synthesized by the PIE, or are they merely transferred from the lumen of the reproductive tract into the PIE? (c) Do the "PIE steroids" control key phenomena during early pregnancy? We wish to emphasize that the mere presence of steroid hormones in the PIE may or may not have important sequelae. An ability of the PIE to synthesize steroid hormones would be very interesting, since the only organs in mammals known to have this ability are ovary, testis, and adrenal [the placenta is considered to be an incomplete steroidogenic organ (Ryan, 1973)]. However, it would be a major advance in developmental biology and reproductive biology if we could produce compelling evidence for our thesis, namely, that the PIE not only contains steroid hormones and makes them, but that these hormones are key factors in the control of early pregnancy.

II. Steroid Hormones in Preimplantation Embryos (PIE's)

Using a competitive protein binding assay, Seamark and Lutwak-Mann (1972) found that day-5 and day-6 rabbit blastocysts contain progesterone, 20α-hydroxypregn-4-en-3-one, and 17α-hydroxyprogesterone. With the exception of 17α-hydroxyprogesterone, which was not studied, the above experiments were repeated and confirmed by Fuchs and Beling (1974). The latter authors found approximately 150 pg of progesterone per day-5 rabbit blastocyst. In our laboratory, we radioimmunoassayed for progesterone in rat (Z. Dickmann, R. J. Baranczuk, S. K. Dey, and J. Sen Gupta, unpublished data) and mouse (J. Sen Gupta, S. K. Dey, J. D. Bast, and Z. Dickmann, unpublished data) blastocysts and found that each contains about 0.1 pg. Since, by volume, the day-5 rabbit blastocyst is roughly one thousand times larger than either the rat or the mouse blastocyst, the amount of progesterone per unit volume is similar in the blastocyst of the three species. The data are convincing that blastocysts contain steroid hormones; however, one should have some reservations about the accuracy of their quantitation. Thus, the average amount of progesterone per day-6 rabbit blastocyst was 135 pg, using radioimmunoassay (J. Bahr, Z. Dickmann, S. K. Dey, and J. Sen Gupta, unpublished data), and 200 pg, using a competitive protein-binding assay (Fuchs and Beling, 1974). Radioimmunoassays have shown that day-6 rabbit blastocysts contain estradiol-17β (Dickmann et al., 1975).

An obvious question is whether the steroids in blastocysts are synthesized by the blastocysts or are transported into them from the uterine lumen, which is known to contain steroids. In Section III, C, we show that the blastocyst can synthesize steroids; however, this does not exclude the possibility that steroids are transported from the lumen into the blastocyst. Along these lines, Dr. R. R. Maurer has suggested (personal communication, 1975) that, in the rabbit, progesterone in the uterine lumen binds to uteroglobin (a protein found during early pregnancy in the uterine secretions of rabbits and some other species), the complex is transported into the blastocyst, where it is unconjugated and then biotransformed into estrogen. This estrogen is later released from the blastocyst and thereby affects implantation. Proper experiments will determine whether this hypothesis is correct *in toto*, in part, or not at all. However, as discussed in Section III, C, the blastocyst most likely has the capacity to synthesize progesterone and therefore would not have to rely on exogenous sources.

We have not said anything about steroids in PIE's younger than blastocysts; the reason for this is that there is no information available. In Section III, A, 2, however, we deduce that morulae also have the capacity to synthesize steroid hormones.

III. Steroidogenesis in the PIE

A. $\triangle^5$-3β-Hydroxysteroid Dehydrogenase (3β-HSD) Activity in PIE's

Since 3β-HSD is a key enzyme in the synthesis of steroid hormones, its presence in a tissue constitutes strong evidence for steroidogenesis (Wiest and Kidwell, 1969). Moreover, positive quantitative correlations have been observed between 3β-HSD activity and steroid hormone production. With this in mind, in our first study (Dickmann and Dey, 1974a) we explored 3β-HSD activity in the rat PIE. 3β-HSD can be determined by a biochemical as well as a histochemical method. For our purposes, the histochemical method offered two distinct advantages: (1) the enzyme can be demonstrated in a very small amount of tissue, and (2) the exact location of the enzyme's activity can be determined. As we have had a number of inquiries about the histochemical method, presently we will expand on the brief description previously published (Dickmann and Dey, 1974a).

1. Histochemical Method for Determining 3β-HSD Activity

The method was originally described by Wattenberg (1958) and later modified by Deane et al. (1962). These authors as well as others used tissue sections. We used whole PIE's, for which the method was again slightly modified. PIE's are obtained by flushing the appropriate section of the reproductive tract with cold (0°–5°C) 0.1 M phosphate buffer (pH 7.5). Five to ten PIE's are then transferred into a depression slide containing 0.5 ml of incubation medium whose composition is: 1.8 mg of dehydro-epiandrosterone (DHA), 4 mg of nicotinamide adenine dinucleotide (NAD), 2 mg of Nitro-Blue tetrazolium (Nitro-BT), 0.4 ml of propylene glycol, and 9.6 ml of 0.1 M phosphate buffer (pH 7.5). The DHA is first dissolved in 0.25 ml of acetone, which is later removed by evaporation. For every experiment, fresh medium is prepared and filtered immediately before use. All the chemicals were purchased from SIGMA. We have noticed that the chemicals from some other companies can yield false results. Controls are treated in the same manner as experimentals except that the substrate (DHA) is omitted from the medium. We consistently obtained conspicuous differences between controls and experimentals. As a general precaution, it should be pointed out that controls could give a positive reaction due to alcohol dehydrogenase activity. This probably can be overcome by replacing propylene glycol with either dimethyl formamide or dimethyl sulfoxide. We have obtained satisfactory results with all three solvents. In all the experiments that we have published so far, we used DHA in the concentration indicated above, i.e., 0.18 mg/ml. However, in additional experiments, we obtained the same level of reaction with 0.05 mg/ml, a somewhat lower reaction with 0.03 mg/ml, and no reaction with 0.01 mg/ml.

The PIE's are incubated at 37°C for 3 hours, after which they are mounted in a small drop of incubation medium between a glass slide and a cover slip supported by four dots of a petroleum jelly–paraffin mixture.

In the presence of 3β-HSD, the Nitro-BT is reduced to a formazan salt, which is seen under a compound microscope as dark blue granules. Thus the location of these granules corresponds to the site of the enzyme's activity. The granules are best seen when the PIE is completely flattened under the cover slip and viewed with bright light. A PIE may appear bluish when viewed with a dissecting microscope, but this does not necessarily mean that the reaction is positive, i.e., that formazan granules have formed.

2. 3β-HSD in Rat PIE's

Details of the following studies have been reported previously (Dickmann and Dey, 1974a; Dey and Dickmann, 1974a). Female rats of the Holtzman strain were mated with fertile males. The morning of finding spermatozoa in the vagina was designated day 1 of pregnancy. 3β-HSD determinations were made in PIE's recovered by flushing the appropriate section of the reproductive tract on days 1 through 6. Day-1 unfertilized eggs were also studied. On day 7, the embryo is already implanted and cannot be recovered by flushing. Hence, the gestation sacs were excised, frozen, sectioned in a cryostat, and the sections were incubated for 3β-HSD determinations. There was no 3β-HSD activity in the day-1 unfertilized eggs and in day-1, -2, and -3 PIE's. Enzyme activity was seen in 43% of day-4 (0800-hour) embryos, in 62% of day-4 (1600-hour) embryos, in 100% of day-5 (0800- and 1600-hour) embryos, and in 89% of day-6 (0800- and 1500-hour) embryos. There was no activity in day-7 embryos. Among the embryos recovered on days 1 through 6, a few were degenerated. None of these degenerated embryos exhibited 3β-HSD activity.

The distribution pattern of the enzyme varied among the stages of embryonic development. In most day-4 PIE's (morulae) which showed a positive reaction, only some of the blastomeres showed activity (Fig. 1). In all the day-5 PIE's (blastocysts), all the blastomeres were positive (Fig. 2). In the day-6 PIE's (blastocysts) which were positive, the enzyme activity was confined to approximately one-half of the embryo, namely, the areas of extraembryonic ectoderm and inner cell mass. The intensity of 3β-HSD activity also varied with embryonic development. It was weak to moderate, moderate to strong, and weak to moderate in day-4, -5, and -6 PIE's, respectively. Taking into account distribution patterns and intensity, we concluded that the enzyme's activities at the various stages of embryonic development were: none in premorula stages, moderate in day-4 morulae, strong in day-5 blastocysts, moderate in day-6 blastocysts, and none in day-7 embryos. It was this particular timing and pattern of enzyme activity that originally gave us (Dickmann and

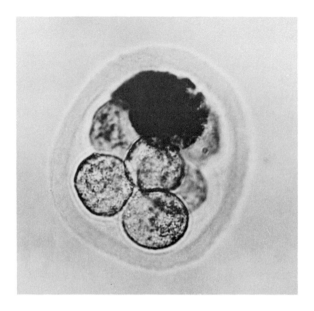

Fig. 1. Rat morula recovered at 08.00 hours on day 4 of pregnancy. Two of eight blastomeres are Δ^5-3β-hydroxysteroid dehydrogenase-positive. $\times$545. From Dickmann and Dey (1974a), by permission of the editor of the *Journal of Reproduction and Fertility*.

Dey, 1974a) the idea that, if 3β-HSD activity is equated with synthesis of steroid hormones, then these hormones may influence morula to blastocyst transformation and implantation of the blastocyst.

3. 3β-HSD in PIE's of Other Species

Once we established the pattern of 3β-HSD activity in rat PIE's, an obvious question was: Is this an exceptional case for the rat, or is this a general phenomenon in mammals? Accordingly, we studied the enzyme activity in PIE's of hamsters (Dickmann and Sen Gupta, 1974), mice (Dey and Dickmann, 1974b), and rabbits (Dickmann et al., 1975). The results in these three species were very similar to the results in rats, namely, enzyme activity began at the early morula stage, peaked at the blastocyst stage, then sharply declined, and disappeared shortly after implantation. There was a minor deviation from this general pattern in the mouse: weak enzyme activity was already seen in 30% of 2-cell embryos, however, the activity became prominent only at the morula stage. Another feature worthy of pointing out is that in most rabbit and mouse blastocysts the enzyme activity was stronger in the inner cell mass than in the trophoblast.

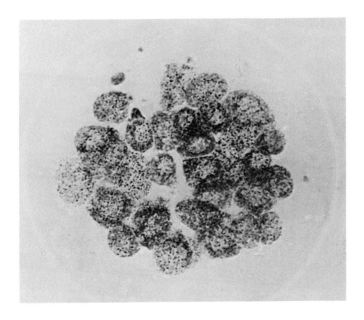

FIG. 2. Rat blastocyst recovered at 08.00 hours on day 5. The blastocyst, which had been flattened under the cover slip, shows formazan granules in all the blastomeres. ×545. From Dickmann and Dey (1974a), by permission of the editor of the *Journal of Reproduction and Fertility*.

In a recent paper, Chew and Sherman (1975) state that they have not detected 3β-HSD activity in preimplantation mouse blastocysts. However, the youngest embryos they assayed were day-4 blastocysts that had been cultured *in vitro* for 2 days, which makes them day-6 embryos. We, too, found no activity in day-6 mouse embryos, but did find some activity in day-5 blastocysts, and peak activity in day-4 blastocysts. Thus, their findings do not contradict our results.

Although our data for 3β-HSD activity in domestic pig PIE's are incomplete (Z. Dickmann, B. N. Day, D. L. Davis, S. K. Dey, and J. Sen Gupta, unpublished data), they are sufficient to permit us to draw the general conclusion that, the pattern of activity in pig PIE's is similar to that which we have described in PIE's of other species. In the pig study, the onset of estrus served as the zero point for timing the age of the PIE's (ovulation in pigs occurs approximately 36–42 hours after the onset of estrus). We have harvested PIE's at the 2- to 4-cell stage on days 3 and 4, and at the 8-cell to blastocyst stage on day 5. So far, we have examined only two 2-cell embryos, one of which was strongly positive and the other negative; a high proportion of the 4- to 8-cell embryos exhibited 3β-HSD activity, but in most cases only some of the blastomeres in a given embryo were positive; the blastocysts were positive. Since Perry *et al.* (1973) have shown that there is no steroidogenic activity in day-10 conceptuses, we tentatively conclude that the enzyme activity disappears some time between days 6 and 9. Whether there is already enzyme activity in the 1-cell PIE remains to be determined.

4. *3β-HSD Activity in Blastocysts under Various Experimental Conditions*

For the sake of discussion, let us assume that the PIE produces steroids that are essential for its own development. Mouse and rabbit 1-cell PIE's can be grown *in vitro* to the blastocyst stage. If the PIE's were to synthesize steroids during their *in vitro* culture, this would suggest that steroidogenesis in the PIE does not depend on maternal factors. However, such *in vitro* experiments have not been done yet. In order to explore the possible influence of maternal factors on steroidogenesis in the PIE *in vivo*, experiments were done to determine whether the uterine environment, pituitary hormones, or ovarian steroid hormones affect 3β-HSD activity in rat blastocysts (Dickmann and Dey, 1974b). 3β-HSD determinations were made in blastocysts obtained under the following experimental conditions: (a) To study the effects of the uterine environment, embryos were prevented from entering the uterus by ligaturing the uterotubal junction on day 1 of pregnancy. On day 5, blastocysts were recovered from the oviducts. (b) To determine the effects of pituitary gonadotropins, rats were hypophysectomized on day 2 of pregnancy. On day 5, blastocysts were recovered from either the oviduct or the uterus. (c) To assess the effects of ovarian hormones, on day 4 of pregnancy rats were ovariectomized and divided into several subgroups: They were either injected daily with 2 mg of progesterone or received no treatment. Blastocysts were recovered from the uterus on either day 5 or 8. Under all the above conditions (a, b, and c), the blastocysts were 3β-HSD positive, although there were some differences in enzyme intensity between the groups. The overall conclusion drawn from these experiments was that, 3β-HSD activity in rat blastocysts is autonomous (Dickmann and Day, 1974b).

5. *3β-HSD Activity During the Postimplantation Period*

Although the purpose of this review is to discuss the PIE as a source of and a target for steroid hormones, we will mention briefly relevant aspects of 3β-HSD activity in postimplantation tissue derived from the fertilized egg. As indicated earlier, shortly after implantation the embryo no longer shows 3β-HSD activity. The absence of activity lasts for a number of days, but then activity is resumed: on day 10 of pregnancy in the rat (Deane *et al.*, 1962), and on day 9 in the mouse (Chew and Sherman, 1975). In both species the enzyme activity is confined to the giant trophoblast cells. For the domestic pig our information is somewhat more fragmentary, but the general pattern seems to be the same as in mice and rats. Thus, 3β-HSD activity was observed in day-3, -4, and -5 PIE's (Z. Dickmann, B. Day, D. Davis, S. Dey, and J. Sen Gupta, unpublished data), there was no activity on day 10, and activity resumed on day 14 (Perry *et al.*, 1973).

The situation in the pig requires some amplification, because the literature is somewhat confusing. The confusion stems from the use of the word "blastocyst." Perry *et al.* (1973) published a paper entitled "Steroid Hormone Production by Pig Blastocysts." These authors examined "blastocysts" recovered at 10, 14, 15, and 16 days post coitum. Steroidogenic activity was found in day-14 through -16 but not in day-10 "blastocysts." It should be pointed out that although they are called "blastocysts," day-14 (or older) "blastocysts" are not comparable to blastocysts of mice, rats, hamsters, guinea pigs, humans, etc. In all of these species, the blastocyst is either the same size or somewhat larger than the embryo during the cleavage stages, it is spherical, and consists of only two types of cells: trophoblast and inner cell mass. In contrast, the day-14 pig "blastocyst" is at a much more advanced stage of development. It is enormously elongated (over 1 meter long), and has a diameter of about 1 mm. The extraembryonic tissue is already differentiated into amnion, yolk sac, and extraembryonic somatopleure, and structures in the embryo include several somites, primitive streak, neural plate, and neural groove. Since we have demonstrated 3β-HSD activity in pig PIE's on day-3, -4, and -5 and Perry *et al.* (1973) observed no activity on day 10, we contend that the steroidogenic activity in day-14 "blastocysts" represents the second wave of steroidogenic activity, which is analogous to the second wave of 3β-HSD activity seen in the postimplantation trophoblast of rats and mice.

B. 17β-Hydroxysteroid Dehydrogenase (17β-HSD) Activity in PIE's

17β-HSD is the enzyme that catalyzes the interconversion of estrone and estradiol. The enzyme activity in PIE's was determined histochemically by the same method as that described for 3β-HSD, but in place of dehydroepiandrosterone, 17β-estradiol was used as the substrate in the incubation medium. In rat (Dey and Dickmann, 1974c) and mouse (S. K. Dey and Z. Dickmann, unpublished) PIE's, 17β-HSD activity was confined to the same developmental stages as was 3β-HSD. In rabbit (Dickmann *et al.*, 1975) and hamster (Dickmann and Sen Gupta, 1974), 17β-HSD activity was observed in blastocysts; earlier stages were not studied.

17β-HSD is present not only in endocrine tissues but also in a variety of other tissues, such as liver, kidney, and intestine. Because it is found in such a variety of tissues, the presence of 17β-HSD, by itself, in PIE's would have had a limited meaning. However, its presence in conjunction with 3β-HSD suggests synthesis of estrogen. This notion is further strengthened by our finding of estrogen in rabbit blastocysts (Dickmann *et al.*, 1975).

C. The Capacity of the PIE to Synthesize Steroids from Steroid and Nonsteroid Precursors

The ovary, testis, and adrenal are known as *the* steroidogenic organs because of their ability to biotransform nonsteroid precursors into steroids; moreover, they have the capacity to make new steroids from existing ones. The placenta is regarded as an incomplete steroidogenic organ because it cannot readily synthesize acetate into steroids, nor can it biotransform C_{21} steroids to androgens or estrogens (Ryan, 1973). A crucial aspect for the support of the "PIE steroids" concept is to demonstrate the PIE's capacity to synthesize steroid hormones. 3β-HSD activity in PIE's indicates but does not prove that there is *de novo* synthesis of steroid hormones. At present, there is only one published study in which the PIE's capacity to synthesize steroid hormones was tested: "Metabolism in vitro of acetate and certain steroids by six-day-old rabbit blastocysts" (Huff and Eik-Nes, 1966). In this carefully planned and executed study, blastocysts were incubated with the following precursors: sodium acetate-1-^{14}C, Δ^5-pregnenolone-7-^{3}H, 17α-hydroxypregnenolone-7-^{3}H, progesterone-4-^{14}C, and androstenedione-4-^{14}C. It was shown that acetate was converted to cholesterol and to pregnenolone, and that each of the steroid precursors used was converted into one or more new steroids. Thus, based on these results we can regard the rabbit blastocyst as a steroidogenic body. Additional experiments should be done to determine the range of steroids that PIE's can synthesize.

D. Tropic Hormones in PIE's

Steroidogenic tissues are known to require tropic hormones to stimulate steroidogenesis in them. Therefore, it is reasonable to postulate that steroidogenesis in the PIE is also dependent upon stimulation by one or more tropic hormones. Such tropic hormones could originate in the pituitary, in the PIE, or in both. Accordingly, experiments were done to determine the effects of pituitary hormones on 3β-HSD activity in rat blastocysts (Dickmann and Dey, 1974b). On day 2 of pregnancy, rats were hypophysectomized. Blastocysts recovered on day 5 showed 3β-HSD activity comparable to that in blastocysts obtained from untreated pregnant rats. Since the time at which the hypophysectomies were done was before the onset of 3β-HSD activity in PIE's, it was concluded that neither the initiation nor the maintenance of 3β-HSD activity in PIE's is dependent on pituitary tropic hormones. Furthermore, it was deduced that the PIE may synthesize its own tropic hormones or else steroidogenesis in the PIE may not require tropic hormone stimulation. Subsequent work by others has shown that the PIE contains and is able to synthesize a luteinizing hormone (LH)- or human chorionic gonadotropin (hCG)-like substance.

LH- or hCG-like Substance in PIE's

Using a radioreceptor assay, Haour and Saxena (1974) determined the presence of an LH- or hCG-like substance in day-6 rabbit blastocysts. This result suggested to them that blastocyst gonadotropin may play a role in maintaining the corpus luteum and that it may protect the embryo during implantation from a maternal immune response. Our interpretation (Dickmann et al., 1975) of their finding was that the gonadotropin they identified is a (the ?) tropic hormone that stimulates steroidogenesis in the blastocyst. Fujimoto et al. (1975) used a double antibody radioimmunoassay to identify an LH-like substance in blastocoelic fluid obtained from day-4, -5, and -6 rabbit blastocysts: all contained an LH-like substance, with the highest concentration in day-6 blastocysts.

Wiley (1974) used an immunocytochemical method to detect an LH- or hCG-like substance in mouse PIE's at various stages of development. The gonadotropic activity found was: 1-cell stage (−), 2-cell (±), 8-cell (+), morula (+++), and blastocyst (±). In a second series of experiments, gonadotropic activity was assayed in PIE's which had been grown in vitro from the 2-cell stage to the blastocyst stage. The gonadotropic activity in these PIE's was similar to that of the PIE's recovered directly from the mother. Thus, the increase in gonadotropic activity in PIE's during their culture in vitro indicated that the LH- or hCG-like substances was synthesized de novo in the PIE. The shape of the curve of gonadotropic activity in mouse embryos during the preimplantation period is similar to the shape of the 3β-HSD activity curve. However, if the two curves are plotted, with the abscissa representing time of pregnancy, the 3β-HSD curve would be to the right of the gonadotropic curve. In other words, the gonadotropic activity appears as well as disappears at slightly earlier stages. This fits our hypothesis that steroidogenesis in the PIE is stimulated by gonadotropin(s) originating in the PIE.

A biological activity of blastocyst gonadotropin has also been demonstrated. It was shown that rabbit blastocoelic fluid caused luteinization of, and progesterone secretion by, monkey granulosa cells grown *in vitro* (Haour *et al.*, 1975). Sundaram *et al.* (1975) used another *in vitro* system in which decapsulated mouse testes, or mouse Leydig cells, showed an increase in testosterone production in the presence of hCG or LH, but not in the presence of day-6 or -7 rabbit blastocoelic fluid. There are obvious explanations for the lack of testosterone production in the above experiment: (a) The particular culture conditions and methodology could have been the cause. (b) The rabbit blastocoelic fluid could contain a substance that has inhibitory effects on mouse male gonadal cells. (c) The mouse cells did not respond, but male gonadal cells of another species might have responded. In addition to the above, there is a more subtle explanation, or rather speculation. It is known that LH and hCG have the capacity to evoke steroidogenesis in both male and female gonads. On the other hand, the blastocyst gonadotropin is a new, unexplored substance; hence, based entirely on the negative results obtained by Sundaram *et al.* (1975), we may suggest that the blastocyst gonadotropin can evoke steroidogenesis in the female gonad and in the PIE, but not in the male gonad.

The discussion in this section has been confined to an LH- or hCG-like substance, because this is the only compound that has been investigated so far. However, we should keep in mind that the PIE may have the capacity to synthesize other known tropic hormones as well as tropic hormones not found in either the pituitary or the placenta. In light of what has been said, we postulate that the PIE tropic hormone or hormones are essential for stimulating steroidogenesis in the PIE.

E. Cyclic AMP in PIE's

It is fairly well established that, when LH stimulates steroidogenesis in cells, cyclic AMP (cyclic adenosine 3′,5′-monophosphate, cAMP) acts as a second messenger, mediating the action of LH (for reviews, see Robison, 1972; Menon and Gunaga, 1974). The sequence of events that have been postulated are: LH interacts with a specific receptor in the cell membrane; this interaction leads to an increase in adenyl cyclase activity; adenyl cyclase causes an increase in intracellular cAMP, which in turn stimulates steroidogenesis. Furthermore, experiments have shown that exogenous cAMP can mimic the effects of LH.

Having said the above, an obvious question is: Does cAMP act as a second messenger in PIE steroidogenesis? Owing to paucity of knowledge in this area, we cannot answer this question definitively. However, the limited information available permits suggesting that cAMP is involved in PIE steroidogenesis. Fisher and Gunaga (1975) have demonstrated (a) that cAMP is present in all stages of mouse PIE's, and (b) that the level of cAMP decreases gradually during the preimplantation period, the blastocyst containing about one-third the amount found in the 1-cell embryo. Moreover, these authors showed that in mouse PIE's grown *in vitro* in medium containing theophylline (theophylline causes increase in cAMP by blocking the activity of phosphodiesterase that degrades cAMP), there was a very significant increase in the levels of cAMP and the development of these PIE's was retarded. We propose that these results can be interpreted in light of steroidogenic activity in the PIE by postulating that (1) the changes in cAMP during the preimplantation period are necessary to permit the proper steroidogenic activity, and (2) the theophylline-caused increase in cAMP had an adverse effect on steroidogenesis in the PIE causing a steroid imbalance, which in turn resulted in retarded development. The above are suggested interpretations whose validity will have to be tested by appropriate experimentation.

F. PROSTAGLANDINS IN PIE's

In the preceding section we pointed out that cAMP acts as a mediator in the process of steroidogenesis. There is a considerable amount of evidence which shows that prostaglandins (PGs), too, act as mediators in steroidogenesis. This subject has been reviewed by Kuehl *et al.* (1973), Kuehl (1974), Silver and Smith (1975), and others. Here, it will suffice to mention some salient points: (a) The mediating action of the PGs works via cAMP. (b) It has been shown that various PGs stimulate synthesis of cAMP, and that among those tested the PGEs were most effective. (c) A number of authors have demonstrated that PGE stimulates steroidogenesis. For example, Speroff and Ramwell (1970) showed that, on a molar basis, PGE_2 was half as effective as LH in stimulating steroid synthesis in bovine corpora lutea slices incubated *in vitro*. (d) Although the point is still controversial, it has been proposed (Kuehl, 1974) that when LH stimulates steroidogenesis, it stimulates first synthesis of PG, which in turn works through cAMP.

Very little can be said about PGs and their relationship to steroidogenesis in the PIE, as only one paper has been published on this subject. Dickmann and Spilman (1975) showed that rabbit blastocysts contain PGF and PGE-A. They speculated that one or more of the PGs found could act as mediators in blastocyst steroidogenesis.

IV. The Function of "PIE Steroids"

A. Evidence from Papers Whose Authors Did Not Evoke the "PIE Steroids" Concept

In the Introduction we postulated that the "PIE steroids" are critical for the control of (1) morula to blastocyst transformation, (2) shedding and dissolution of the zona pellucida, (3) implantation of the blastocyst, and (4) a variety of as yet undefined metabolic activities in morulae and blastocysts. We will now discuss indirect evidence that can be used to support the "PIE steroids" concept. The evidence is taken from published papers whose authors probably were not aware of the "PIE steroids" concept and therefore did not evoke it.

1. Morula to Blastocyst Transformation

During the cleavage stages, many biochemical changes take place in the PIE. It is possible that some researchers may refer to some of these changes as "differentiation" simply because the word differentiation has many nuances. However, if we define differentiation as a process that leads to morphological, biochemical, and functional distinction between cells, then the first time the fertilized egg undergoes differentiation is during morula to blastocyst transformation. This is manifested in that the blastocyst, but not the morula, has two types of cells—trophoblast and inner cell mass (see Gardner, 1972). We do not think that it is a mere coincidence that 3β-HSD activity begins at the morula stage, and therefore postulate that the process of morula to blastocyst transformation is regulated, at least in part, by steroid hormones synthesized by the morula. If this postulate is correct, then disturbing the normal hormonal balance within the morula should impede development. Actually, there are a few published experimental results that tend to support this line of reasoning. Dickmann (1970) showed that rat morulae degenerated subsequent to their transfer into the uteri of ovariectomized recipient rats treated with progesterone (2 mg/day). It should be remembered that in the intact pregnant rat, the ovaries secrete progesterone and estrogen. Thus, under the experimental conditions, the progesterone had deleterious effects on the morula. When, under the same conditions, instead of morulae, blastocysts were transferred, they suffered no ill effects. An explanation for this drastic difference in response between morulae and blastocysts is as follows: (1) The considerably greater steroidogenic capability of the blastocyst enabled it to cope with the exogenous steroid. (2) Blastocyst development depends to a much smaller degree on steroid stimulation.

(3) During the blastocyst stage, the function of the "PIE steroids" is primarily that of preparing the uterus for implantation, and the exogenous dose of progesterone used was compatible with uterine preparation for implantation.

In the present discussion, we have been assuming that the morulae were affected directly by the exogenous progesterone. But, we cannot exclude the possibility that the effect of the progesterone was not direct but was mediated via the uterus. However, it has been shown that progesterone can have direct toxic effects on mouse morulae grown *in vitro* (Whitten, 1957; Kirkpatrick, 1971). Treating intact pregnant rats with a combination of 6α-methyl-17α-hydroxyprogesterone acetate (Provera) and estrone also prevented morulae from developing into blastocysts (Dickmann, 1973). The deleterious effects of the exogenous steroids in all the above cases can be explained in terms of disturbance of the normal balance of steroid hormones within the morula. In other words, we propose that the morula synthesizes steroid hormones at certain rates and in certain proportions which are essential for the normal development of the morula. At this juncture it would be premature to speculate which steroids are involved; they could be sex steroids, corticosteroids, or even new steroids that hitherto have not been identified.

2. *Shedding and Dissolution of the Zona Pellucida*

After the blastocyst stage is reached, the next major event in pregnancy is implantation. The beginning of implantation is marked by the attachment of the blastocyst's trophoblast to the uterine epithelium. This attachment cannot take place as long as the blastocyst is enclosed in the zona pellucida (zona). Therefore, removal (shedding) of the zona is a *sine qua non* for implantation. On the basis of experimental evidence, three mechanisms for zona shedding were proposed (Dickmann, 1969): (1) The entire zona is lysed by an agent originating in either the uterus or the blastocyst, or in both. (2) The blastocyst actively escapes from the zona through a narrow passage, leaving behind an intact zona. (3) A wide crack is formed in the zona through which the blastocyst is released; the crack results from increased pressure in the perivitelline space and/or a lytic agent emanating from the blastocyst. In the rat, there is good evidence that the second mechanism is operating, but mechanisms (1) and (2) cannot be excluded (Dickmann, 1969). Under normal pregnancy conditions, most rat blastocysts lose their zonae between 14.00 and 18.00 hours on day 5 of pregnancy (Dickmann, 1967). Dissolution of the zona seems to occur very shortly after shedding, as attested by the finding that very few empty zonae are recovered when uteri are flushed in the afternoon of day 5 (Dickmann, 1967). If pregnant rats are ovariectomized on day 4 or earlier and are then given no further treatment, or are treated with progesterone, estrogen, or both, one can induce premature shedding (Wu, 1973), delay shedding (Dickmann, 1969, 1972; Dickmann and De-Feo, 1967), and have empty zonae persist *in utero* for days after shedding had occurred (Dickmann, 1969, 1972). From these results it was deduced that the ovarian hormones regulate, at least in part, both shedding and dissolution of the zona (Dickmann, 1972).

Regardless of the mechanism by which shedding and dissolution is achieved, a lytic agent must be involved, which very likely is an enzyme or enzymes. We propose that the *de novo* synthesis of the lytic agent is induced by one or more steroid hormones that originate in either the ovary or the blastocyst, or in both. Because of the close proximity of the blastocyst to the zona, we tend to assign a more important role to the "blastocyst steroids." Evidence in support of this contention are the findings that mouse blastocysts transferred into a variety of extrauterine sites lost their zonae regardless of the hormonal status of the hosts, which were pregnant and nonpregnant females, intact and castrated males, and immature males and females (see Dickmann, 1969).

3. *Implantation of the Blastocyst*

Since the hormonal control of implantation has been studied more extensively in rat and mouse than in any other species, we use the rat as our primary model for discussion.

The basic requirements for implantation in the rat are a mature, zona-free blastocyst and a uterus which had been primed with progesterone and is then stimulated with estrogen. The estrogen stimulation occurs in the form of an "estrogen surge" that occurs about 24 hours before the onset of implantation. For many years it had been universally accepted that the progesterone and estrogen required for implantation originate in the ovaries and reach the uterus via the circulation. Dickmann and Dey (1974a) proposed that this is only part of the story and that *"After the embryo settles on a prospective site for implantation, it exerts a local hormonal effect on the endometrium which is critical for implantation. . . . In other words, the two sources of steroid hormones, the ovary and the preimplantation embryo, complement each other and implantation cannot occur in the absence of either source."* This hypothesis can be expanded as follows. The relative importance of the hormonal contribution by the ovary vs the blastocyst may vary from species to species. For example, in the rat, it is well established that ovarian progesterone and estrogen are indispensable for implantation. Based on experimental evidence (see Section IV, B), we maintain that the ovarian estrogen (or exogenous estrogen given systemically to ovariectomized pregnant rats), although necessary, is not sufficient, and that local "blastocyst estrogen" is also required for the induction of implantation.

In the rabbit, the hormonal conditions are somewhat different. Implantation occurs in ovariectomized does which receive substitution therapy of progesterone only, although a slightly higher percentage of blastocysts implant when estrogen is added to the progesterone (Kwun and Emmens, 1974). It was shown that rabbit blastocysts contain estrogen (Dickmann et al., 1975). We propose that in the rabbit, as in the rat, both progesterone and estrogen are required for the induction of implantation. In the rabbit, however, the blastocyst is the all-important source of the estrogen, and therefore implantation can occur in the absence of ovarian estrogen. However, implantation cannot occur in the absence of ovarian progesterone.

Many studies in which hormonal substitution therapy was given to pregnant ovariectomized mammals indicate that the ovary contributes progesterone, which is critical for the induction of implantation, and estrogen, which may or may not be critical, depending on the species. It seems that progesterone and estrogen are the only ovarian hormones involved in the control of implantation. However, since the exploration of "blastocyst steroids" is still in its infancy, we should consider the possibility that "blastocyst steroids" other than progesterone and estrogen could be involved in the induction of implantation.

Various studies have shown that preceding implantation, the uterus undergoes local changes in the area adjacent to the blastocyst. The authors of some of these studies suggested that these local changes are caused by a substance released from the blastocyst, but none suggested what this substance might be. As already stated, we think that the substance contains one or more steroids. Examples of studies concerned with local uterine changes follow.

a. *Autolysis of the Uterine Luminal Epithelium.* El-Shershaby and Hinchliffe (1975), working with mice, described deterioration and death of uterine epithelial cells adjacent to the blastocyst. They suggested that this phenomenon is caused by ". . . self digestion, rather than by trophoblast attack or secretion." They offered no explanation as to what initiates autolysis. Abraham et al. (1970) observed that in rabbit uterine epithelium adjacent to the blastocyst, there was a sharp increase in the number and size of lysosomes and an increase in acid phosphatase activity. It seemed to these authors that ". . . the lysosomes in the epithelial cells play a distinct role in destroying their cytoplasm just prior to and during implantation. . . ." We concur with their suggestion as it is well established that, lysosomes and lysosomal enzymes such as acid phosphatase play a significant role in autolytic processes of cells. There is evidence that certain steroid hormones labilize whereas others stabilize lysosomes (Weissmann, 1969). Furthermore, it was shown that estrogen can regulate development and digestive activity of lysosomes in rabbit uterine mucosa (Henzl et al., 1968). On the basis of all the above findings, we propose that the disintegration of the uterine epithelium is brought about by epithelial lysosomes whose activity is regulated by steroid hormones. Since the phenomenon occurs only around the blastocyst, the steroid or steroids involved most likely originate in the blastocyst.

b. *Leukocytic Response.* Smith and Wilson (1974) observed in mice that during the period from before until after shedding of the zona, there was a significant increase in the number of leukocytes in the uterine luminal epithelium surrounding the blastocyst as compared with epithelium from interimplantation areas or from pseudopregnant uteri. Although this seems to have been an obvious effect caused by the blastocyst, the authors explain the leukocytic increase as being ". . . due to an increased secretion of estrogen, which takes place at the time of implantation." We agree that estrogen can cause a leukocytic response. If estrogen was the causative agent, then, because of its local effect, it most probably was "blastocyst estrogen."

c. *"Implantation Material."* Implantation in the rat begins in the evening of day 5 of pregnancy. It was shown that when afternoon day-5 blastocysts were transferred into the uteri of suitable recipients, their survival rate was significantly lower than that of morning day-5 blastocysts. The interpretation given for these results was that the blastocyst may have a limited supply of "implantation material," and, when this is used up, the blastocyst can no longer implant (Dickmann and Noyes, 1960). Our present interpretation of these results is as follows. The "implantation material" contains steroid hormones. By the afternoon of day 5, the blastocyst has already released onto the uterine epithelium a considerable portion of the total steroids it would eventually release. After it is removed from its native uterus, this relatively old blastocyst may no longer have the capacity to synthesize sufficient quantities of steroids to affect implantation in the uterus of the host rat.

The experimental results by Bitton-Casimiri et al. (1971) support the above postulate. By using time-lapse photography, they recorded changes in afternoon day-5 rat blastocysts cultured *in vitro*. They observed blastocyst contractions that eventually led to the expulsion of a large portion of the blastocoelic fluid plus several vesicles. They suggested that the released material may provide the stimulus for the endometrial vascular changes that precede implantation. They did not comment on the chemical identity of these expelled materials.

d. *Synthesis of Nucleic Acids in the Uterus.* Heald et al. (1975) compared pregnant with pseudopregnant rat uteri and found that, during day

5, the increase in RNA and DNA synthesis was markedly greater in the pregnant uteri. They attributed the increase in synthesis to a stimulus by the blastocysts, but did not suggest what the nature of the stimulus might be. However, the evidence that the blastocysts were the causative agents was inconclusive, because of the specific experimental design Heald *et al.* used. They unilaterally ovariectomized rats, and mated them 3 to 4 weeks later. For the assays, they compared the nonpregnant (pseudopregnant) with the pregnant uterus taken from the same rat. It is possible that the differences they observed resulted from disturbance of the blood supply to the pseudopregnant uterus, and/or from local hormonal effects on the pregnant uterus by the remaining ovary. These possibilities could be ruled out by using the following experimental design. Recover morulae (day-4 embryos) from donor rats and transfer them into one of the uteri of a day-4 pseudopregnant recipient, and to the contralateral uterus transfer controls: either transfer medium, transfer medium containing unfertilized eggs, or premorula embryos. On day 5, by which time the morulae will have developed into blastocysts, compare RNA and DNA synthesis in the experimental and control uteri. Should such experiments demonstrate that the blastocysts do cause an increase in synthesis of nucleic acids, we would then suggest that the nature of the stimulus was "blastocyst estrogen," as estrogen is known to have the capacity to stimulate synthesis of nucleic acids (e.g., Billing *et al.*, 1969).

4. *Metabolic Activities in Morulae and Blastocysts*

It is well established that steroid hormones have a wide range of effects on metabolism. For example, in specific target tissues, estrogen is known to stimulate RNA, DNA, protein, lipid, and carbohydrate synthesis. This being the case, steroid hormones could regulate, at least in part, metabolic activities in the PIE, providing the PIE has steroid hormone receptors. There is evidence, but not complete proof, that the cytoplasm of rabbit blastocysts contains receptors for estrogen (Bhatt and Bullock, 1974). Receptors for other steroids may also be present in PIE's, but so far no attempts have been made to identify them.

The currently widely accepted theory for the mode of action of steroid hormones is that the hormone enters the cell and binds to a cytoplasmic receptor; this is followed by a chain of reactions that lead to synthesis of nuclear RNA, which, in turn, leads to synthesis of new proteins (Jensen and DeSombre, 1972; O'Malley and Means, 1974). Although currently not considered very popular, we should entertain the possibilities that a steroid hormone may exert its effects by altering the properties of the cell membrane (Willmer, 1961) or by interacting directly with enzymes, nucleic acids, and lysosomes (Thompson and Lippman, 1974).

In the mouse, RNA and protein synthesis (Mintz, 1964; Monesi and

Salfi, 1967; Graves and Biggers, 1970) and carbon dioxide output (Brinster, 1967) increase considerably during the morula through blastocyst stages. These changes in metabolic activity could be caused by "PIE steroids," as 3β-HSD activity becomes prominent at the morula stage. Metabolic activities in rat and mouse blastocysts have been studied by recording changes in production of carbon dioxide (Menke and McLaren, 1970; Torbit and Weitlauf, 1974) and synthesis of RNA and DNA (Dass et al., 1969; Sanyal and Meyer, 1970; Jacobson et al., 1970) and protein (Weitlauf and Greenwald, 1968). Using these parameters, it was shown that in pregnant females ovariectomized and treated with progesterone, the metabolic activity in blastocysts was very low, but it rose sharply when estrogen was superimposed on progesterone. In these in vivo experiments, it could not be determined whether the estrogen effects on the blastocyst were direct or mediated via a uterine product. A direct effect of estrogen on the metabolism of mouse blastocysts cultured in vitro was shown: the estrogen caused an increase in synthesis of protein (Smith and Smith, 1971), RNA (Lau et al., 1973; Harrer and Lee, 1973), and DNA (Harrer and Lee, 1973). The experiments cited show that estrogen can affect metabolic activities in the blastocyst. This suggests, but does not prove, that steroid hormones affect metabolism of the PIE in the untreated animal. Should it be demonstrated that steroid hormones do play a role in regulating the metabolism of the PIE, the source of the steroids could be the PIE, the ovary, or both. However, the primary role would probably be carried by the "PIE steroids" because of their close proximity to target. Moreover, if the steroids originating in the ovary played a role, it probably would not be obligatory, since embryos can develop in vitro from the 1-cell stage to the blastocyst in media not containing any steroids.

Throughout Section IV, A, we have given examples of experimental results that can be explained in light of the "PIE steroid" concept. In the next section, we will turn our attention to more direct evidence in support of the concept.

B. Experiments Specifically Designed to Explore the Functional Significance of "PIE Steroids"

1. Local Increase in Uterine Capillary Permeability

Our discussion will refer to rats and mice, because most of the work on local increase in capillary permeability (ICP) in the uterus has been done in these two species (e.g., in mice: Finn and McLaren, 1967; McLaren, 1968; in rats: Psychoyos, 1960, 1961). The ICP is the earliest macroscopic indication that the uterus has reacted to the presence of the blastocyst. The reaction can be demonstrated experimentally by injecting intravenously a high-molecular-weight dye (e.g., Pontamine Sky Blue, Evans Blue, Chicago Blue) and inspecting the uteri 15 minutes later. In the area where each blastocyst is located, a discrete blue band will be seen across the uterus. Apparently, the macromolecular dye leaves the circulation only in loci where ICP had occurred. Psychoyos (1967) proposed, and we agree, that the ICP is a necessary preliminary for the decidual reaction; and it is well established that in rats and mice (and in other species) the decidual reaction is a prerequisite for implantation. It seems obvious that the blastocyst provides the stimulus for the induction of ICP, since the reaction occurs only in the vicinity of the blastocyst. Nevertheless, we have not encountered in the literature any suggestion as to what the nature of the stimulus by the blastocyst might be. However, it has been demonstrated that in castrated rats and rabbits (Hechter et al., 1941) and in immature rats (Ham et al., 1970), systemic injection of estrogen induces ICP throughout the length of the uterus.

When we designed the experiments described below (Z. Dickmann, J. Sen Gupta, and S. K. Dey, unpublished), our working hypothesis was the following: *The stimulus for the ICP in the intact pregnant rat is "blastocyst estrogen." This stimulus is effective only in a uterus which had been properly primed with systemic progesterone and estrogen.* As background controls, we used day-5 pregnant rats which, between 22.00 23.00 hours, were injected intravenously with a solution of Chicago Blue. Fifteen minutes later the rats were killed; the uteri were excised and inspected for blue bands. The number of blue bands per rat corresponded to the expected number of blastocysts. Experiments were then done to test our hypothesis. Day-5 pseudopregnant rats were used. At various times between 10.00 and 16.00 hours, the rats were anesthetized, the uteri were exteriorized, and by going through the uterine wall, a minute quantity of estrogen in water was instilled into each lumen at three separate loci. As in the controls, between 22.00 and 23.00 hours, the rats were injected with Chicago Blue and later killed and checked for blue bands. The procedure did induce blue band formation. However, when we instilled into uteri water not containing estrogen, and when we inserted the pipette without instilling anything, blue bands also formed. These results could have been predicted, since trauma induces ICP. However, we were hoping that the trauma would be sufficiently mild not to induce ICP, as we employed the method used for egg transfer (Dickmann, 1971), which is gentle enough not to induce deciduomata. At any rate, our next task was to find a way by which to deliver estrogen to local areas in the uterine lumen without physically traumatizing these same areas. This problem was resolved in the following manner.

Fertilized eggs were recovered from pregnant rats on day 3 between

12.00 and 14.00 hours. The eggs were incubated for 2 hours in a balanced salt solution containing estrodiol-17β (2 μg/ml) and were then transferred into the uteri of day-5 pseudopregnant recipients. For reasons which will be clarified below, the uteri were punctured and the transfer pipette was inserted into the ovarian quarter of the uterus. On the same day, between 22.00 and 23.00 hours, the recipients were injected with Chicago Blue; 15 minutes later they were killed and the uteri were checked for blue band formation. Normally, during day 5 of pregnancy, blastocysts are distributed throughout the length of the uterus; therefore, we were hoping that the transferred day-3 eggs would also be distributed, and once they settled on a particular spot, they would lose there the estrogen that they had picked up during the *in vitro* incubation. Then, if our hypothesis was correct, the estrogen released from an egg would result in the induction of a blue band. The presence of one or more blue bands in the ovarian quarter of the uterus would be interpreted as having been induced by the physical trauma of the puncture needle and the transfer pipette, but blue bands in the other three quarters of the uterus would be regarded as resulting from a stimulus by the transferred eggs. Control transfers were done in the same way as experimentals, except that the eggs were incubated in estrogen-free balanced salt solution. Nine recipients for experimental transfers and ten recipients for control transfers were used. In the controls, blue bands were present only in the ovarian quarter of the uterus, whereas in the experimentals, blue bands were present in all four quarters. Thus, the estrogen-carrying eggs, but not the estrogen-free eggs, induced ICP. We conclude, therefore, that our working hypothesis had been correct. The local estrogen most likely works by inducing local release of uterine histamine (Spaziani and Szego, 1958; Szego, 1965), or some other vasoactive substance which in turn causes ICP. A more remote interpretation could be that the estrogen stimulated the release of a vasoactive substance from the egg itself, and that this is also what happens with blastocysts. At present, we have no information whether blastocysts can synthesize and release vasoactive substances. However, as pointed out in Section III, F, rabbit blastocysts contain prostaglandins, which are vasoactive substances.

2. Effects of CI-628 and Estrogen on the Development of Mouse PIE's Grown in Vitro

Estrogen has the capacity to affect a wide range of metabolic activities (see Section IV, A, 4). Rabbit blastocysts seem to contain estrogen receptors (Bhatt and Bullock, 1974), and they also contain estrogen, which is probably synthesized by the blastocyst itself (Dickmann et al., 1975). On the basis of this information, we formulated the following working hypothesis. "PIE estrogen" plays a major role in the regulation of the metabolism of mouse PIE's. If this is correct, then an antiestrogen would interfere with the development of the PIE. The experiments presented below (J. Sen Gupta, S. K. Dey, and Z. Dickmann, unpublished) were designed to test this hypothesis.

Embryos of 4–8 cells were recovered from random-bred Swiss mice, which were killed in the morning of day 3 of pregnancy. The PIE's were cultured in tubes for 48 hours according to the procedures described by Whitten (1971). For the experimental groups, the culture media contained various concentrations of the nonsteroidal antiestrogen CI-628 (1,2-$(p$-α-$(p$-methoxyphenyl)-β-nitrostyrylphenoxy) ethylpyrrolidine, monocitrate). This compound has been shown to displace estradiol-17β from receptor sites (Callantine et al., 1968, 1969). Concurrently with each experimental group, control PIE's were cultured in CI-628-free media. The end point in these experiments was the formation of normal blastocysts. The results are presented in Table I. At the concentration of 1.5 μg/ml, CI-628 prevented development in all the PIE's tested. Additional experiments showed that the inhibitory action took place during the transformation period from morula to blastocyst.

Like other antiestrogens, CI-628 is also a weak proestrogen. However, in these experiments, CI-628 is unlikely to have acted as a proestrogen, as we have observed no inhibitory effects with estradiol-17β at a concentration of 10 μg/ml. Callantine and his associates have carried out many studies wtih CI-628 and concluded (Callantine et al., 1969) that this compound exerts its effects by virtue of its antiestrogenic properties, not by virtue of an antimetabolic action. We therefore conclude that the development of the embryos was inhibited because "PIE estrogen" was displaced from the PIE receptors by the CI-628. This, in turn, suggests

TABLE I

RESULTS OF CULTURING 4- TO 8-CELL MOUSE EMBRYOS FOR 48 HOURS[a]

	Experimental			Control		
Group	No. of PIE's	CI-628/ml (μg)	% Developed to blastocysts	No. of PIE's	CI-628/ml	% Developed to blastocysts
1	106	0.5	61	89	None	84
2	49	1.0	45	46	None	98
3	60	1.5	0	56	None	89

[a] Each experimental group was cultured concurrently with a control group. PIE, preimplantation embryo.

that the "PIE estrogen" plays a crucial role in the development of the mouse PIE.

A tissue that is responsive to, and dependent on, stimulation by one or more steroid hormones, will not function properly if it is either understimulated or overstimulated. We have seen that estrogen understimulation (by use of CI-628) of the mouse PIE results in its demise. Thus, as would have been expected, overstimulation with estrogen also caused degeneration of mouse PIE's grown *in vitro* (Kirkpatrick, 1971; J. Sen Gupta, S. K. Dey, and Z. Dickmann, unpublished).

3. Effects of CI-628 on the Development of Rabbit Blastocysts in Vivo

Bhatt and Bullock (1974) studied the effects of CI-628 on implantation of the rabbit blastocyst. Three kinds of experiments were done. (1) On day 5 of pregnancy, in each rabbit, the uteri were exteriorized and one was instilled with saline and the other with saline containing CI-628. On day 12, the rabbits were relaparotomized and checked for the presence of implantations. On the saline-treated sides, which had 18 corpora lutea, there were 15 implantations, whereas the CI-628-treated sides had 27 corpora lutea, but only one implantation. (2) In the second experiment, day-5 control blastocysts were incubated *in vitro* for 1 hour in TC medium 199, and experimental blastocysts were incubated in TC medium 199 containing CI-628. The control and experimental blastocysts were then transferred into opposite uteri of day-5 pseudopregnant recipient rabbits. The percentages of blastocysts implanting was 83% for controls and 13% for experimentals. (3) In the third experiment, it was shown that ^{3}H-labeled estradiol binds to blastocyst cytosol, and that this estradiol is displaced by CI-628. In interpreting these results, the authors suggested that in the intact pregnant rabbit ". . . estradiol bound to the blastocyst may act as a local signal to the uterus." And by acting directly on the blastocyst, the CI-628 displaced the estrogen and thereby prevented implantation. The authors did not opine whether the estrogen bound to the blastocyst originated in the ovary or in the blastocyst.

We utilized the above results for designing experiments (S. K. Dey, Z. Dickmann, and J. Sen Gupta, unpublished) whose purpose was to explore the function(s) of "blastocyst estrogen." We argued that if an antiestrogen inhibits implantation, it follows that estrogen must be playing a critical role in implantation. In the intact pregnant rabbit the source for this estrogen could be the blastocyst, the ovary, or both. By ovariectomizing the rabbit, we can eliminate the ovaries as a possible source of estrogen. If under such conditions the CI-628 still inhibits implantation, this would indicate that the blastocyst is the source of the estrogen needed for implantation. The adrenals are an unlikely source of "nidatory estrogen," since implantation occurs in ovariectomized–adrenalectomized rabbits treated with progesterone (Kwun and Emmens, 1974).

In experiment I, we repeated the first experiment of Bhatt and Bullock and confirmed their results. In experiment II, rabbits were ovariectomized on day 1 of pregnancy (i.e., 24 hours after mating), injected twice daily with 1 mg of progesterone on days 1 through 5 and 2 mg of progesterone twice daily on days 6 and 7. On day 5, the rabbits were laparotomized, and saline was instilled into one uterus (control) and saline containing CI-628 into the other (experimental). On day 8 they were killed, and the uteri were inspected for implantations and were then flushed to recover possible unimplanted eggs or blastocysts. In six rabbits, the ovaries on the control side had 29 ovulation points, and the uteri contained 19 implantations and one collapsed, degenerating blastocyst; on the experimental side, there were 31 ovulation points, 2 implantations, and 8 collapsed, degenerating blastocysts. It appeared, therefore, that CI-628 prevented the action of "blastocyst nidatory estrogen." However, this interpretation needs to be broadened in light of the results obtained in experiment III. In this experiment, the same procedures as in experiment II were followed, except that the rabbits were killed 6 days after mating. No implantations were expected at this time, since implantation in the rabbit begins 6.5–7 days post coitum. Accordingly, the uteri were flushed in order to assess the fate of the PIE's. In five rabbits, on the control side, the ovaries had 23 ovulation points, and the uteri yielded 20 good and 3 collapsed, degenerating blastocysts; on the experimental side, there were 30 ovulation points, 1 good and 13 collapsed, degenerating blastocysts. We maintain that CI-628 exerted its inhibition by preventing the action of "blastocyst estrogen." This estrogen may be needed for direct stimulation of the blastocyst for its own growth and development. Alternatively, the estrogen may stimulate the uterus, which, in turn, may secrete products essential for blastocyst survival and development. Moreover, the action of "blastocyst estrogen" during days 5 and 6 may prime the uterus in preparation for implantation. Thus, at present, we have to consider that "blastocyst estrogen" may act on either the blastocyst or the uterus, or on both.

C. Evidence from Papers Whose Authors Evoked the "PIE Steroids" Concept

Van Hoorn and Denker (1975) have shown that there is strong arylamidase activity in rabbit uterine epithelium on days 5 through 8 post coitum and that this enzyme is secreted into the uterine lumen. Studies on days

6 through 8 showed that the epithelium adjacent to blastocysts contained significantly less arylamidase than epithelia in interimplantation areas or pseudopregnant uteri. The authors suggested that the depletion of the enzyme from the epithelium could have been caused by steroid hormones released from the blastocyst.

Boshier (1975) studied rat uteri on day 5 of pregnancy and found that the neutral lipids were absent from the epithelium in the area adjacent to the blastocyst. The author suggested that the local loss of neutral lipids resulted ". . . from localized increase in esterase activity stimulated by estrogen released from the blastocyst."

At the time of writing this review, the above were the only two publications we encountered, other than our own, whose authors evoked the "PIE steroids" concept.

V. Concluding Remarks

In this review we have presented a new concept—the "PIE steroids" concept—which is fundamental for developmental biology and reproductive biology. The concept states that, starting at the morula stage (possibly at an earlier stage in the mouse and in some other species which hitherto have not been studied) and continuing through the blastocyst stage, the PIE has the capacity to synthesize steroid hormones. These "PIE steroids," whose targets are the PIE itself and the uterus, are essential for the maintenance of early pregnancy. In our opinion, the broad range of evidence we have presented throughout the review is adequate to permit us to state with confidence that the foundation for this concept has been established. This, then, is a beginning. On this foundation, a whole new structure will have to be built, which will require many years of investigation by scientists in various disciplines.

ACKNOWLEDGMENTS

The research work quoted from our laboratory was supported by grants from NIH (1 R01 HD08644-01A1), The National Foundation (1-406), and the Ford Foundation. Our thanks are due to Ms. Shirley Harrelson for typing the manuscript.

REFERENCES

Abraham, R., Hendy, R., Dougherty, W. J., Fulfs, J. C., and Goldberg, L. (1970). *Exp. Mol. Pathol.* **13,** 329.
Bhatt, B. M., and Bullock, D. W. (1974). *J. Reprod. Fertil.* **39,** 65.
Billing, R., Barberali, B., and Smellie, R. (1969). *Biochim. Biophys. Acta* **190,** 60.
Bitton-Casimiri, V., Brun, J. L., and Psychoyos, A. (1971). *J. Reprod. Fertil.* **27,** 461.
Boshier, D. P. (1975). *Annu. Conf. Soc. Study Fertil.* Abstract No. 35.

Brinster, R. L. (1967). *Exp. Cell Res.* **47**, 271.

Callantine, M. R., Clemens, L. E., and Shih, Y. (1968). *Proc. Soc. Exp. Biol. Med.* **128**, 382.

Callantine, M. R., Clemens, L. E., and Shih, Y. (1969). *Am. J. Physiol.* **216**, 1241.

Chew, N. J., and Sherman, M. I. (1975). *Biol. Reprod.* **12**, 351.

Dass, C. M. S., Mohla, S., and Prasad, M. R. N. (1969). *Endocrinology* **85**, 528.

Deane, H. W., Rubin, B. L., Driks, E. C., Lobel, B. L., and Leipsner, B. (1962). *Endocrinology* **70**, 407.

Deanesly, R. (1966). *In* "Marshall's Physiology of Reproduction" (A. S. Parkes, ed.), 3rd ed., Vol. 3, pp. 891–1063. Little, Brown, Boston, Massachusetts.

Dey, S. K., and Dickmann, Z. (1974a). *Endocrinology* **95**, 321.

Dey, S. K., and Dickmann, Z. (1974b). *7th Annu. Meet., Soc. Study Reprod.* Abstract No. 150.

Dey, S. K., and Dickmann, Z. (1974c). *Steroids* **24**, 57.

Dickmann, Z. (1967). *J. Exp. Zool.* **165**, 127.

Dickmann, Z. (1969). *Adv. Reprod. Physiol.* **4**, 187.

Dickmann, Z. (1970). *Fertil. Steril.* **21**, 541.

Dickmann, Z. (1971). *In* "Methods in Mammalian Embryology" (J. C. Daniel, Jr., ed.), pp. 133–145. Freeman, San Francisco, California.

Dickmann, Z. (1972). *J. Endocrinol.* **54**, 39.

Dickmann, Z. (1973). *J. Reprod. Fertil.* **32**, 65.

Dickmann, Z. (1975). *Res. Reprod.* **7**, 3.

Dickmann, Z., and DeFeo, V. J. (1967). *J. Reprod. Fertil.* **13**, 3.

Dickmann, Z., and Dey, S. K. (1973). *J. Reprod. Fertil.* **35**, 615.

Dickmann, Z., and Dey, S. K. (1974a). *J. Reprod. Fertil.* **37**, 91.

Dickmann, Z., and Dey, S. K. (1974b). *J. Endocrinol.* **61**, 513.

Dickmann, Z., and Noyes, R. W. (1960). *J. Reprod. Fertil.* **1**, 197.

Dickmann, Z., and Sen Gupta, J. (1974). *Dev. Biol.* **40**, 196.

Dickmann, Z., and Spilman, C. H. (1975). *Science* **190**, 997.

Dickmann, Z., Dey, S. K., and Sen Gupta, J. (1975). *Proc. Natl. Acad. Sci. U.S.A.* **72**, 298.

El-Shershaby, A. M., and Hinchcliffe, J. R. (1975). *J. Embryol. Exp. Morphol.* **33**, 1067.

Finn, C. A., and McLaren, A. (1967). *J. Reprod. Fertil.* **13**, 259.

Fisher, D. L., and Gunaga, K. P. (1975). *Biol. Reprod.* **12**, 471.

Frankel, L. (1903). *Arch. Gynaekol.* **68**, 438.

Fuchs, A. R., and Beling, C. (1974). *Endocrinology* **95**, 1054.

Fujimoto, S., Euker, J. S., Riegle, G. D., and Dukelow, W. R. (1975). *Proc. Jpn. Acad.* **51**, 123.

Gardner, R. L. (1972). *J. Embryol. Exp. Morphol.* **28**, 279.

Graves, C. N., and Biggers, J. D. (1970). *Science* **167**, 1506.

Ham, K. N., Hurley, J. V., Lopata, A., and Ryan, G. B. (1970). *J. Endocrinol.* **46**, 71.

Haour, F., and Saxena, B. B. (1974). *Science* **185**, 444.

Haour, F., Channing, C. P., and Saxena, B. B. (1975). *57th Annu. Meet. Endocrine Soc.* Abstract No. 114.

Harrer, J. A., and Lee, H. H. (1973). *J. Reprod. Fertil.* **33**, 327.

Heald, P. J., O'Grady, J. E., O'Hare, A., and Vass, M. (1975). *J. Reprod. Fertil.* **45**, 129.

Hechter, O., Krohn, L., and Harris, J. (1941). *Endocrinology* **29**, 386.

Henzl, M., Smith, R. E., Magoun, R. E., and Hill, R. (1968). *Fertil. Steril.* **19**, 914.

Huff, R. L., and Eik-Nes, K. B. (1966). *J. Reprod. Fertil.* **11**, 57.

Jacobson, M. A., Sanyal, M. K., and Meyer, R. K. (1970). *Endocrinology* **86**, 982.

Jensen, E. V., and DeSombre, R. E. (1972). *Annu. Rev. Biochem.* **41**, 203.

Kirkpatrick, J. F. (1971). *J. Reprod. Fertil.* **27**, 283.

Kuehl, F. A., Jr. (1974). *Prostaglandins* **5**, 325.

Kuehl, F. A., Jr., Cirillo, V. J., Ham, E. A., and Humes, J. L. (1973). *Adv. Biosci.* **9**, 155–172.

Kwun, J. K., and Emmens, C. W. (1974). *Aust. J. Biol. Sci.* **27**, 275.

Lau, N. I. F., Davis, B. K., and Chang, M. C. (1973). *Proc. Soc. Exp. Biol. Med.* **144**, 333.

McLaren, A. (1968). *J. Endocrinol.* **42**, 453.

Marshall, F. H. A., and Jolly, W. A. (1905). *Philos. Trans. R. Soc. London, Ser. B* **198**, 123.

Menke, T. M., and McLaren, A. (1970). *J. Endocrinol.* **47**, 287.

Menon, K. M. J., and Gunaga, K. P. (1974). *Fertil. Steril.* **25**, 732.

Mintz, B. (1964). *J. Exp. Zool.* **157**, 85.

Monesi, V., and Salfi, V. (1967). *Exp. Cell Res.* **46**, 632.

O'Malley, B. W., and Means, A. R. (1974). *Science* **183**, 610.

Perry, J. S., Heap, R. B., and Amoroso, E. C. (1973). *Nature (London)* **245**, 45.

Psychoyos, A. (1960). *C. R. Seances Soc. Biol. Ses. Fil.* **154**, 1384.

Psychoyos, A. (1961). *C. R. Hebd. Seances Acad. Sci.* **252**, 1515.

Psychoyos, A. (1967). *Adv. Reprod. Physiol.* **2**, 257.

Robison, G. A. (1972). *Am. J. Pharm. Educ.* **36**, 723.

Ryan, K. J. (1973). *Handb. Physiol., Sect. 7: Endocrinol.* **2**, Part 2, 285–293.

Sanyal, M. K., and Meyer, R. K. (1970). *Endocrinology* **86**, 976.

Seamark, R. F., and Lutwak-Mann, C. (1972). *J. Reprod. Fertil.* **29**, 147.

Silver, M. J., and Smith, J. B. (1975). *Life Sci.* **16**, 1635.

Smith, A. F., and Wilson, I. B. (1974). *J. Reprod. Fertil.* **38**, 307.

Smith, D. M., and Smith, A. E. S. (1971). *Biol. Reprod.* **4**, 66.

Spaziani, E., and Szego, C. M. (1958). *Endocrinology* **63**, 669.

Speroff, L., and Ramwell, P. W. (1970). *J. Clin. Endocrinol.* **30**, 345.

Sundaram, K., Connell, K. G., and Passantino, T. (1975). *Nature (London)* **256**, 739.

Szego, C. M. (1965). *Fed. Proc., Fed. Am. Soc. Exp. Biol.* **24**, 1343.

Thompson, E. B., and Lippman, M. E. (1974). *Metabolism* **23**, 159.

Torbit, C. A., and Weitlauf, H. M. (1974). *J. Reprod. Fertil.* **39**, 379.

Van Hoorn, G., and Denker, H. W. (1975). *J. Reprod. Fertil.* **45**, 359.

Wattenberg, L. W. (1958). *J. Histochem. Cytochem.* **6**, 225.

Weissmann, G. (1969). *Lysosomes Biol. Pathol.* **1**, 276–295.

Weitlauf, H. M., and Greenwald, G. S. (1968). *J. Exp. Zool.* **169**, 463.

Whitten, W. K. (1957). *J. Endocrinol.* **16**, 80.

Whitten, W. K. (1971). *Adv. Biosci.* **6**, 129–139.

Wiest, W. G., and Kidwell, W. R. (1969). *In* "The Gonads" (K. W. McKerns, ed.), pp. 295–325. Appleton, New York.

Wiley, L. D. (1974). *Nature (London)* **252**, 715.

Willmer, E. N. (1961). *Biol. Rev. Cambridge Philos. Soc.* **36**, 368.

Wu, J. T. (1973). *J. Reprod. Fertil.* **33**, 331.

Subject Index

A

A-Betalipoproteinemia, vitamin E
deficiency in, 59–60
Abortion, vitamin E in therapy of, 68–69
Acetate synthesis, methyl B_{12}
requirement by, 6
Amino acids, conversions of, folic acid in,
12–13
Androgens
germ cell stimulation of, 206–209
peritubular cell stimulation by, 198–199
Leydig cell stimulation of, 193–195
Sertoli cell stimulation by, 203–206
Antioxidants, tocopherols as, 83–84
Apes, chemical communication in, 140
Athletic performance, vitamin E effects
on, 69

B

Baboon, sex-attractant acid changes in,
177–178
Beta thalessemia, major vitamin E
therapy of, 69
Blastocyst
implantation of, PIE steroid effect on,
230–233
metabolic activities in, 233–234
Blood coagulation, vitamin E and, 68

C

Cancer, progression from bad to worse,
127
Capillary permeability, PIE steroid
studies on, 234–236
Carcinogenesis, prolactin role in, 107–136
Chemical communication
human sexuality and, 181
in primates, 137–186
in rhesus monkeys, 141–155
CI-628, effects on PIEs, 236–239
Claudication, intermittent, peripheral
vasular disease with, 67–68
Cobalamin, reactions requiring, 6
Coenzyme B_{12}, reactions requiring, 6

Cyclic AMP, in preimplantation embryo,
227
Cystic fibrosis, vitamin E deficiency in,
48–52
Cystic mastitis, vitamin E therapy of, 69

D

5'-Deoxyadenosylcobalamin, see
Coenzyme B_{12}
Diet, mammary tumors and, 123
Dimethyltocols, methyltocols as
precursors of, 87–88
Dioldehydrase, cobalamin requirement
by, 6

E

Ejaculate, effects on vaginal fatty acids,
171
Estradiol, effects on vaginal fatty acids,
166–167
Estrogens
carcinogenesis and, 130
effect on monkey communication,
144–146
intravaginal, 147
effects on PIEs, 236–238
Leydig cell stimulation of, 191–193
Ethanolamine deaminase, cobalamin
requirement by, 6

F

Fatty acids
unsaturated, vitamin E relationship to,
38–40
in vaginal secretions, as sex attractants,
161–166
Flowering, tocopherols in initiation of, 85
Folic acid
in amino acid conversions, 12–13
in cell poiesis, 1–30
coenzymes of, role in one-carbon-unit
transfers, 11–13
derivatives of, structures and
nomenclature of, 9